Preventing Dance Injuries

SECOND EDITION

Ruth Solomon, Professor Emerita

John Solomon, PhD

Sandra Cerny Minton, PhD

EDITORS

HUMAN KINETICS

Cataloging-in-Publication Data

Solomon, Ruth (Ruth L.)
 Preventing dance injuries / Ruth Solomon, John Solomon, Sandra Cerny Minton.-- 2nd ed.
   p. cm.
 Includes bibliographical references and index.
 ISBN 0-7360-5567-3 (soft cover)
 1. Dancing injuries. 2. Dancing injuries--Prevention. I. Solomon, John. II. Minton, Sandra Cerny, 1943- III. Title.
 RC1220.D35S64 2005
 617.1'02--dc22

                  2004030395

ISBN: 0-7360-5567-3

This book is a revised edition of *Preventing Dance Injuries: An Interdisciplinary Perspective,* published in 1990 by the American Alliance for Health, Physical Education, Recreation & Dance.

Acquisitions Editor: Judy Patterson Wright, PhD; **Developmental Editor:** Jacqueline Eaton Blakley; **Assistant Editors:** Kathleen Bernard and Derek Campbell; **Copyeditor:** Joyce Sexton; **Proofreader:** Jim Burns; **Permission Manager:** Dalene Reeder; **Graphic Designer:** Nancy Rasmus; **Graphic Artist:** Yvonne Griffith; **Photo Manager:** Kelly J. Huff, **Cover Designer:** Keith Blomberg; **Photographer (cover):** Don Fukuda; **Photographers (interior):** Rosalind Newmark, Robert E. Stephens, Lyle Micheli, Bruce Berryhill, Randy Bradley; **Art Manager:** Kelly Hendren; **Illustrators:** Accurate Art, Barry LaPoint, Mary Cosenza, David Petrie; **Printer:** Versa Press

Printed in the United States of America   10 9 8 7 6 5 4 3 2 1

Human Kinetics
Web site: www.HumanKinetics.com

United States: Human Kinetics; P.O. Box 5076; Champaign, IL 61825-5076
800-747-4457
e-mail: humank@hkusa.com

Canada: Human Kinetics; 475 Devonshire Road Unit 100; Windsor, ON N8Y 2L5
800-465-7301 (in Canada only)
e-mail: orders@hkcanada.com

Europe: Human Kinetics; 107 Bradford Road; Stanningley; Leeds LS28 6AT, United Kingdom
+44 (0) 113 255 5665
e-mail: hk@hkeurope.com

Australia: Human Kinetics; 57A Price Avenue; Lower Mitcham, South Australia 5062
08 8277 1555
e-mail: liaw@hkaustralia.com

New Zealand: Human Kinetics; Division of Sports Distributors NZ Ltd.; P.O. Box 300 226 Albany
North Shore City; Auckland
0064 9 448 1207
e-mail: blairc@hknewz.com

To Jean Erdman, who taught me to teach so that the individual artist in each of us could emerge without damage to the body or psyche.

R.S.

Contents ⌒

Contributors   vi

Credits   viii

Introduction   x

Part I   Screening for Common Dance Injuries

Chapter 1   **Determinants of Injuries in Young Dancers**   3
Anthony C. Luke, MD, MPH; Susan A. Kinney, PT; Pierre A. d'Hemecourt,
MD; Jessica Baum, MSPT, MM; Michael Owen; and Lyle J. Micheli, MD

Chapter 2   **Physical Screening Procedures**   19
Janice Gudde Plastino, PhD

Chapter 3   **A Somatic Screening Procedure Using
Bartenieff Fundamentals**   29
Sandra Kay Lauffenburger, BEd, MSc, Dip (psych) CMA

Part II   Diagnosing, Treating, and Rehabilitating Dance Injuries

Chapter 4   **Common Foot and Ankle Injuries in Dancers**   39
Richard N. Norris, MD

Chapter 5   **Knee Problems in Dancers**   53
Carol C. Teitz, MD

Chapter 6   **Iliopsoas Tendinitis in Dancers**   73
Ruth Solomon, Professor Emerita, and Lyle J. Micheli, MD

Chapter 7   **Spinal Problems in Dancers**   79
Elly Trepman, MD; Arleen Walaszek, PT; and Lyle J. Micheli, MD

Chapter 8   **Stress Fractures in Dancers**   97
Lyle J. Micheli, MD, and Ruth Solomon, Professor Emerita

Part III   Preventing Dance Injuries Through Biomechanically Efficient Training

Chapter 9   **An Efficient Warm-Up Based on Anatomical Principles**   **111**
Ruth Solomon, Professor Emerita

Chapter 10   **A Biomechanical Approach to Aerobic Dance Injuries**   **129**
Stephen P. Baitch, PT

Chapter 11   **Biomechanical Considerations in Turnout**   **135**
Karen S. Clippinger, MSPE

Chapter 12   **The Neuroanatomical and Biomechanical Basis of Flexibility Exercises in Dance**   **151**
Robert E. Stephens, PhD

Chapter 13   **Strengthening and Stretching the Muscles of the Ankle and Tarsus**   **165**
Sally Sevey Fitt, EdD

Chapter 14   **Pronation As a Predisposing Factor in Overuse Injuries**   **185**
Steven R. Kravitz, DPM

Part IV   Psychological Concerns

Chapter 15   **Stress, Performance, and Dance Injuries**   **193**
Raymond W. Novaco, PhD

Chapter 16   **The Role of Dance Teachers in the Prevention of Eating Disorders**   **201**
Niva Piran, PhD

Chapter 17   **The Female Athlete Triad in Dancers**   **211**
Bonnie E. Robson, MD, D.Psych, DCP, FRCP(C)

Dance Glossary   217
Medical Glossary   219
Index   230
About the Editors   243

Contributors

Stephen P. Baitch, PT, is coordinator of the foot and biomechanics program, Sports Medicine Center, Union Memorial Hospital, Baltimore, and has a private physical therapy practice in Lutherville, MD, specializing in treatment of foot-related problems. He is a frequent presenter on lower extremity biomechanics and foot-related abnormalities at various meetings on both national and local levels.

Jessica Baum, MSPT, MM, is a physical therapist with Performing Arts Therapy in Boston. She treats students at the Walnut Hill School, the New England Conservatory, and the Boston Conservatory. She also holds bachelor's and master's degrees from the Eastman School of Music in viola performance.

Karen S. Clippinger, MSPE, is an associate professor of dance at California State University at Long Beach, and prior consultant to the Pacific Northwest Ballet. She has presented over 350 lectures/workshops throughout the United States and in Canada and Japan, including at the annual conferences of the International Association of Dance Medicine & Science, the American College of Sports Medicine, and the International Association of Biomechanics in Sports. She has authored numerous articles and chapters focusing on optimizing technique and preventing injury in dancers, and is currently coeditor in chief of the *Journal of Dance Medicine & Science.*

Pierre A. d'Hemecourt, MD, is a primary care sports medicine physician at Children's Hospital, Boston, and Boston College. He has a clinical interest in spinal biomechanics and rehabilitation in the dancer. He has worked with the Boston Ballet as well as adolescent and beginning dancers since 1996.

Sally Sevey Fitt, EdD, is professor emerita from the department of modern dance at the University of Utah, where she taught from 1976 to 2001. She is the author of *Dance Kinesiology* (1988, 1996) and coauthor of the book *Diet: A Complete Guide to Nutrition and Weight Control,* as well as numerous

articles. She is presently working on a manuscript tentatively titled *Muscular Wellness.*

Susan Kinney, PT, is the founder and owner of Performing Arts Therapy, an on-site physical therapy clinic located at the Walnut Hill School, New England Conservatory, and Massachusetts College of Art. She is also co-owner of Arts Medicine Collaborative, a physical therapy clinic located at the Boston Conservatory, that specializes in performing arts injuries.

Steven R. Kravitz, DPM, is assistant professor in the department of orthopedics, Pennsylvania College of Podiatric Medicine. He is a past consultant to the Pennsylvania Ballet Company and the School of Dance at Philadelphia University of the Performing Arts. He has authored articles in both medical and dance publications.

Sandra Kay Lauffenburger, BEd, MSc, Dip (psych) CMA, is a registered movement therapist and psychotherapist in private practice based in Canberra, Australia. She currently specializes in the rehabilitation of chronic pain and chronic illness. Her work combines Laban Movement Analysis, Bartenieff Fundamentals, Pilates method, and psychodynamic psychotherapeutic techniques.

Anthony Luke, MD, MPH, is a primary care staff physician at the Fowler Kennedy Sports Medicine Clinic, University of Western Ontario, London, Ontario, Canada. Dr. Luke received PAMA's 2001 Alice G. Brandfonbrener Young Investigator Award and the 2002 NETWORK Research Award, International Network of Performing and Visual Arts Schools.

Lyle J. Micheli, MD, is associate clinical professor of orthopaedic surgery, Harvard Medical School, and director of the Division of Sports Medicine at Children's Hospital, Boston. He is an associate editor of *Medicine and Science in Sports and Exercise.* For the last 22 years he has been attending physician to the Boston Ballet and the School of the Boston Ballet, and he is a former president of the American College of Sports Medicine.

Richard N. Norris, MD, is a specialist in physical medicine and rehabilitation, with a subspecialty in performing arts medicine. He studied jazz dance and ballet for many years and directed several dance medicine clinics. He is now with Pioneer Spine and Sports Physicians in Northampton, MA, where he is active in treating and educating members of the local dance community.

Raymond W. Novaco, PhD, is a professor of psychology and social behavior at the University of California at Irvine. His primary research concerns the assessment and treatment of anger- and stress-related disorders. He serves on the editorial board of *Clinical Psychology: Science and Practice*. In 2000 he received the Distinguished Contributions to Psychology Award from the California Psychological Association.

Michael Owen is the artistic director and head of the dance department at the Walnut Hill School. He was a principal dancer and administrator at the American Ballet Theatre for over 20 years.

Niva Piran, PhD, is professor of education at the University of Toronto and a practicing clinical psychologist. She consults to schools, including the National Ballet School, in the area of body image development and the prevention of eating disorders. Dr. Piran has published two books on eating disorders, *Preventing Eating Disorders: A Handbook of Interventions and Special Challenges* and *A Day Hospital Program for the Treatment of Anorexia Nervosa and Bulimia Nervosa*. Her research studies have appeared in many professional journals and as chapters in books, and she has presented at scientific forums in North America and elsewhere. She is the prevention editor of *Eating Disorders: The Journal of Treatment and Prevention*.

Janice Gudde Plastino, PhD, is a professional performer and choreographer of ballet, opera, musicals, and modern dance. She codirected Penrod Plastino Movement Theater, a modern dance company, for 12 years. Her publications include numerous articles and the book *The Dancer Prepares* (with James Penrod). She is professor of dance at the University of California at Irvine and heads the dance medicine/science program on that campus.

Bonnie E. Robson, MD, D. Psych, DCP, FRCP(C), is a child psychiatrist who has 20 years experience in performance arts medicine. Currently a consultant to the Quinte Ballet School of Canada, and previously consultant to the National Ballet School of Canada, she has through her research provided material for field-related publications, workshops, seminars, and several multidisciplinary educational videotapes on dance injury prevention and anxiety. She has served on the boards of the Performing Arts Medicine Association and International Network of Performing and Visual Arts Schools, and recently was only the third person ever honored with that organization's Lifetime Achievement Award.

Ruth Solomon is professor emerita of theater arts and former director of the dance theater program at the University of California at Santa Cruz. Her approach to teaching has been documented in an hour-long video, *Anatomy as a Master Image in Training Dancers* (1988). She is widely published in the field of dance medicine.

Robert E. Stephens, PhD, is professor and chair of anatomy and the associate dean for biomedical sciences at the Kansas City University of Medicine and Biosciences in Kansas City, Missouri. He is coauthor of *Dance Medicine: A Comprehensive Guide* (1987) and *The Dancer's Complete Guide to Health Care and a Long Career* (1988).

Carol C. Teitz, MD, is professor of orthopaedics and sports medicine at the University of Washington. She studied dance for 11 years before entering the School of Medicine at Yale University. Her work related to dancers' musculoskeletal problems has been published in *Foot and Ankle*, *JOPERD*, *Pediatric Clinics of North America*, *American Journal of Sports Medicine*, *Journal of Musculoskeletal Medicine*, *Clinical Journal of Sport Medicine*, *Journal of Dance Medicine & Science*, and a number of textbooks. Dr. Teitz is team physician for the UW dance department as well as for UW Husky athletes.

Elly Trepman, MD, is an associate professor in the section of orthopaedic surgery, department of surgery, University of Manitoba, Winnipeg, Manitoba, Canada. He was a fellow in sports and dance medicine under the guidance of Dr. Lyle J. Micheli at Children's Hospital, Boston, and a consultant to the Harkness Center for Dance Injuries in New York City, and is currently an associate editor of the *Journal of Dance Medicine & Science* and assistant editor of *Foot and Ankle International*.

Arleen Walaszek, PT, formerly staff physical therapist, Children's Hospital, Boston, was physical therapist to the Boston Ballet Company for 15 years.

Credits

Figure 3.1 Photos courtesy of Randy Bradley. Reprinted by permission.

Figure 3.2 Photos courtesy of Randy Bradley. Reprinted by permission.

Figure 3.3 Photos courtesy of Randy Bradley. Reprinted by permission.

Figure 4.1 Reprinted, by permission, from R.S. Behnke, 2001, *Kinetic anatomy* (Champaign, IL: Human Kinetics), 224.

Figure 4.2 Illustration by Barry LaPointe.

Figure 4.7 Reprinted, by permission, from R.S. Behnke, 2001, *Kinetic anatomy* (Champaign, IL: Human Kinetics), 219.

Figure 5.1 Reprinted, by permission, from R.S. Behnke, 2001, *Kinetic anatomy* (Champaign, IL: Human Kinetics), 207.

Figure 5.2 Reprinted, by permission, from R.S. Behnke, 2001, *Kinetic anatomy* (Champaign, IL: Human Kinetics), 209.

Figure 5.6 Reprinted, by permission, from R.S. Behnke, 2001, *Kinetic anatomy* (Champaign, IL: Human Kinetics), 207.

Figure 5.7 Reprinted, by permission, from C.C. Teitz, 1982, "Sports medicine concerns in dance and gymnastics," *Pediatric Clinics in North America* 29(6): 1402.

Figure 5.8 Reprinted, by permission, from C.C. Teitz, 1982, "Sports medicine concerns in dance and gymnastics," *Pediatric Clinics in North America* 29(6): 1405.

Figure 5.9 Reprinted, by permission, from C.C. Teitz, 1982, "Sports medicine concerns in dance and gymnastics," *Pediatric Clinics in North America* 29(6): 1410.

Figure 5.11 Reprinted, by permission, from C.C. Teitz, 1983, "Office management of common knee problems," *Current Concepts in Pain* 1(4): 14.

Figure 5.12a Reprinted, by permission, from C.C. Teitz, 1983, "Office management of common knee problems," *Current Concepts in Pain* 1(4): 14.

Figure 5.12b Reprinted, by permission, from C.C. Teitz, 1988, "Ultrasonography in the knee: Clinical aspects," *Radiographic Clinics in North America* 26(1): 55.

Figure 6.1a Reprinted, by permission, from J.E. Donnelly, 1990, *Living anatomy,* 2nd edition (Champaign, IL: Human Kinetics), 143.

Figure 6.1b Reprinted, by permission, from J.E. Donnelly, 1990, *Living anatomy,* 2nd edition (Champaign, IL: Human Kinetics), 116.

Figure 6.2 Photo courtesy of Dr. Lyle Micheli.

Figure 6.3 Photo courtesy of Dr. Lyle Micheli.

Figure 6.4 Photo courtesy of Dr. Lyle Micheli.

Figure 7.1 Illustration by Elly Trepman, M.D.

Figure 7.2 Illustration by Elly Trepman, M.D.

Figure 7.3 Illustration by Elly Trepman, M.D.

Figure 7.4 Illustration by Elly Trepman, M.D.

Figure 9.1 Reprinted, by permission, from L.J. Micheli, and R. Solomon, 1987, Training the young dancer. In *Dance medicine: A comprehensive guide,* edited by A.J. Ryan and R.E. Stephens (Chicago and Minneapolis: Pluribus Press/The Physician and Sportsmedicine), 70.

Figure 9.2 Reprinted, by permission, from L.J. Micheli, and R. Solomon, 1987, Training the young dancer. In *Dance medicine: A comprehensive guide,* edited by A.J. Ryan and R.E. Stephens (Chicago and Minneapolis: Pluribus Press/The Physician and Sportsmedicine), 70.

Figure 9.3 Reprinted, by permission, from L.J. Micheli, and R. Solomon, 1987, Training the young dancer. In *Dance medicine: A comprehensive guide,* edited by A.J. Ryan and R.E. Stephens (Chicago and Minneapolis: Pluribus Press/The Physician and Sportsmedicine), 63. Photographer: Bruce Berryhill. Models: Greg Lizenbery and Sharon Cullen.

Figure 9.4 Reprinted, by permission, from L.J. Micheli, and R. Solomon, 1987, Training the young dancer. In *Dance medicine: A comprehensive guide,* edited by A.J. Ryan and R.E. Stephens (Chicago and Minneapolis: Pluribus Press/The Physician and Sportsmedicine), 64. Photographer: Bruce Berryhill. Models: Ruth Solomon and Sativa Saposnek.

Figure 9.5 Reprinted, by permission, from L.J. Micheli, and R. Solomon, 1987, Training the young dancer. In *Dance medicine: A comprehensive guide,* edited by A.J. Ryan and R.E. Stephens (Chicago and Minneapolis: Pluribus Press/The Physician and Sportsmedicine), 60. Photographer: Bruce Berryhill. Model: Sativa Saposnek.

Figure 9.6 Photos courtesy of Bruce Berryhill. Model: Martha Curtis.

Figure 9.7 Photos courtesy of Bruce Berryhill. Model: Ruth Solomon.

Figure 9.8 Photos courtesy of Bruce Berryhill. Model: Martha Curtis.

Figure 9.9 Photos courtesy of Bruce Berryhill. Model: Ruth Solomon.

Figure 9.10 Photos courtesy of Bruce Berryhill. Model: Ruth Solomon.

Figure 9.11 Photos courtesy of Bruce Berryhill. Model: Martha Curtis.

Figure 9.12 Photos courtesy of Bruce Berryhill. Model: Ruth Solomon.

Figure 9.13 Photos courtesy of Bruce Berryhill. Model: Ruth Solomon.

Figure 9.14 Photos courtesy of Bruce Berryhill. Model: Martha Curtis.

Figure 9.15 Photos courtesy of Bruce Berryhill. Models: Martha Curtis and Ruth Solomon.

Figure 9.16 Photos courtesy of Bruce Berryhill. Model: Martha Curtis.

Figure 9.17 Photos courtesy of Bruce Berryhill. Models: Martha Curtis and Ruth Solomon.

Figure 9.18 Photos courtesy of Bruce Berryhill. Model: Martha Curtis.

Figure 9.19 Photos courtesy of Bruce Berryhill. Model: Ruth Solomon.

Figure 9.20 Photos courtesy of Bruce Berryhill. Model: Ruth Solomon.

Figure 10.1 Illustrations courtesy of David Petrie. Reprinted by permission.

Figure 10.2 Illustrations courtesy of David Petrie. Reprinted by permission.

Figure 10.3 Illustrations courtesy of David Petrie. Reprinted by permission.

Figure 11.1 Illustration courtesy of Mary Cosenza. Reprinted by permission.

Figure 11.2 Illustration courtesy of Karen Clippinger.

Figure 11.3 Photo courtesy of Karen Clippinger.

Figure 11.4 Photo courtesy of Karen Clippinger.

Figure 11.5 Photo courtesy of Karen Clippinger.

Figure 11.6 Photo courtesy of Karen Clippinger.

Figure 11.7 Photo courtesy of Karen Clippinger.

Figure 11.8 Photo courtesy of Karen Clippinger.

Figure 11.9 Illustration courtesy of Karen Clippinger.

Figure 11.10 Photo courtesy of Karen Clippinger.

Figure 11.11 Photo courtesy of Karen Clippinger.

Figure 11.12 Photo courtesy of Karen Clippinger.

Figure 11.13 Photo courtesy of Karen Clippinger.

Figure 11.14 Photo courtesy of Karen Clippinger.

Figure 12.8 Photo courtesy of Robert Stephens. Model: Jessica Stulik.

Figure 12.9 Photo courtesy of Robert Stephens. Model: Jessica Stulik.

Figure 12.10 Photo courtesy of Robert Stephens. Model: Jessica Stulik.

Figure 12.11 Photo courtesy of Robert Stephens. Model: Jessica Stulik.

Figure 13.1 Reprinted, by permission, from R.S. Behnke, 2001, *Kinetic anatomy* (Champaign, IL: Human Kinetics), 227.

Figure 13.6 Photos courtesy of Rosalind Newmark. Reprinted by permission.

Figure 13.7 Photo courtesy of Rosalind Newmark. Reprinted by permission.

Figure 13.8 Photo courtesy of Rosalind Newmark. Reprinted by permission.

Figure 13.9 Photo courtesy of Rosalind Newmark. Reprinted by permission.

Figure 13.10 Photo courtesy of Rosalind Newmark. Reprinted by permission.

Figure 13.11 Photos courtesy of Rosalind Newmark. Reprinted by permission.

Figure 13.12 Photo courtesy of Rosalind Newmark. Reprinted by permission.

Figure 13.13 Photo courtesy of Rosalind Newmark. Reprinted by permission.

Figure 13.14 Photo courtesy of Rosalind Newmark. Reprinted by permission.

Figure 13.15 Photo courtesy of Rosalind Newmark. Reprinted by permission.

Figure 13.16 Photo courtesy of Rosalind Newmark. Reprinted by permission.

Figure 13.17 Photo courtesy of Rosalind Newmark. Reprinted by permission.

Figure 13.18 Photo courtesy of Rosalind Newmark. Reprinted by permission.

Figure 14.1 Illustration courtesy of Barry LaPoint. Reprinted by permission.

Figure 14.2 Illustration courtesy of Barry LaPoint. Reprinted by permission.

Introduction

When this book appeared in 1990 it took its place in what future historians of dance medicine and science will inevitably identify as the first generation of texts in the field. Other members of that august company included D. Arnheim, *Dance Injuries*, 1986; C. Shell, *The Dancer as Athlete: The 1984 Olympic Scientific Congress Proceedings*, 1986; A. Ryan and R. Stephens, *Dance Medicine: A Comprehensive Guide*, 1987; and P. Clarkson and M. Skrinar, *Science of Dance Training*, 1988. With the exception of Arnheim's, these books were all of a piece—collections of chapters authored by various experts in some aspect of what was then considered to be the appropriate subject matter of dance medicine and science. This model has withstood the test of time quite well in the sense that the information produced has remained, for the most part, germane and useful. However, the extreme eclecticism it fostered has proven to be something of a double-edged sword. On the positive side it illustrated how representatives of an extremely broad range of constituencies—from MDs and PTs, through somaticists and biomechanists and kinesiologists, to artistic directors and dance teachers and individual dance students—might contribute to, and benefit from, participation in the field. Conversely, by offering something for everyone it tended to obscure the interrelationships among diverse interests that lend the field its depth.

In this revised edition we have used a number of new devices to help ameliorate this kind of problem. First, we have in many cases regrouped the chapters to create blocks of material that more clearly than in the original edition build logically on one another. Thus, part I is now composed of three chapters that have to do primarily with techniques for identifying the potential for injury in dancers. The five chapters of part II describe those injuries that are most common to dancers, by site of injury, with attention to their etiology, diagnosis, treatment, and rehabilitation. Part III has six chapters that are unified by a common concern for preventing dance injuries through the application of biomechanical principles that promote relatively safe and efficient training methods. Finally, part IV is a self-contained unit of three chapters devoted to various aspects of what has become in recent years the "hottest" of dance medicine and science subjects, dance psychology.

Throughout this edition we have added editorial "signposts" of various sorts—introductory editorial comments, section headings, highlight boxes, and so on—to aid the reader in finding specific subjects quickly and grasping their relationship to surrounding material. There is also a much enlarged, cross-referenced index. We anticipate that these reader-friendly additions will especially enhance the book's usefulness as an academic text for students and reference guide for health care practitioners.

Beyond these structural changes there is new substance totaling approximately 25% of the text. This is embodied primarily in four new chapters, each of which updates or augments material from the original edition. Thus, chapter 1, by Dr. Anthony Luke and associates, not only represents an epidemiologic study of dance injuries (as did the chapter it replaces, by Schafle et al.), but also discusses problems resulting from the diversity of methods used in earlier studies of this sort and suggests possible solutions. Our own chapter (chapter 6) deals with "snapping hip," a condition that has commanded a good deal of attention at recent conferences in both dance medicine and sports medicine. The other new chapters (chapters 16 and 17), by Drs. Niva Piran and Bonnie Robson, respectively, introduce several interrelated topics—eating disorders, body image, and the female athlete triad—that are at the core of dance psychology, thus enlarging our coverage of what we previously identified as the field's currently most popular subject.

Virtually all of the original chapters have undergone some revision by their authors to enhance their accuracy and timeliness. We have supported this effort by adding a total of 137 recommended readings from the current literature to the references at the end of each chapter. The glossary of medical terms appended to the text has been significantly enlarged.

As the first-generation books in dance medicine and science have aged and in some cases, no doubt, reached "remainder" status, one wonders when, or if, the next generation will arrive. In the intervening years, opportunities to publish in the periodical literature have proliferated; most essentially the *Journal of Dance Medicine & Science* has become a major new resource, but also journals in allied fields and in other coun-

tries have opened their pages to dance-oriented subjects. Hence, even as the knowledge in our field becomes broader and deeper, one must look harder to find it. There is, perhaps, a decreasing sense of where we have come from, and what we share in common. This revised edition of *Preventing Dance Injuries* guarantees that at least one of the classic texts will be available to provide a sense of continuity into the foreseeable future.

—*The editors*

Part I

Screening for Common Dance Injuries

Since the publication of Dr. Ernest Washington's groundbreaking effort to identify and quantify the most common dance injuries ("Musculoskeletal Injuries in Theatrical Dancers." *American Journal of Sports Medicine* 6[2]: 75-98, 1978), numerous subsequent studies have enriched our understanding of the subject. Augmenting this line of investigation is the increasingly popular practice among individual dance medicine researchers, academic dance departments, professional companies, and even private studios of screening dancers to record their injury histories and physiological predisposition to further injuries. The three chapters of part I illustrate this development by way of a sample epidemiological study, the description of an institutionalized screening procedure, and an example of what somatic (body therapy) techniques have to contribute.

Chapter 1

Determinants of Injuries in Young Dancers

Anthony C. Luke, MD, MPH; Susan A. Kinney, PT; Pierre A. d'Hemecourt, MD; Jessica Baum, MSPT, MM; Michael Owen; Lyle J. Micheli, MD

We begin with a chapter on the epidemiology of dance injuries, as it is our belief that the prevention of injuries properly originates in a clear understanding of the what, where, when, and how of their occurrence. There is by now a fairly substantial body of such material, as indicated by the references at the end of this chapter and our Recommended Readings, which supplement them. The work of Dr. Luke and associates is particularly useful for our purposes because it not only represents an epidemiologic study, but also raises interesting questions about problems that have arisen because no effort has yet been made to standardize the practices used in gathering and analyzing data that result from screening dancers for injuries.

The objectives of the work explored in this chapter were to develop and pilot-study tools to identify injuries and risk factors for injury in young dancers. The injuries described were determined using a survey approach. By identifying self-reported (self-perceived) and reported (medically assessed) injuries, we hoped to understand the development of dance injuries better in order to support implementation of strategies for injury prevention and to improve the awareness of dancers concerning appropriate medical care.

Primary prevention of dance injuries is needed, especially in younger dancers, as the aesthetic movements of turnout, pointe work, and jumping put repetitive stresses on the body. The incidence of injury to members of professional companies has been reported at 40% to 55.5% in a performance season (Bronner and Brownstein 1997; Evans et al. 1996; Garrick and Requa 1993). A study of high school and college dancers showed 352 injuries occurring in 84.9% of 218 dancers in one school year (Rovere et al. 1983).

Adapted by permission from A.C. Luke, S.A. Kinney, P.A. D'Hemecourt, J. Baum, M. Owen, and L.J. Micheli, 2002, "Determinants of injuries in young dancers," *Medical Problems of Performing Artists* (Philadelphia: Hanley & Belfus) 17: 105-112. Supported in part by a research grant from the Massachusetts Governor's Committee on Physical Fitness and Sports.

Dance injuries most commonly occur in the lower extremities (52%), back (22%), and neck (12%) (Evans et al. 1996; Garrick and Requa 1993). In the lower extremities, ankle and foot problems are most prevalent, followed by the knee and then the hip. Many of these injuries are considered preventable (Evans et al. 1996).

Injury Survey

The definition of injury and the means of gathering data are major challenges in studies of this sort, as they determine the number of cases used to estimate injury rates. Injuries cannot be defined accurately in terms of missed practice or class, because dancers often dance through injuries. Examples of definitions that identify early injuries are "any damaged body part that interfered with training" (Sands, Schultz, and Newman 1993) and "any complaint about which dancers have questions" (Garrick 1999). The method of acquiring information on injuries can be either self-report or report by an objective party, usually a therapist or health professional.

The incidence of dance injuries is probably underreported, as dancers may not present with "minor" injuries to a health professional (Garrick 1999). These injuries can then play a role in the development of "major" injuries. Hence, identifying those injuries that the dancer self-perceives can help prevent them from worsening, which translates into less time away from dance and decreased health care costs.

Intrinsic and Extrinsic Risk Factors

Intrinsic risk factors for injury can be considered to remain relatively constant, while extrinsic factors put the dancer at risk for injury over transient periods. Intrinsic risk factors include anatomical characteristics (Reid et al. 1987), medical history, previous injuries (DuRant et al. 1992), menstrual history (Hamilton, Brooks-Gunn, and Warren 1985), and dance experience (Evans et al. 1996). Extrinsic risk factors include type and duration of training, fatigue, stress (Hamilton et al. 1989), shoes, floor surface, and nutrition (Yannakoulia and Matalas 2000; Micheli 1984). The challenge in research related to risk factors is that injuries are multifactorial, and isolating causative factors is difficult because of the number of confounding variables.

Study Design and Methods

The work described in this chapter was a prospective cohort study. Its protocol was reviewed by the Internal Review Board at the Children's Hospital of Boston, Boston, Massachusetts. The subjects were preprofessional dancers aged 14 to 18 years at a liberal arts high school in Natick, Massachusetts. Signed dancer and parental informed consent forms were obtained in all cases.

The assessment instruments used in this study included (1) a history and physical exam at the start of the season (figure 1.1), (2) biweekly surveys to identify self-reported injuries (SRIs)

Some Concerns in the Epidemiologic Study of Dance Injuries

- How is "injury" to be defined?
- Who is to determine whether an injury has occurred?
- How are injuries to be reported and classified?
- How should unreported injuries be classified?
- What about matters of confidentiality?
- How are "new" and "recurrent" injuries to be differentiated?
- Can the language used to describe such matters as the "severity," "location," "rate," and "duration" of injuries be standardized?
- How could standardized screening procedures inform the collection and use of injury data?

HISTORY

Age _____   Sex ❏ M ❏ F Any trouble reading/writing English? ❏ Yes ❏ No

How many years of dancing so far _____   Years of ballet training _____   Started pointework at _____

Dance type preferred   Modern _____   Ballet _____   Both equally _____   Other _____

Any medical problems? _____

Any surgeries: (Indicate year) _____

_____

Common ones:

    Asthma _____   Diabetes _____   Heart problems _____

    Arthritis _____   Scoliosis (curved spine) _____

Medications:

_____

_____

Birth control pills ❏ Yes ❏ No

Age at menarche _____   Have you missed any periods in the last year? ❏ Yes ❏ No

Irregular periods ❏ Yes ❏ No   Cycle _____   Duration _____

Do you play other sports? ❏ Yes ❏ No   Which ones? _____

Handedness ❏ Left ❏ Right

Do you want to become a professional dancer? ❏ Yes ❏ No

How much do you sleep at night? _____ (in hours)

How much sleep do you need to feel refreshed the next day? _____ (in hours)

Any previous injuries (saw doctor and was treated, or had to take time off from dance)? ❏ Yes ❏ No

Injured body part	*Diagnosis*
❏ Head (includes ears, eyes, nose, and mouth)	_____
❏ Neck	_____
❏ Back	_____
❏ Chest	_____
❏ Abdomen	_____
❏ Pelvis	_____
❏ Arms (shoulder, elbow, wrist, hands) ❏ Left or ❏ right	_____
❏ Hip (thigh, knees, calf/Achilles, ankles, feet) ❏ Left or ❏ right	_____
❏ Knees ❏ Left or ❏ right	_____
❏ Calves or lower leg ❏ Left or ❏ right	_____
❏ Ankles ❏ Left or ❏ right	_____
❏ Feet ❏ Left or ❏ right	_____

(continued)

Figure 1.1 History and physical exam tool.

ID number _____

STATION 1

    a. Weight _____ in kg

    b. Height _____ in cm

    c. Marshall/Micheli score ___/5 (flexibility)

Back

    a. Scoliosis ❑ Yes ❑ No   If yes _____° max reading level of apex _____

    b. Swayback ❑ Yes ❑ No

Ankle and foot

    a. Plantarflexion _____ in degrees

    b. Dorsiflexion _____ in degrees

    c. Foot arch ❑ Flat foot ❑ Normal arch ❑ Cavus

    d. Foot type ❑ Egyptian ❑ Grecian ❑ Morton's

    e. Bunion (1st metatarsal phalangeal angle) N<15 _____ in degrees

STATION 2

Lower extremity

    a. Q angle _____ in degrees

    b. Leg lengths (ASIS to medial malleoli)   Left _____   Right _____ in cm

    c. External/Internal rotation (Staheli) _____ in degrees

    d. Popliteal angle _____ in degrees

    e. Thomas   R Grade _____   L Grade _____

    f. Ober sign   R Grade _____   L Grade _____

    g. Foot thigh angle _____ in degrees

Figure 1.1 *(continued).*

and extrinsic risk factor information (figure 1.2), and (3) physical therapy summaries of reported injuries (RIs, figure 1.3). These study tools were developed based on examination of the literature.

Subject Population

Thirty-nine dancers participated in the study. Thirty-four were females and five males. Their average age was 15.8 years (±1.0 year, range 14 to 18 years). They had an average of 10.0 years of dance experience (±2.7 years) and averaged 6.0 years of ballet training (±2.4 years). Females started pointe work at 10.9 years of age (±1.1

years). Seventy-four percent of the dancers preferred ballet, 10% preferred modern dance, and 15% enjoyed both equally. Dance training at the school in question consisted mostly of classical ballet.

Preparticipation Physicals

A screening history and physical exam were obtained for each subject, providing information concerning intrinsic risk factors. A physician took standardized medical histories. The orthopedic exam was divided into three stations and was performed by two physical therapists and a physician (table 1.1). Each screening history

Important: Please enter your identification number at the end of the survey first!
If there is a line, fill in the blank if it applies. If there is a box, check off the appropriate box. If the answer is "yes" or "no," circle whichever is correct.

1. Do you have any injuries at present?   Yes   No
2. Have you had any injuries in the last 2 weeks?   Yes   No

    (If you answered yes, continue. If you answered no, then go to question 12.)
3. Date of onset of the injury _____ (month) / _____ (day) [example Sep/15]
4. Did you see a therapist, doctor, or other health professional?   Yes   No
5. If you answered yes, was the doctor or therapist at school?   Yes   No
6. If you have an injury **at present,** check the injured body part (check any that apply):

    ❏ Head (includes ears, eyes, nose, and mouth)

    ❏ Neck

    ❏ Back

    ❏ Chest

    ❏ Abdomen

    ❏ Pelvis

    (Indicate left or right for the following)

    ❏ Arms (shoulder, elbow, wrist, hands)   L   R

    ❏ Hip or thigh   L   R

    ❏ Knees   L   R

    ❏ Calves or lower leg   L   R

    ❏ Ankles   L   R

    ❏ Feet   L   R

    What do you think the injury/problem is? _____   ❏ No idea

    [For example "ankle sprain, tendinitis"; be as specific as possible]
7. How bad is/are the injuries?   (Not bad)   1   2   3   4   5   (Terrible)

    My injury causes no problems dancing at all.   Yes   No

    I can feel my injury when dancing, but I can dance fully.   Yes   No

    My injury causes me to alter my technique.   Yes   No

    My injury causes me to avoid certain techniques.   Yes   No

    I don't feel I can dance properly because of my injury.   Yes   No
8. How did you get your recent injury? (Check any that apply.)

    ❏ Barre   ❏ Practicing on own

    ❏ Center   ❏ Performance

    ❏ Jumping   ❏ Other/outside dance

    ❏ Fell

    In one line, please explain how (Remember, this is a confidential survey.)

    _____
9. Did you finish class the day you were injured?   Yes   No

    If no, hours danced before injury _____

(continued)

Figure 1.2   Dance injury biweekly survey.

10. Have you missed a class because of your injury?   Yes   No

    How many days of class missed? _____

11. Do you have to modify your activities?   Yes   No

    Back to dance class?   Yes   No   _____ total length of this injury in days

    Back to full dance?   Yes   No   _____ total length of this injury in days

12. How long have you used the *present* ballet shoes you use *most*?   _____ weeks

13. How stressed are you? (Circle one number.)   (Not at all) 0 1 2 3 4 (Very)

14. Are you rehearsing for something?   Yes   No

    When is your performance (from today) _____ wks and _____ days

15. On average over the last two weeks, how many hours are you dancing a day?

    _____ (in complete hours)

16. How many minutes of stretching or warming up do you do? _____

17. How many hours did you dance yesterday? _____

18. If you are female, when did your last period start? _____ weeks ago or ❑ now

19. How many dairy products did you have yesterday? _____ servings

    (1 serving = 1 glass of milk, 1 yogurt, 1 slice of cheese)

Thank you for filling out this survey.

Please enter your ID number here _____

Figure 1.2   *(continued).*

took approximately 5 minutes, while each physical exam required approximately 5 to 10 minutes to complete. No counseling was provided to the dancers.

Biweekly Surveys

The biweekly questionnaire was revised after test sampling of 20 age-specific patients visiting a sports medicine clinic. At the initial survey session the principal investigator explained instructions for the survey to the study participants and answered any questions. Subsequently, the school's dance director administered the survey every two weeks (except for holidays). The surveys were immediately sent to the principal investigator, and the information was not made available to dance teachers. For purposes of confidentiality, each individual subject was identified by a three-digit number known only to the dancer and the principal investigator.

Injury Summaries

Injuries were categorized by history, location, mechanism of injury, severity, and stage of development. They were divided into new and recurrent injuries. A "new" injury was one that the dancer had not previously experienced, as determined by the investigator based on the dancer's medical history, the location of the injury, the diagnosis by the physical therapist, and the report of onset in the participant's surveys. A "recurrent" injury was one that the dancer had reported on previous biweekly surveys or during the preparticipation history. The investigator classified the injuries by type (table 1.2), using a system that was modified

Name _____

Diagnosis _____

_____

Duration of injury _____

Previous history of similar injury   Y   N   Number of episodes _____

Duration of symptoms _____   Menstrual history   LMP _____   Regular _____

How bad is the injury?   1   2   3   4   5
     Able to dance, no restrictions, no treatment needed
     Able to dance, no restrictions, treatment needed
     Able to dance, with some restrictions
     Able to dance, with severe limitations
     Unable to dance

Recommendations
    ❑ Return to dance, no modification of activities or therapy required
    ❑ Return to dance with modification of activities and/or therapy required
    ❑ Avoid dance/rest recommended for up to 2 weeks
    ❑ Avoid dance for more than 2 weeks/or patient requires surgery/casting

Duration of injury _____

_____

Final diagnosis _____

_____

_____

Figure 1.3   Dance injury biweekly survey. Injury form.

from one developed by Dr. James Garrick (1999). Overuse injuries encompassed pathology caused by repetitive stress from dance, including tendinitis, shinsplints, "tight" muscles, patellofemoral pain, os trigonum irritation, and spondylolysis. Soft-tissue injuries included traumatic bursitis, contusion, and laceration.

Outcomes

1. **Self-reported injuries.** The biweekly surveys provided information on SRIs and extrinsic risk factors. If no injury was reported, or no survey was submitted, the dancer was considered to have been injury free during that period.

2. **Reported injuries.** Information on RIs was gathered by the physical therapists at each dancer's visit. The diagnosis by the therapist, the duration of injury, the mechanism of injury, the severity of injury (five-point Likert scale), and the recommended treatment were recorded.

3. **Duration of injury.** The duration of injury was determined based on the number of biweekly surveys on which the dancer reported the injury. The date of onset that the student

Table 1.1   Preparticipation Physical Examination Tests

Test for	Methods used	Results*
Weight	Measured in pounds using a digital scale.	118.5 lb ± 19.4
Height	Measured with a tape measure affixed to the wall (in centimeters).	164.8 cm ± 8.4
Marshall test/Micheli score (1999) Scored 4 or 5	Measured left thumb abduction to forearm to assess ligamentous flexibility: 3/5 for a 90° to 135° bend, 4/5 for 135° thumb almost touching, 5/5 for thumb touching forearm.	92.3%
Scoliosis	Measured at 60° and 90° of lumbar flexion with a scoliometer, as described by Liederbach et al. (1997).	15.4% greater than 7°
Ankle dorsiflexion	Measured using a goniometer (Norkin and White 1995). The head of the fibula was palpated and marked with a sticker to facilitate alignment of the proximal arm of the goniometer. The distal arm was aligned parallel to the fifth metatarsal, and the fulcrum of the goniometer was aligned with the lateral aspect of the lateral malleolus.	R = 8.8° ± 3.7° L = 7.0° ± 4.9°
Ankle plantarflexion	Measured using a goniometer (Norkin and White 1995).	R = 76.2° ± 7.0° L = 75.4° ± 8.0°
Foot arch	Determined using the Feiss line as a guide (Magee 1997). The navicular bone of the right foot was palpated in both sitting and standing. If the navicular dropped from sitting to standing, the subject was determined to have a flat foot type. If there was no drop, the arch type was normal. If there was no drop and the arch appeared high, the foot type was cavus.	53.9% flat foot 33.3% normal 12.8% cavus
Foot type (Magee 1997)	The second toe was compared to the first toe. If the second toe was greater than 0.5 cm shorter than the first toe, the foot type was Egyptian. If the second toe was greater than 0.5 cm longer than the first toe, the foot type was Morton's. Otherwise, the foot type was square.	69.2% square 20.5% Egyptian 10.3% Morton's
First MTP angle	Subjects stood with their first metatarsophalangeal (MTP) joint on the center of a protractor, and the center of their Achilles tendon aligned with the center line of the protractor. The angle was measured from first MTP joint through the center of the first toe.	R = 12.2° ± 4.9° L = 13.9° ± 5.8°
External rotation of the hip	Using the Staheli method (1985), the subject was asked to lie prone on table (pillow under head). The non-test leg remained straight and flat. The tested leg was bent 90° at the knee, and the subject was instructed to keep pelvis flat on table while internally or externally rotating the femur. Angle of the tibia from vertical was measured using a goniometer.	R = 54.9° ± 6.4° L = 54.7° ± 5.7°
Internal rotation of the hip	See external rotation of the hip.	R = 40.6° ± 8.2° L = 41.0° ± 9.1°
Popliteal angle	The subject lay supine on table with head on a pillow. Non-test leg was straight and flat on table. The tested leg was passively brought to a 90° angle at hip, with knee bent. Knee was then passively straightened and knee extension was measured with a goniometer, with one arm of the goniometer on the long axis of the thigh and the other on the long axis of the lower leg.	R = 9.9° ± 7.9° L = 10.0° ± 8.2°

Test for	Methods used	Results*
Hip flexor flexibility (Thomas test)	The subject was placed in the supine position with the pelvis near the end of the examination table. The non-test hip and knee were held in maximal flexion by the subject, and the test hip and knee were taken passively from the fully flexed position to an extended position off the table. The ipsilateral anterior superior iliac spine (ASIS) was palpated during the full range of motion. The test was considered positive if the ipsilateral ASIS/ilium began to nutate before the thigh reached an angle of 20° in relation to the table.	Positive bilaterally in 64.1%
Iliotibial band tightness: Ober's test (Reid et al. 1987)	The subject was asked to lie on one side while the hip and knee away from the table were tested. The non-test hip and knee was placed in full flexion and held by the subject. The testing knee was flexed to 90° and the hip was passively abducted and extended behind the subject. The examiner supported the subject's foot to maintain knee flexion at 90°, and the leg was allowed to drop passively with gravity. The long axis of the thigh was categorized as neutral (at the level of the horizontal parallel to the table), positive (knee above neutral), or negative (knee below neutral).	Positive bilaterally in 71.8%
Q-angle (Magee 1997)	Subject supine on the table. The center of the patella was determined by the examiner and marked with a pen. Using a tape measure, the axis from the ASIS to the center of the patella was identified, and a point proximal to the knee along the axis was marked. The center of the tibial tubercle was then marked. The Q-angle was determined with a goniometer measuring the angle between the line from the ASIS to the center of the patella and the axis of the patellar tendon (identified by the line between the center of the patella and the tibial tubercle).	R = 14.7° ± 3.7° L = 14.2° ± 4.1°
Leg lengths	Measured from the ASIS to the inferior tip of the medial malleolus, using a tape measure (Magee 1997).	L = 85.3 ± 5.6 cm R = 85.4 ± 5.7 cm
Foot/thigh angle	The subject sat at edge of table with a good upright trunk and hands holding on to sides of table. Subject was asked to relax lower legs and feet. One arm of goniometer was aligned along axis from ASIS to the mid patella. Other arm of a goniometer was aligned down midline of foot. The measurement was read with the examiner's dominant eye lined over the center of the goniometer and the other eye closed.	R = 54.9° ± 6.4° L = 54.7° ± 5.7°

*Numbers represent average values ± SD or percentage values in the population tested.

Table 1.2 Types of Injury

Mechanism	SRI	% of SRI	RI	% of RI
Overuse	61	56.1	35	49.3
Sprain	8	8.8	5	7.0
Acute strain	20	14.0	28	39.4
Fracture	3	5.3	0	0
Soft-tissue injury	3	3.5	2	2.8
Neurologic	0	0	1	1.4
Concussion	0	0	0	0
Other	13	8.8	0	0
Missing	4	3.5	0	0

SRI = Self-reported injury; RI = Reported injury

provided was used as the starting date of injury if it occurred within the two-week period that the survey represented. Otherwise, the date of the survey on which the injury was first reported was used.

4. **Severity of injury.** The severity of injury was rated on a five-point Likert scale by the dancers for SRIs and by the physical therapist in cases of RIs (table 1.3). An injury was considered to be "worsening" if the student reported increasing levels of severity over time, if multiple injuries occurred in the area (e.g., an ankle sprain followed by tendinopathy), or if the injury persisted for more than six weeks.

Table 1.3 Comparison of Severity Ratings

Dancer rating	Physical therapist rating
Self-reported injuries (SRI)	*Reported injuries (RI)*
My injury causes:	How bad is the injury?
1 = No problems	1 = Dance, no restrictions, no treatment
2 = Can feel injury but can dance fully	2 = Dance, no restrictions, treatment needed
3 = Causes me to alter technique	3 = Dance, some restrictions
4 = Causes me to avoid certain techniques	4 = Dance, severe limitations
5 = Unable to dance at all	5 = Unable to dance

Statistical Analysis

The data were entered into Microsoft Access and Excel 2000 (Microsoft Corp., Redmond, WA) and analyzed using SPSS 9.0 (SPSS Inc., Chicago, IL). Descriptive statistics were calculated on demographic information and intrinsic and extrinsic risk factors. Univariate tests were performed on intrinsic risk factors. T-tests and Pearson correlations were used to identify associations between the binomial, categorical, and continuous variables, and the SRIs and RIs. Injury rates were estimated using the sum of the average reported hours of dance per two-week block and the number of SRIs and RIs.

Four surveys with no identification number were discarded. One subject left the dance program within the first month of the study and was dropped.

Results

The past medical history revealed that only two of 39 dancers had reported no previous musculoskeletal injury. Five dancers had undergone lower extremity surgery. The surgeries included ankle ligament reconstruction (Chrisman-Snook), resection of an avulsion fracture in the first toe phalanx, os trigonum removal in two patients, and anterior cruciate ligament reconstruction. Twenty-seven of the 39 dancers had previous unilateral or bilateral ankle problems (69%); 10 had previous back problems (25.6%); six had a history of asthma (which in five cases was exercise-induced asthma); and three females reported hormone-related metabolic disorders, namely anorexia, "hormonal imbalance," and osteopenia. The average age of menarche was 13.1 years (±1.4 years, range 10 to 17 years). Eight women reported irregular periods. Four were taking oral contraceptives.

Self-Reported Injuries

The return rate for the biweekly surveys was 90% (range 77-100% response per survey session). Six hundred thirty-three surveys were collected over 18 reporting days. One hundred twelve SRIs were identified; 90% of the students listed an SRI. The mean number of SRIs per dancer was three, with one dancer reporting seven. Of the SRIs, 56.3% were new injuries and 43.7% were recurrent. The most common types of SRIs were overuse (54%), acute strain (39.4%), and ligament sprain (18%). The majority of the SRIs were in the lower extremities, followed by the back. Ankles had the highest number of injuries (figure 1.4).

Reported Injuries

There were 71 RIs identified in 77% of the students by the physical therapy reports. Fifteen RIs were not identified in the biweekly surveys (12 missing, 3 absent during survey). The ankle and the back were the most common areas for RIs. The clinical diagnoses of these injuries are presented in table 1.4. The average numbers of RIs were 2.8 RIs/male and 1.6 RIs/female student.

Duration of Injuries

The median period between the onset of an SRI and reporting the injury to the physical therapist was 13 days. Self-reported injuries were recorded over an average of 2.8 ± 2.3 weeks, or median of two surveys. Eighty percent of the SRIs were no longer being reported by six weeks, and 90% appeared to be resolved by 12 weeks.

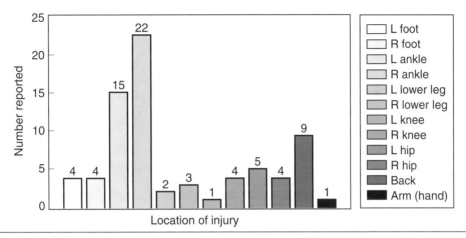

Figure 1.4 Location of self-reported injuries.

Table 1.4 Diagnoses of Reported Injuries

Ankle	
Achilles tendinopathy/strain	7
Ankle sprain	4
Os trigonum/post-op os trigonum removal	3
Flexor hallucus longus tendinopathy/strain	3
Plantar fasciitis	2
Peroneal strain	1
Anterior tibialis tendinopathy	1
Posterior tibialis tendinopathy	1
Total	22
Back	
Lumbar strain	9
Mechanical low back pain	6
Spondylolysis	2
Rib injury	2
Disc problem with right radicular pain	1
Thoracic spine pain	1
Total	21

Severity of Injuries

The average severity for an SRI was 2.8 ± 1.1 on a Likert scale of 5 with a median value of 3. This level of severity corresponded to injuries that required the dancer to begin altering his or her technique. The severity ratings by the dancers

and by the physical therapists had fair correlation ($r = 0.52$ [$p < 0.01$]). Twelve of 14 dancers who self-reported injuries of severity 4 or 5 were temporarily removed from dance. Two dancers had surgery performed during the study period (left ankle os trigonum resection and left knee lateral release). Twenty-eight of the 112 SRIs (24.8%) met the criteria for "worsening injuries."

Injury Rates

The dancers reported an average of 3.2 hours of dance per day during each two-week block. The estimated SRI rate was 4.7 SRIs per 1,000 dance hours (95% confidence interval [CI] = 3.8-5.6), and the RI rate was 2.9 RIs per 1,000 dance hours (95% CI = 2.2-3.6).

Risk Factors

The measurements assessing intrinsic biomechanical risk factor variables (table 1.1) produced values similar to those in other studies. Only three of these values demonstrated a positive correlation with SRIs or RIs: sex, age as a continuous variable (with SRI $r = 0.453$, $p = 0.004$, and with RI $r = 0.455$, $p = 0.004$), and left popliteal angle (with SRI $r = 0.340$, $p = 0.03$). The males self-reported a mean difference of approximately 1.5 injuries/dancer more than the females, which was statistically significant ($p = 0.02$).

Analysis of extrinsic risk factors demonstrated an average warm-up time of 22 minutes (±15 minutes). Stress levels of dancers averaged 2.2 on a five-point Likert scale from 0 (none) to 4 (most). Women reported a slightly higher dairy intake

(2.9 products/day) than the men (2.4 products/day). Twenty-seven percent of the students took calcium tablets.

Discussion

This study identifies some of the important issues in conducting injury survey research. As a pilot study, it demonstrates a feasible means of acquiring data from a larger, similar population in a prospective manner, avoiding "retrospective contamination" of data (Kolt and Kirkby 1999). The prospective approach decreases the amount of bias, particularly with regard to the reporting of minor injuries, duration of problems, and "worsening" severity of injuries. Primary prevention of dance injuries requires reliable determination of injury rates and risk factors, plus useful measures of prediction, in order that effective prevention strategies can be designed.

Limitations

The small sample size of this study and the possibility of confounding variables make it difficult to identify associations between risk factors and injury. As is typical of survey studies, responses by the dancers are subject to recall, reporting, and classification biases. Validating an efficient tool to describe injuries, with adequate attention to frequency and medical detail, would help to minimize these problems.

The data relating to SRIs are likely underestimated. Absent students were considered to be uninjured. Multiple injuries occurring in a single dancer were treated as one injury, as the tool could not track multiple injuries. New tools need to be developed that can perform this function.

Other variables could be considered in future studies. Assessments of functional testing and strength testing could be added. Objective isokinetic strength testing has not yet demonstrated a clear function in assessing young dancers (Solomon, Micheli, and Ireland 1993).

Self-Reported Injuries and Reported Injuries

Distinguishing between SRIs and RIs in this study was useful for understanding the development of injuries in students and their use of health services. Significant SRIs, such as fractures, would not be identified if the student sought treatment

from someone other than the physical therapists. Recording both RIs and SRIs can facilitate detection of all injuries.

As noted previously, we calculated the incidence rate of SRIs to be 4.7 injuries/1,000 hours of dance exposure (95% CI = 3.8-5.6). By way of comparison, young elite and sub-elite gymnasts in one study (Kolt and Kirkby 1999) were found to have 3.64 injuries per gymnast, 2.63 injuries per 1,000 training hours in elite gymnasts, and 4.11 injuries per 1,000 hours for the sub-elite athletes (hours of training and injuries were self-recorded weekly by each gymnast in an injury diary). Other studies in gymnastics show injury rates from 0.5 (Lindner and Caine 1990) to 22.7 (Sands, Schultz, and Newman 1993) injuries per 1,000 hours. Obviously a standardized method of defining, classifying, and rating the severity of injuries needs to be widely adopted so that results from different studies can be compared.

Severity of Injury

Dancers in general tend to have a good sense of their bodies. As dancers start to feel significant discomfort, they often alter their technique to avoid aggravation of the injury. The threshold of pain is distinct for each individual. Understanding the threshold at which the dancer seeks medical attention can help in providing medical services. To avoid using a subjective pain scale we graded the severity of SRIs in relation to their influence on the dancer's technique. Both the dancer and the physical therapist rated the severity of injury, again based on their assessment of the effect the injury was having on what the dancer could perform. We defined a "worsening injury" as one with a chronic duration (greater than six weeks), increasing severity, or recurrence of injury at a joint. These injuries made up one-fourth of the SRIs, and were differentiated as potentially warranting evaluation by a health professional.

The correlation between the dancers' (SRI) and the physical therapists' (RI) ratings of severity was fair (r = 0.52). This was due mainly to the fact that the dancers assessed injuries between the third and fourth categories of severity as more severe than the therapists; the therapist often felt that the dancer could return to limited activities (rating 3), while the dancer was more hesitant and conservative (rating 4). We feel this is a positive result, as dancers should modify their technique until they are examined by a health professional rather than risk aggravating an injury. Apparently the dancers in our group had a good understanding of the severity of their injuries, and were more cautious in their dance activities when they were experiencing a serious injury.

Education

Education is a key element in preventing dance injuries, for both dancers and the medical professionals who care for them. Developing increased understanding of injury in dancers is important as it may allow for early detection and modification of routines to avoid worsening injuries. As more research-based information becomes available, health care professionals and teachers can better perform specific interventions in the preseason and during activities to decrease the risk of injury. The dancers enrolled in our study high school attend workshops at the beginning of the school year related to matters of health and injury prevention. The teachers promote a healthy class environment and encourage early detection of injuries through open communication with their associated health care professionals.

Preparticipation Dance History and Exam

Standardization of dance screening exams, with follow-up longitudinal studies, are needed to determine what benefits can be derived from these procedures (Clippinger 1997). The preparticipation examination should include a detailed medical history. In our study we identified higher prevalence of asthma variants, lower extremity surgery, and female hormonal disorders than expected, findings that warrant attention by health professionals. Almost 70% of the dancers studied had previous ankle injuries, and one-fourth had previous back problems. Orthopedic injuries are often recurrent sources of frustration for dancers, and identifying such problems from the injury history is one of the best means of avoiding reinjury (Strong et al. 1994; Lysens, Steverlynck, and van den Auweele 1984).

Intrinsic Risk Factors

Age and sex were the only risk factors that significantly affected injury. The remaining intrinsic risk factors, including anatomical measurements, showed no obvious associations, although the study was underpowered to detect small differences. The association between popliteal angle and SRI may be due to statistical multiple testing rather than a true biomechanical cause. Intrinsic anatomical risk factors (e.g., range of motion at the ankle or hip) may not be alterable to any clinically or functionally significant extent (Khan et al. 2000). The senior dancers often had the more demanding roles in productions, which may explain the significance of the age factor.

Health professionals must be aware of specific issues for young female and male dancers. Female dancers should be screened for disordered eating, menstrual irregularities, calcium intake, and bone health. Injury rates in male dancers may be underestimated. Our sample size is too small to justify a definitive statement, but the males had an injury rate twice as high as the female dancers. The few male dancers typically had less dance experience, yet they had to perform demanding dance maneuvers, including lifts. Furthermore, the male dancers may not have reached full physical maturity.

Extrinsic Risk Factors

Analysis of extrinsic risk factors, which tend to be transient in nature, requires an appropriate statistical approach. One such approach is suggested by Maclure (1991) and Mittleman et al. (1993, 1995). When looking at a brief exposure to a risk factor, it is necessary to identify short-effect periods. This requires more frequent reporting—for example, on a daily basis—of risk factors such as volume and duration of training.

Conclusion

Standardization of the definition and classification of dance injuries is needed in order to make future study results more comparable. Self-reported and reported injuries should be considered as outcomes in the design of injury survey studies. If dance programs utilized similar injury surveillance tools, a database could be developed that would greatly enhance the capabilities of researchers studying the epidemiology of dance injuries. A multicenter study based on this pilot study could generate a larger sample size of dancers, producing more statistically significant results due to its greater power to detect trends. The Internet provides a means of acquiring data, with dancers potentially inputting their information via e-mail survey. More specific studies on particular risk factors or special populations could be conducted with smaller subgroups responding to surveys on a more frequent basis for shorter periods of time. Prevention strategies could then be formulated based on the results.

References

Bronner, S., and B. Brownstein. 1997. Profile of dance injuries in a Broadway show: A discussion of issues in dance medicine epidemiology. *Journal of Orthopedic and Sports Physical Therapy* 26(2): 87-94.

Clippinger, K.S. 1997. Dance screening. *Journal of Dance Medicine & Science* 1(3): 84.

DuRant, R.H., R.A. Pendergrast, C. Seymore, G. Gaillard, and J. Donner. 1992. Findings from the preparticipation athletic examination and athletic injuries. *American Journal of Diseases of Children* 146(1): 85-91.

Evans, R.W., R.I. Evans, S. Carvajal, and S. Perry. 1996. A survey of injuries among Broadway performers. *American Journal of Public Health* 86(1): 77-80.

Garrick, J.G. 1999. Early identification of musculoskeletal complaints and injuries among female ballet students. *Journal of Dance Medicine & Science* 3(2): 80-83.

Garrick, J.G., and R.K. Requa. 1993. Ballet injuries: An analysis of epidemiology and financial outcome. *American Journal of Sports Medicine* 21(4): 586-590.

Hamilton, L.H., J. Brooks-Gunn, and M.P. Warren. 1985. Sociocultural influences on eating disorders in professional female ballet dancers. *International Journal of Eating Disorders* 4(4): 465-477.

Hamilton, L.H., W.G. Hamilton, J.D. Meltzer, P. Marshall, and M. Molnar. 1989. Personality, stress, and injuries in professional ballet dancers. *American Journal of Sports Medicine* 17(2): 263-267.

Khan, K.M., K. Bennell, S. Ng, B. Matthews, P. Roberts, C. Nattrass, S. Way, and J. Brown. 2000. Can 16-18-year-old elite ballet dancers improve their hip and ankle range of motion over a 12-month period? *Clinical Journal of Sport Medicine* 10(2): 98-103.

Kolt, G.S., and R.J. Kirkby. 1999. Epidemiology of injury in elite and subelite female gymnasts: A comparison of retrospective and prospective findings. *British Journal of Sports Medicine* 33(5): 312-318.

Liederbach, M., J. Spivak, and D.J. Rose. 1997. Scoliosis in dancers: A method of assessment in quick-screen settings. *Journal of Dance Medicine & Science* 1(3): 107-112.

Lindner, K.J., and D.J. Caine. 1990. Injury patterns of female competitive gymnasts. *Canadian Journal of Applied Sports Science* 15(4): 254-261.

Lysens, R., A. Steverlynck, and Y. van den Auweele. 1984. The predictability of sports injuries. *Sports Medicine* 1: 6-10.

Maclure, M. 1991. The case-crossover design: A method for studying transient effects on the risk of acute events. *American Journal of Epidemiology* 133(2): 144-153.

Magee, D. 1997. *Orthopedic physical assessment.* 3rd ed. Philadelphia: Saunders.

Micheli, L.J. 1984. *Pediatric and adolescent sports medicine.* Boston: Little Brown.

Micheli, L.J., H.S. Greene, M. Cassella, J. Gruber, and D. Zurakowski. 1999. Assessment of flexibility in young female skaters with the modified Marshall Test. *Journal of Pediatric Orthopedics* 19(5): 665-668.

Mittleman, M.A., M. Maclure, and J.M. Robins. 1995. Control sampling strategies for case-crossover studies: An assessment of relative efficiency. *American Journal of Epidemiology* 142(1): 91-98.

Mittleman, M.A., M. Maclure, G.H. Tofler, J.B. Sherwood, R.J. Goldberg, and J.E. Muller. 1993. Triggering of acute myocardial infarction by heavy physical exertion. *New England Journal of Medicine* 1(329): 1677-1683.

Norkin C.C., and D.J. White. 1995. *Measurement of joint motion: A guide to goniometry.* Philadelphia: Davis.

Reid, D.C., R.S. Burnham, L.A. Saboe, and S.F. Kushner. 1987. Lower extremity flexibility patterns in classical ballet dancers and their correlation to lateral hip and knee injuries. *American Journal of Sports Medicine* 15(4): 347-352.

Rovere, G.D., L.X. Webb, A.G. Gristina, and J.M. Vogel. 1983. Musculoskeletal injuries in theatrical dance students. *American Journal of Sports Medicine* 11(4): 195-198.

Sands, W.A., B.B. Schultz, and A.P. Newman. 1993. Women's gymnastics injuries. *American Journal of Sports Medicine* 21(2): 271-276.

Solomon, R., L.J. Micheli, and M.L. Ireland. 1993. Physiological assessment to determine readiness for pointe work in ballet students. *Impulse* 1(1): 21-38.

Staheli, L.T., M. Corbett, C. Wyss, and H. King. 1985. Lower-extremity rotational problems in children: Normal values to guide management. *Journal of Bone and Joint Surgery* 67A(1): 39-47.

Strong, W.B., C.L. Stanitski, R.E. Smith, and J.H. Wilmore. 1994. Athletic preparticipation examinations for adolescents: Report of the board of trustees. *Archives of Pediatric and Adolescent Medicine* 148: 93-98.

Yannakoulia, M., and A. Matalas. 2000. Nutrition intervention for dancers. *Journal of Dance Medicine & Science* 4(3): 103-108.

Recommended Readings (Editors)

Bennell, K., and P. Brukner. 1997. Epidemiology and site specificity of stress fractures. *Clinics in Sports Medicine* 16(2): 179-196.

Bronner, S., S. Ojofeitimi, and D. [J] Rose. 2003. Injuries in a modern dance company: Effect of comprehensive management on injury incidence and time loss. *American Journal of Sports Medicine* 31(3): 365-373.

Byhring, S., and K. Bo. 2002. Musculoskeletal injuries in the Norwegian national ballet: A prospective cohort study. *Scandinavian Journal of Medicine and Science in Sports* 12(6): 365-370.

Caine, C.G., and J.G. Garrick. 1996. Dance. In *Epidemiology of sports injuries,* edited by D.J. Caine, C.G. Caine, and K.J. Lindner. Champaign, IL: Human Kinetics, 124-160.

Carvajal, S., R.I. Evans, R.W. Evans, S.G. Nash, and T.W. Carvajal. 1998. Risk factors for injury in the career female dancer: An epidemiologic study of a Broadway sample of performers. *Medical Problems of Performing Artists* 13(3): 89-93.

Mainwaring, L.M., D. Krasnow, and G. Kerr. 2001. And the dance goes on: Psychological impact of injury. *Journal of Dance Medicine & Science* 5(4): 105-115.

Miller, C., and G. Moa. 1998. Injury characteristics and outcomes at a performing arts school clinic. *Medical Problems of Performing Artists* 13(3): 120-124.

Ramel, E.M., U. Moritz, and G-B. Jarnlo. 1999. Recurrent musculoskeletal pain in professional ballet dancers in Sweden: A six-year follow-up. *Journal of Dance Medicine & Science* 3(3): 93-100.

Scharff-Olson, M.R., H.N. Williford, and J.A. Brown. 1999. Injuries associated with current dance-exercise practices. *Journal of Dance Medicine & Science* 3(4): 144-150.

Solomon, R., L.J. Micheli, J. Solomon, and T. Kelley. 1995. The "cost" of injuries in a professional ballet company: Anatomy of a season. *Medical Problems of Performing Artists* 10(1): 3-10.

Solomon, R., L.J. Micheli, J. Solomon, and T. Kelley. 1996. The "cost" of injuries in a professional ballet company: A three-year perspective. *Medical Problems of Performing Artists* 16(3): 67-74.

Solomon, R., J. Solomon, L.J. Micheli, and E. McGray. 1999. The "cost" of injuries in a professional ballet company: A five year study. *Journal of Dance Medicine & Science* 3(1): 34-35.

Chapter 2

Physical Screening Procedures

Janice Gudde Plastino, PhD

The preceding chapter makes mention of the kind of physical examination to which dancers at all levels of the field are now frequently being exposed, usually at the beginning, and sometimes again at the end, of a dance season. The purpose of such procedures is to promote safer practices by alerting dancers (and those who train them) to aspects of their medical history, anatomic alignment, and habitual movement patterning that might increase their susceptibility to injury. This chapter explores in detail the screening process being used in a major university dance program.

This chapter introduces a basic screening model to teachers, choreographers, directors, and health professionals who care for dancers' well-being. The procedure described can be used to increase the artistic ability of dancers in any technique or at any level in the dance world.

Physical evaluation of student and professional dancers before actual participation in dance programs has increased in the United States and many other parts of the world over the last 10 years. For example, Rachel Rist, director of dance at the Arts Educational School in Tring, England, has established a very rigorous screening program for dancers that begins with the audition for acceptance to the school and continues throughout their course of study (Plastino 2003b). Similar screening programs exist in Israel and the Netherlands (Plastino 2003a).

Physical screening is the process of evaluating dancers for general health and anatomic parameters and for existing and previous injuries that might eventually affect their dance career. This process is a well-established requirement in the athletic world; no self-respecting amateur or professional sport program would begin a training season without a preparticipation examination of all performers.

The screening program in dance at the University of California at Irvine was developed to reduce dance injuries and teach student dancers more about their bodies. It originated with this author (who is a kinesiologist), in collaboration with the athletic department trainer and his staff, and an orthopedic surgeon who, as a sports medicine specialist, was seeing all injured dancers at the University Student Health Service. We believe that this plan, modeled after successful athletic screening programs, is the best available to us for screening large numbers of dancers in the limited time allowed. Due to budget and personnel changes, the program has undergone major modifications over the years.

With the cooperation of the physician just mentioned and qualified faculty and students in the dance department, the physical exam is completed in one intense afternoon session at the beginning of the university year, before the students start technique classes. Auditions are held the previous day, so the results of the screening and the audition can be used to place each student at the proper level of technique class.

The Screening Process

There are two basic parts to the screening: (1) taking an injury history and (2) analyzing posture and body type as they relate to various types of dance, with specific evaluation of the feet, ankles, knees, hips, and spine. For testing, women should be dressed in a two-piece bathing suit, men in trunks, and both should be barefoot. It is desirable that the dancers bring with them any shoes and orthotics used daily or in class, rehearsal, and performance. An exam progresses faster if the examiner has a recorder; also, for liability protection, more than one person should be present during the process. Other tests can be carried out in the studio, with medical problems referred to a health professional.

The main problem facing the faculty at Irvine, given the large dance population (170 majors), was the amount of time needed to advise the dancers based on the audition or placement

The Screening Exam

- Health and injury forms
- Evaluation by health professional
- Foot and ankle evaluation
- Posture evaluation
- Evaluation by dance advisor

exam and the results of the screening. The last station of the screening process is a consultation with the dance kinesiologist, who is a technique teacher, choreographer, and ex-professional performer. Any problem found by the examiners is conveyed to the kinesiologist, who in turn brings it to the attention of the dancer. On the basis of this information the kinesiologist may recommend alternative or additional training procedures, alteration of the level or number of technique classes to be taken, or both. For the student dancer, rehearsal and performance schedules are an integral part of the evaluation, though the pressing need to complete university requirements for graduation often takes priority over other considerations (in the private school or professional company situation the dancer's rehearsal and performance commitments carry more weight).

Ultimately, the appropriate advisor must have access to the findings of the screening; follow-up with proper advising of each dancer regarding his or her physical and aesthetic progress is a necessity. It takes less time to evaluate each body than it does to assess each examination and then advise each dancer, yet there is no doubt that the time spent in this way can help dancers know more about their bodies and how they may help themselves to become stronger and healthier in their craft.

History Form

The most important aspect of the screening process is the health and injury history form that is completed by each dancer. (For an example of this type of form see figure 1.1, pp. 5-6.)

The form should be brief and organized so that it can be completed by the dancer in a short period of time. It should include questions that reveal all aspects of the dancer's present health. The form should contain the following information, organized for easy interpretation by the dance professional who advises the dancer:

1. Name, current and permanent address, and telephone number; the identity of and appropriate information about someone who is responsible for the dancer (parent, spouse, significant other, friend); the dancer's age, date of birth, and status in the school (e.g., junior) or the company (e.g., corps member three years).

2. The next section should briefly question the dancer, requiring simple yes or no answers, about histories of heart disease, diabetes, bladder problems, epilepsy, extraordinary menstrual irregularities, eating disorders, psychological issues, or recent surgeries. This type of information is usually available in more detail from the student health service or the dancer's private physician (in both cases with a signed patient consent), and is needed in case of emergency only.

3. The most important part of the form asks for identification of all significant injuries: date, recurrence, treatment, specific diagnosis, person who diagnosed the injury, and current status of the injury. This is most easily accomplished by a form that lists the specific parts of the body (toes, foot, ankle, etc.) and has appropriate boxes to be checked by the dancer to indicate the injuries and the care received.

4. Finally, the form asks for the number of hours spent in technique class, rehearsal, performance, and additional physical conditioning activities in the last two months, and the type and level of dance technique(s) used.

Posture Exam and Body Type Analysis

The evaluator should be sure to scan the history form before starting the posture exam. Any current, former, or recurrent injury should be inquired about and any existing medical protocol noted. Other medical problems, such as diabetes, should be briefly discussed and noted. It is important to be aware of the amount of time the dancer has spent in dance activities and associated physical exercise in the past six weeks. This indicates how fast the dancer can get into "performing shape. "

Side View

Each dancer should be viewed from the side in the "normal stance." This procedure, which must be completed by a teacher or health professional trained in dance and proper dance alignment, reveals potential or existing problems and is the easiest way to bring them to the attention of the dancer. If a posture grid is available, this part of the exam can proceed faster and more accurately. These grids can easily be purchased from medical supply houses.

The imaginary (plumb) line used to evaluate posture as seen from the side descends from the mastoid process, through the center of the shoulder joint, slightly in front of the greater trochanter of the hip, just behind the center of the knee joint, and slightly anterior to the lateral malleolus. Perhaps the greatest single problem facing dancers is some degree of spinal lordosis (swayback), and this can readily be seen in relation to the plumb line. Verbal and manipulative instructions can be used to indicate how the problem is to be corrected.

Another common problem in dance posture is hyperextension of the knee. This is actually a desirable trait in some styles of ballet, yet the dancer needs to be made aware of the condition and told that it can contribute to a weak knee if proper strengthening does not occur. The dancer in figure 2.1 is exaggerating the posture with which she came to dance four years ago as a freshman. By now she has mastered advanced ballet, modern, and jazz techniques and has assumed a new alignment (figure 2.2).

Back View

Following evaluation from the side, the dancer is viewed from the back. A discrepancy in the height of the two shoulders can be an indication of scoliosis (curvature of the spine), though many humans have one shoulder higher than the other (figure 2.3). After observing the level of the shoulders and noting it either mentally or verbally to the recorder, the evaluator has the dancer bend forward toward the knees with the hands touching in front of the body and the feet together in parallel position. One side of the back may disclose a slight hump, which would indicate some degree of curvature. Usually the hump will be more pronounced on the side where the shoulder is higher. In the young dancer this

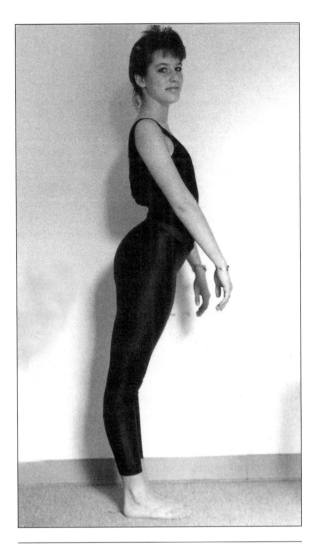

Figure 2.1   Exaggerated posture.

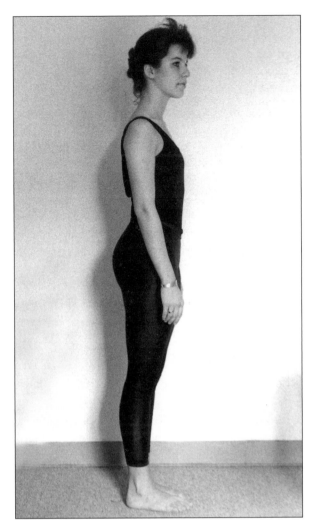

Figure 2.2   Corrected posture.

curvature may indicate problems of sufficient seriousness to have the student referred to an orthopedic physician before proceeding with technique classes. The dancer should be made aware that one side is likely to be stronger or preferred over the other.

Front View

The dancer is next asked to face the evaluator with the feet in parallel position. The anterior superior iliac crests are palpated, and should be level. If the evaluator has noticed a spinal curvature, the iliac crests may not be level. Measuring with a small steel tape measure from the iliac spines to the medial malleolus can usually pinpoint the discrepancy. If this measurement shows that the two legs are the same length, the evaluator can have the dancer lie flat on the back, with knees bent, and check to see if

the knees are level. If the knees are not level, a difference in length of the femurs may be indicated. The addition of an orthotic in the street shoe, character or jazz shoe, and in extreme cases the soft ballet shoe can help balance the dancer. These devices are prescribed by an orthopedist or podiatrist, and must be professionally and individually constructed for each dancer. In most cases orthotics cannot be worn on stage in pointe or soft ballet shoes, or with bare feet for modern dance.

Knees are one of the easiest areas to evaluate because the dance population understands genu valgus (knock-knees), genu varum (bowlegs), genu recurvatum (hyperextended knees), and femoral anteversion (lack of external rotation). In this author's experience, many advanced students and professional female dancers have some degree of genu varum. Whether this re-

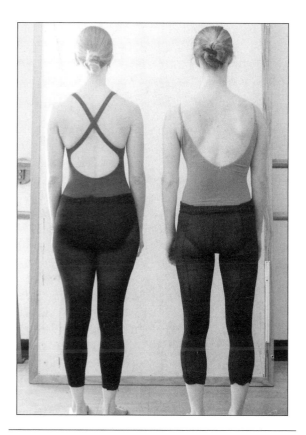

Figure 2.3 Note the curvature, shoulder height, and scapulae discrepancy in dancer on right, as compared to dancer on left.

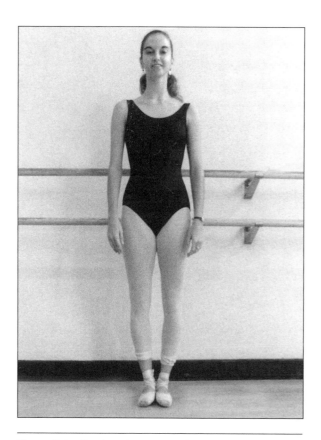

Figure 2.4 Bowlegs (genu varum).

sults from training or from genetics is unknown, but it is common (figure 2.4). This outward (lateral) curvature of the femur or tibia (or both) must be brought to the attention of the dancer, as it can be mitigated, if not completely corrected. With genu varum the natural weight of the body descends through the lateral side of the foot rather than through the tarsus bones, where it should end in line with the second toe (figure 2.5). This alignment problem can lead to ankle sprains and to peroneus longus or brevis tendinitis.

The propensity to genu valgus is more natural in the female population because of the width of the hips, and can lead to poor turnout, as can the problem of femoral anteversion. Often "squinting kneecaps" can indicate a lack of hip external rotation (figure 2.6). These are common occurrences in the less trained dancer and may require additional strength training of the lower body.

Continuing down the body, the position of the ankles, feet, and toes in parallel position is evaluated. The ankles should not supinate (roll out,

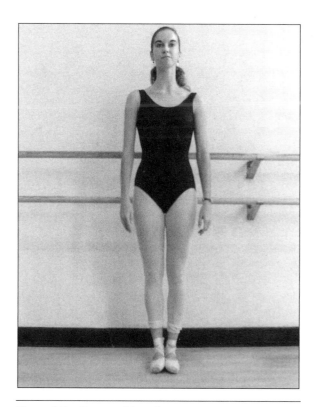

Figure 2.5 Corrected leg alignment.

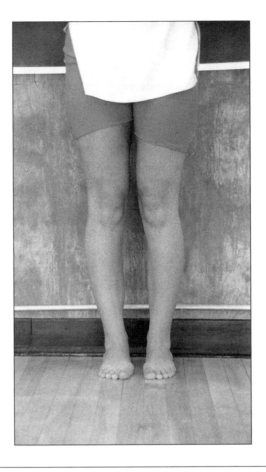

Figure 2.6 "Squinting" kneecaps (internal hip rotation).

figure 2.7; corrected alignment, figure 2.8) or pronate (roll in, figure 2.9). From the rear, the Achilles tendon should ascend in a straight line, curving neither to the lateral nor to the medial side.

Turnout

As many forms of dance use both parallel and rotated hip positions, it is important to view the dancer in both stances. After the knees have been examined in parallel, the dancer should stand in turnout. The natural turnout is easily assessed starting with the feet and continuing upward. (For a more complete discussion of techniques for measuring turnout see chapter 11, pp. 140-142.) The second toe should be in line with the center of the kneecap. The tibia (shinbone) may curve laterally as the evaluator gently glides a finger along it toward the center of the patella. The weight of the body should be distributed evenly through the tarsus and forefoot (figure 2.10). Make sure the dancer understands the correct basic alignment for dance. Careful continuous work can almost always correct or adjust lordosis, hyperextended knees, and the pronated or supinated foot. These alignment problems are common in dance, and all this information should be brought to the attention of the dancer verbally and with some hands-on adjustments.

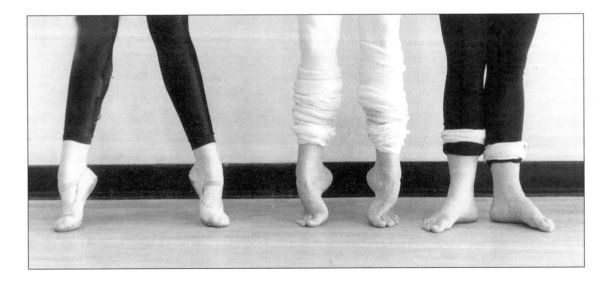

Figure 2.7 Supination (rolling out).

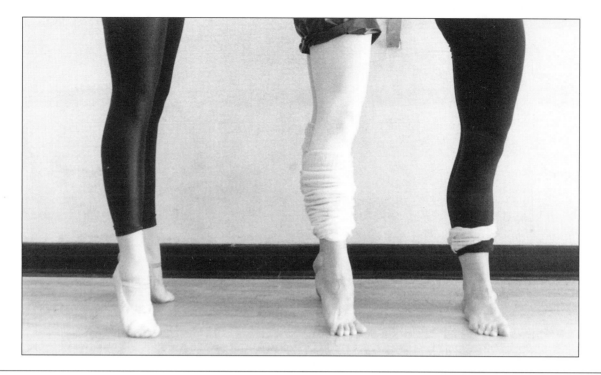

Figure 2.8 Corrected foot and ankle alignment.

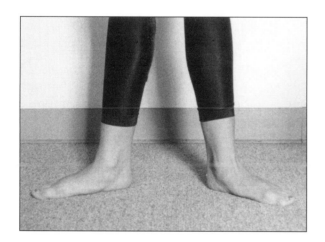

Figure 2.9 Pronation (rolling in).

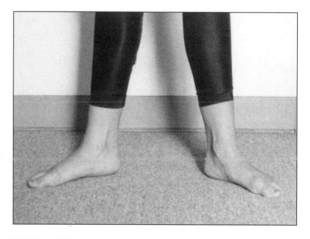

Figure 2.10 Corrected foot alignment.

The use of caliper measurements and the podiascope (figure 2.11) at Irvine has been extremely helpful in two ways (Plunk 1986). First, indications are that the depth of the forefoot at the first metatarsal head as measured by standard calipers is important in the correct fitting of toe shoes. Second, the placement of the bare foot on the podiascope may show foot placement problems not caught in the visual exam. The negative aspect of the podiascope is the inordinate amount of time required to evaluate each foot individually. It is most valuable for examining extreme cases, or to further evaluate those dancers with the most difficult or puzzling problems.

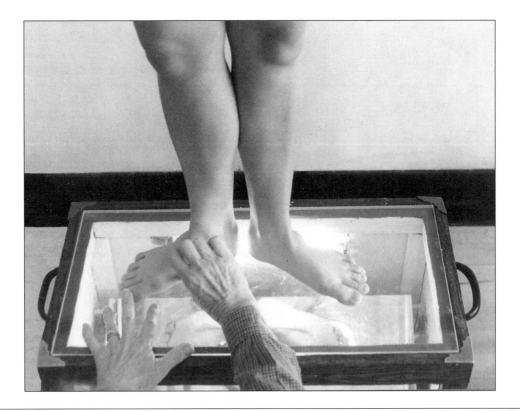

Figure 2.11 The podiascope.

Additional Concerns

It is important that all information concluded from the exam be held in the strictest confidentiality. Only the evaluator, the dancer, and an appropriate health professional should have access to the information. It is also important that the evaluator be very gentle and positive in conveying any findings, especially before consultation with a licensed health professional.

Conclusion

It is important that the dancer be viewed in all of the ways described, the relevant information recorded, and potential problems and appropriate corrective measures brought to the dancer's attention. Ideally, following the initial screening process the dancer should be carefully observed while performing any dance movements or positions that are commonly used by the choreographer, school, or company. Particular areas of stress resulting from the demands of the technique on body parts that are not well adapted to them can then be identified. Special exercises might have to be incorporated into or added to the technique class to increase the dancer's strength, flexibility, or endurance and improve alignment. Part III contains many exercises for enhancing the dancer's strength, flexibility, and alignment. Chapter 9, for example, addresses all of these issues, while chapter 12 takes a holistic approach to increasing flexibility. For more body-part-specific exercises see chapter 11 (hip), chapter 13 (ankle), and chapter 14 (foot).

References

Plastino, J.G. 2003a. Notes from correspondence with Margot Rijven, physical therapist for the theatre school, Amsterdam School of the Arts, Amsterdam, Netherlands. In possession of Janice Plastino, Dance Department, University of California at Irvine, CA.

Plastino, J.G. 2003b. Notes from correspondence with Rachel Rist, director of dance, Arts Educational School, Tring, England. In possession of Janice Plastino, dance department, University of California at Irvine, CA.

Plunk, B.B. 1986-present. Evaluation of the ballet foot for the fitting of the pointe shoe. Unpublished study, University of California, Irvine.

Recommended Readings (Author)

Amheim, D.D. 1991. *Dance injuries: Their prevention and care.* 3rd ed. St. Louis: Mosby.

Fitt, S.S. 1996. *Dance kinesiology.* 2nd ed. New York: Schirmer Books.

Hardaker, W.T., L. Erickson, and M. Myers. 1986. The pathogenesis of dance injury. In *The dancer as athlete,* edited by C.G. Shell. Champaign, IL: Human Kinetics.

Plastino, J.G. 1987. The university dancer: Physical screening. *Journal of Physical Education, Recreation and Dance* 58(5): 49-50.

Stephens, R.E. 1987. The etiology of injuries in ballet. In *Dance medicine: A comprehensive guide,* edited by A.J. Ryan and R.E. Stephens. Chicago and Minneapolis: Pluribus Press/Physician and Sportsmedicine.

Recommended Readings (Editors)

See the preceding chapter in this book by Luke et al.

Bonbright, J.M. 1995. Developing screening and education programs for detecting and preventing eating disorders at the subclinical level in dancers. *Impulse* 3(4): 303-311.

Clippinger, K.S. 1997. Dance screening. *Journal of Dance Medicine & Science* 1(3): 84.

Garrick, J.G. 1991. Orthopedic participation screening examination of the young athlete. In *Sports medicine: Second edition,* edited by R.H. Strauss. Philadelphia: Saunders, 453-463.

Liederbach, M. 1997. Screening for functional capacity in dancers: Designing standardized, dance-specific injury prevention screening tools. *Journal of Dance Medicine & Science* 1(3): 93-106.

Molnar, M., and J. Esterson. 1997. Screening students in a pre-professional ballet school. *Journal of Dance Medicine & Science* 1(3): 118-121.

Plastino, J.G. 1997. Issues encountered in the screening process. *Journal of Dance Medicine & Science* 1(3): 85-86.

Schon, L.C., K.R. Biddinger, and P. Greenwood. 1994. Dance screen programs and development of dance clinics. *Clinics in Sports Medicine* 13(4): 865-882.

Siev-Ner, I., A. Barak, M. Heim, M. Warshavsky, and M. Azaria. 1997. The value of screening. *Journal of Dance Medicine & Science* 1(30): 87-92.

Solomon, R. 1997. A pro-active screening program for addressing injury prevention in a professional ballet company. *Journal of Dance Medicine & Science* 1(3): 113-117.

Chapter 3

A Somatic Screening Procedure Using Bartenieff Fundamentals

Sandra Kay Lauffenburger, BEd, MSc, Dip (psych) CMA

The dance community has for generations made abundant use of so-called body or somatic therapies as alternatives or adjuncts to mainstream medicine. While the primary thrust of these modalities—including Alexander Technique, Bartenieff Fundamentals, Body-Mind Centering, Feldenkrais Method, Ideokinesis, Laban Movement Analysis, and Rolfing—is therapeutic, they also serve a diagnostic function. Thus, much of the injury prevention information provided to dancers in group screening sessions like those described in chapters 1 and 2 is also available through one-on-one work with a knowledgeable somatics practitioner. This chapter offers an example of such work. The strong emphasis here on movement patterning is echoed in chapter 9.

Most dance injuries are not sudden or traumatic; they are commonly chronic, stemming from carefully cultivated but inefficient movement patterns developed by the dancer during years of training. These inefficient patterns appear as an unprepared or unaware body tries to cope with technique or choreography. The patterns manifest themselves in improper muscle sequencing, misfiring of unneeded muscles, overuse of certain muscles, and muscle tone imbalance.

In non-dancers (or nonathletes), injury potential resulting from these inefficient movement patterns may not cause concern. However, given the degree of repeated usage required during dance training, rehearsals, and performances, in dancers it deserves serious attention. Inefficient patterns produce muscle misuse or overdependence on inappropriate muscles. As training continues this can lead to overuse of the muscles being engaged, as well as lack of use and subsequent weakening of the more appropriate ones. Finally, muscle imbalance results; and when this is added to excessive stress (repetitive use) and fatigue, all the ingredients for injury are present.

The best place to break this potentially destructive chain is at the beginning; the dancer will benefit from early detection of inefficient movement patterns and increased awareness of other movement possibilities. Thus, injury prevention depends greatly on the teacher's or trainer's ability to spot incorrect muscle usage and inappropriate motor patterning. Inefficient body usage is easiest to observe and correct if one looks at simple joint functions. However, given the range and complexity of most dance movement, the teacher or trainer needs a method for organizing, understanding, breaking down, and observing movement patterns.

Bartenieff Fundamentals are an effective way of organizing an evaluation of muscle use and motor patterns. The Fundamentals are a series of exercise concepts that are now an integral part of the Laban Movement Analysis System in the United States. These exercise concepts embody the basic internal and external processes that underlie all movement, from athletics and dance to life-supporting pedestrian tasks. Most of the basic exercises involve simple lifting and lowering or flexing and extending of limbs or segments of limbs or trunk.

Any aspect of technique or choreography can be broken into components that relate directly to one or more specific Fundamentals. A list of the Fundamentals is given in table 3.1. This chapter focuses on the use of some of these Fundamentals to identify inefficient motor function and the consequent potential for chronic injury. I illustrate this with one example for the lower body, one for the upper body, and one example for integrated full body movement.

Lower Body Movement Analysis

One of the simplest Fundamentals is the "thigh lift." The exercise procedure, as outlined in figure 3.1*a* and *b*, is as follows: Lie back in a "hook lie" position (3.1*a*). Exhale and hollow the abdomen to initiate the movement of leading with the top of the knee to lift the thigh toward the chest (3.1*b*). Return to the starting position while maintaining the same amount of flexion in the knee. What we commonly call the "dancer experience" can be described thusly: The lumbar extensor muscles begin to lengthen (i.e., tension diminishes in them). The gluteal muscles gradually relax so that the whole sacrum settles on the floor. This allows the iliopsoas to function. The whole process will be experienced as a changing of tension around the greater trochanter. Anchoring of the rest of the body occurs in the opposite (nonworking) leg from ischium to heel, and in the utmost width across the back and front of the chest. The kinesiologic action is pure flexion and extension at a single hip joint.

Table 3.1 Basic Eight Bartenieff Fundamentals

Fundamental exercise	Associated kinesiologic action
Heel rock	Flexion/extension of spine
	Breath support
Thigh lift	Flexion of hip
Forward pelvic shift	Extension of hip
Lateral pelvic shift	Abduction/adduction of hip (minor rotation)
Body half	Abduction/adduction/rotation of proximal joints (and minor spine)
Knee reach	Rotation of spine and right and left hip joints
Arm circles	Rotation/abduction/adduction/flexion/extension of shoulder joint
	Protraction/retraction/upward and downward rotation of scapula
	Flexion/extension (small) of the glenoid-humeral joint as well as mobilization of the sternoclavicular, acromioclavicular, and scapulo-thoracic joints
"X" rolls	Rotation/circumduction of the shoulder and hip joints

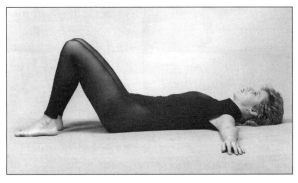

a

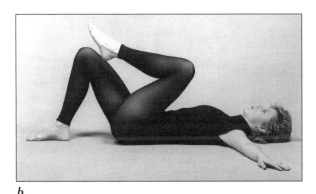

b

Figure 3.1 Thigh lift.

Hip flexion and extension are components of dance technique and choreography (plié, passé, walking, running, etc.). Through this exercise the teacher or trainer has a chance to observe the dancer's motor pattern and possible muscle imbalances and to draw the dancer's attention to problems before repetitive use causes chronic pain with the potential for injury. When performed correctly and with awareness, the same exercise can be used to train for a safer and more efficient motor action.

There are three main injury-prone locations related to simple hip flexion and extension: the spine, the hip joint, and the knee joint.

Spine

One can detect the potential for spinal injury by observing the relationship of the sacrum to the floor as the degree of flexion increases. An anterior tilt of the pelvis (particularly to initiate the movement) or a loss of full sacral contact with the floor (by rolling onto the coccyx or the lumbar spine) should not occur. Either indicates an inability to stabilize the pelvis during hip flexion, and true articulation at the hip joint is

lost. Often shortening rather than lengthening of the lumbar area (usually as a result of anterior pelvic tilt, but also possibly through hyperextension of the lumbar spine) is observed. This signals misuse or overuse of the lumbar erector spinae and quadratus lumborum muscles to perform the action, and a concurrent lack of use or weakness in the abdominal muscles (pyramidalis and transversus abdominis, in particular) and pelvic floor. This shortening creates compression on the vertebrae, while the misuse of the erector spinae and quadratus lumborum can lead to hypercontraction, spinal asymmetry, and muscle spasm. Also, poor articulation of the hip joint results. These are all symptoms indicating potential low back problems.

Hip Joint

The hip is a second site to evaluate for injury potential. The action of flexion should involve only the rectus femoris and iliopsoas of the working leg, with the rectus and transversus abdominal muscles stabilizing the pelvis and the balanced usage of the hamstrings and quadriceps stabilizing the knee in its flexed position. However, careful observation of this exercise often reveals excessive involvement of the tensor fascia latae and gluteal muscles. A shortening along the lateral side of the working hip, or abduction of the thigh, or both, are key indicators of this muscular involvement.

Actual hip joint injuries are not so common, but continuance of this rotary tension leads to spinal misalignment. Muscle spasm and pain in the sacral area and hip joint often occur from hypercontracted gluteals. Overused abductors can result in overall thigh muscle imbalance, which is a precursor of knee problems.

Knee Joint

The potential for knee injury as a result of hip flexion and extension is less obvious, but it exists and can be detected by examination of the performance of this exercise. As the knee moves toward the chest it should maintain a constant distance from the body's midline. Deviation toward the midline signals too much adductor or gracilis tension, or both; deviation away can indicate overuse of the abductors (tensor fascia latae, gluteus medius). Imbalance of the lateral and medial thigh muscles can cause pain and potential for injury by distorting the alignment of the knee. Tight or overactive adductors can cause a medial distortion in alignment and put strain on the medial ligaments and meniscus. Overuse of the abductors leads to lateral distortion in alignment. The knee joint's healthy functioning is dependent on the maintenance of pure tracking in its movement. Strain on ligaments is the first step in weakening or tearing these important support fibers.

Injury potential resulting from muscle imbalance or misuse can be found when this action is performed in parallel position. Any inappropriate muscle functioning will be intensified when working in outward rotation, and particularly during weight bearing.

Other Bartenieff Fundamentals also address movement patterns of the lower limbs; however, let us now consider the potential for injury in the upper body. Although dance injuries in this area tend not to be as frequent or severe, the potential for problems still exists. This potential may manifest itself in later life as arthritis or limited shoulder mobility, or in relatively benign ways such as unattractive form and line in dance movement.

Upper Body Analysis

The upper body is a complex system of joints, the shoulder joint forming only one small part. The whole shoulder area is a remarkably mobile arrangement of bones connected by a number of synovial joints. The scapulohumeral joint is the major ball and socket joint. However, the sternoclavicular joints, and the joints where the ribs meet the sternum, can be imaged as very shallow ball and socket joints. This imaging facilitates fuller mobilization. Movement in the upper body results from an integrated function of all these joints. Injury potential arises from the fixing, holding, or overstabilization of one or more joints, or from the improper sequencing of the combination of these joints.

The Bartenieff Fundamental termed "arm circles" addresses the functioning of the upper body. Fixing, holding, overstabilization, and improper sequencing can be evaluated by the arm circle exercise (figure 3.2, a-d). The basic actions of this exercise are as follows. Lie back in a "hook lie" position with arms horizontally spread (figure

3.2a). Let the knees drop to the right side without moving the feet; the arms establish a strong diagonal plane (figure 3.2b). Allow the left arm to extend into the diagonal pull (figure 3.2c). From there the left arm moves into a large counterclockwise circle. Allow the eyes to follow the hand with a slight movement of the head. When the hand returns to the starting position, rest (figure 3.2d). Then reverse the direction of circling. (Repeat the whole sequence to the opposite side.) As soon as the circling movement begins, feel a gradual outward rotation of the arm, noticing how the palm changes its facing. The pelvis must remain anchored. As the arm crosses the body's midline to the opposite side, feel the scapula come "around the side" of the body with the arm. Also, a holding or softening sensation is felt in the sternum area. Thus, movement is experienced on the front and back of the body. The Laban Movement Analyst (a qualified teacher of Bartenieff Fundamentals) looks for scapula mobility, folding and opening in the sternum, and gradated rotation throughout the arm circle. Each of these items may uncover a potential for injury.

Scapula Mobility

Although shoulder dislocations have been uncommon in dance, the increased popularity of aerobic dance and of athleticism in modern choreography may yield a greater potential for this type of injury. During an arm movement, the head of the humerus must stay in its socket, which is located on the lateral edge of the scapula. The range of motion available to the humerus means that the scapula must also have concurrent movement. This synchronized movement, called scapulohumeral rhythm, supports the humeral movement and provides connection between these two bones. In the arm circle the scapula should float smoothly, with control, on the posterior and lateral surfaces of the torso. Overstabilization of the scapula, or nonsynchronized movement, will begin to weaken the ligaments that keep this joint intact. Continued use of a non-synchronized pattern can lead to tearing of the small muscles of the rotator cuff that support this joint.

Muscle interaction in scapulohumeral rhythm is complex. A constant involvement of all three main muscle groups of the shoulder joint (flexors

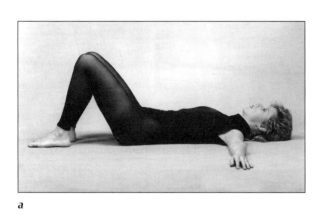

a

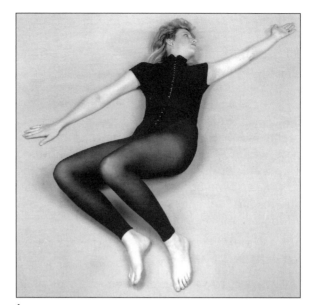

b

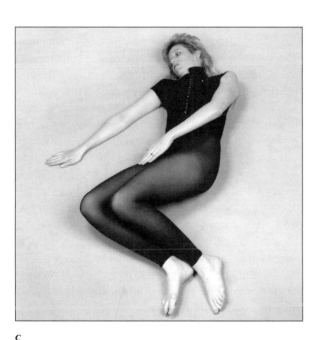

c

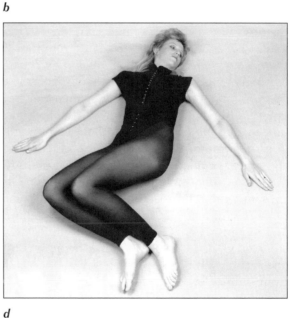

d

Figure 3.2 Arm circles.

and extensors, abductors and adductors, internal and external rotators) must occur (Bartenieff and Lewis 1980). In the arm circle exercise, an unbalanced involvement of these three groups manifests as a lopsided or irregular circle. For example, often a circle that has more height than width indicates an overuse of the upper trapezius and a weakness of the lower trapezius fibers and serratus anterior. The potential for injury begins with neck-shoulder tension and ultimately shifts to lower back and neck problems.

Sternoclavicular Mobility—Chest Folding and Opening

Sternoclavicular mobility is a subtle problem because our Western culture generally places a high value on jutting the chest forward and holding it there, which is not functional. It is identified in the dancer by having the dancer do the arm circle, and the teacher then looks for discomfort or difficulty when the arm enters the portion of the circle where it crosses the midline of the body to the opposite side. The circle will probably lose width at this moment, and often the arm appears detached at the shoulder. Kinesiologically, the dancer needs to become aware of the availability of movement in the sternoclavicular joint as well as in the rib-sternum joints. The dancer also must learn to synchronize the actions of the middle trapezius, the rhomboids, and the pectoralis major. The injury potential identified here is related to humeral detachment from the scapula. However, immobility in the chest can also lead to problems with breathing and breath support of movement.

Gradated Rotation

There are circles within circles in the arm circle exercise. In addition to the humerus and scapula describing full circular paths during this activity, the head of the humerus must rotate within the joint. This action is called gradated rotation. If there is no internal rotation, bony and muscular impingements can occur. This is particularly a problem under the coracoacromial arch. Several tendons (the supraspinatus in particular) and bursa lie in this area. If the head of the humerus does not rotate properly during abduction or elevation, problems can occur. These include (1) chronic microtrauma and damage to the tissues under the coracoacromial arch; (2) vascular impairment, which in turn can lead to swelling and inflammation; (3) partial tear of the rotator cuff; and (4) distortion of the bones or joints (Roy and Irvin 1983). These problems may not result from simple port de bras work; but when heavy handheld props are used, or active upper body choreography is demanded, the potential for problems exists if gradated rotation is lacking.

Neuromuscular Connectivity—Whole Body Analysis

Even if upper and lower body activities have been analyzed and found to utilize acceptable movement patterns, there is still potential for injury when the dancer has to integrate the upper and lower body in full body activity. Again, Bartenieff Fundamentals provide a context for assessing the injury potential in the integrated movement pattern. There are several "exercises" that address full body integration. I will discuss the "body half" exercise, and use a case example to show the need for analyzing full body coordination for injury potential.

The body half exercise, as illustrated in figure 3.3*a* and *b*, addresses the dancer's awareness of the midline division of the body. Lie on your back in a symmetrical and large "X" position (3.3*a*). Exhale as you simultaneously draw the elbow and right knee toward each other on the floor. The right side of the torso may shorten slightly and the head can tilt to the side (3.3*b*). Reverse this action by retracing the original path back to the starting position, leading with the fingers and toes. (Repeat on the left side.) Feel the midline of the body separating the major activities of the two sides. The body should stay as flat (in the vertical plane) as possible, thus using primarily the abduction and rotational muscles of the working joints. The opposite (nonmoving or stabilizing) side is anchored by a counterbalancing outward rotation in the hip joint, initiated by the deep lateral rotator muscles. The nonmoving side stays open and extended, undisturbed during the movement of the other side.

It is often important in movement to be able to stabilize one part of the body in order to free up movement of the other side. This exercise gives the dancer a clear sense of which part of the body is operating, and which is stabilizing (however, within this stabilization there must not be a holding or nonfunctional muscle activity that inhibits full or needed movement). It is done primarily in the frontal plane, thus identifying muscle actions that support lateral movement. Any forward–back movement signals the nonfunctional muscle activity that is the precursor of misuse or overuse injury.

The Case of the "Functionally Inflexible" Dancer

I worked with a client who complained of left hamstring pain and adductor tightness, as well as a gluteal spasm. The concern was prevention of both muscle tearing and decreased mobility from sciatic pain. After checking for hamstring flexibility (which was excellent) and hip joint patterning using the "thigh lift" (pure and functional), I observed the dancer in rehearsal.

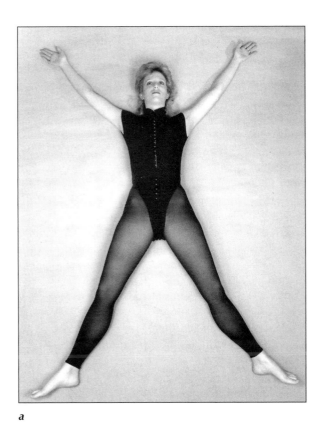

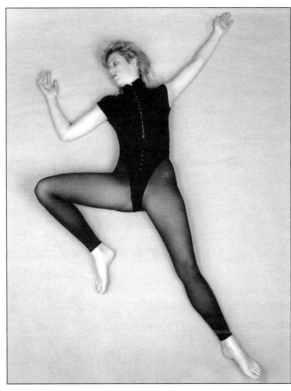

a   *b*

Figure 3.3   Body half.

I noticed a subtle loss of support on the left side when both the right arm and leg were actively gesturing. I recognized the body half exercise as a component of this choreographic movement, and thus examined the dancer doing the body half exercise.

In performing the body half exercise on the right side (with the left side as "stabilizer"), rotation in the right hip joint must occur in order to keep the body in the frontal plane. Rotation must also occur in the anchoring (left) side's hip joint as a counterbalance. In this dancer, however, this subtle action of the deep lateral rotators was not activated. Instead, the hamstrings (and gluteals to some extent) contracted to an exaggerated degree, thus signaling the beginning of a nonfunctional "misuse" pattern.

When this action is performed in the standing position, the hip joint serves several functions: The body's weight must be supported, and the counterbalancing discussed earlier must be achieved. When the hamstrings and gluteals "grip" too strongly, the beginnings of overuse are set in motion. Ultimately, in the course of

this performer's choreography, the stabilizing side may be called upon to provide stability during locomotor activities. If the hamstrings and gluteals are in a state of frozen contraction, and action at that hip joint is required (i.e., flexion in a plié or forward motion), the rectus femoris must work against those "frozen" hamstrings and gluteal muscles. The likelihood of microtearing or even major tears exists. I call this type of muscular holding "functional inflexibility" because the muscle is capable of sufficient flexibility in a passive mode; however, when certain neuromuscular patterns are activated this flexibility ceases to exist. In this case the hamstrings lacked the ability to lengthen when asked to function in the eccentric mode while supporting the body.

By guiding the dancer through a correct performance of the body half exercise on the floor I alerted her to the complex and inefficient way she was organizing her body's actions. Once her attention was drawn to what was occurring she was better able to understand a correction. We used the body half exercise in a variety of formats to re-pattern this neuromuscular action.

Conclusion

Screening for injury potential can be done through use of one or more of the Bartenieff Fundamentals. However, Bartenieff Fundamentals assess more than just kinesiological action. They help to organize the body's understanding of efficient movement patterns and aid the teacher or trainer in drawing the dancer's attention to an inefficient pattern, "interrupting" it, *and* facilitating the development of functional usage. Knowledgeable, trained usage of the full spectrum of Bartenieff Fundamentals allows the teacher or trainer to work on any movement problem.

Training in Bartenieff Fundamentals is available through the Laban/Bartenieff Institute for Movement Studies (New York City, Seattle, and several regional extensions), or through individual Certified Movement Analysts (graduates of these training programs).

References

Bartenieff, I., and D. Lewis. 1980. *Body movement: Coping with the environment.* New York: Gordon and Breach.

Roy, S., and R. Irvin. 1983. *Sports medicine: Prevention, evaluation, management and rehabilitation.* Englewood Cliffs, NJ: Prentice Hall.

Recommended Readings (Editors)

Chatfield, S.J., and S. Barr. 1994. Towards a testable hypothesis of training principles for the neuromuscular facilitation of human movement. *Dance Research Journal* 26(1): 8-14.

Eddy, M. 1995. Holistic approaches to dance injury assessment and intervention. *Impulse* 3(4): 270-279.

Hackney, P. 1998. *Making connections: Total body integration through Bartenieff Fundamentals.* Amsterdam, Netherlands: Gordon and Breach.

Lauffenburger, S.K. 1994. Bartenieff Fundamentals: Preventing dance injuries through early detection and retraining of key movement patterns. In *Kindle the fire: Proceedings of the 1994 conference of dance and the child: International.* Sydney: Macquarie University, Dance and the Child International, 217-225.

Minton, S.C. 2003. *Dance mind and body.* Champaign, IL: Human Kinetics.

Scott, M. 1996. Laban movement analysis and Bartenieff Fundamentals. In *Dance kinesiology: Second edition,* edited by S.S. Fitt. New York: Schirmer, 357-364.

Solomon, R., and J. Solomon, eds. 1995. Selected papers from the third symposium on the science and somatics of dance, February 10-12, 1995, Salt Lake City. *Impulse* 3(4): 227-311.

Part II

Diagnosing, Treating, and Rehabilitating Dance Injuries

Part II views dance injuries within the context of anatomy. Chapters 4, 5, and 7 are surveys of common injuries at three of the most vulnerable anatomic sites in dancers: the foot and ankle, knee, and spine, respectively. The most distinguishing feature of these chapters is that each is authored by a physician who has extensive experience in treating dancers and is therefore accustomed to addressing their unique concerns in a language they can understand. Chapter 6 is anomalous in that, rather than taking the survey approach to hip injuries (several studies designed in this manner are referenced in the Recommended Readings at the end of the chapter), it focuses on one all-too-common injury in dancers, iliopsoas tendinitis. Chapter 8 deals with a type of injury, stress fracture, that occurs in dancers at anatomic sites throughout the upward progression of the other chapters from foot to spine.

As an aid to those readers with limited background in anatomy and medicine, a table that defines terms used to describe anatomical locations and directions is located near the beginning of each chapter in part II.

Chapter 4

Common Foot and Ankle Injuries in Dancers

Richard N. Norris, MD

While this chapter provides a sound introduction to the anatomy of the foot and ankle, its primary focus is on the treatment, and especially the rehabilitation, of some of the most common dance injuries at that region. Hence, it should be of special interest to practitioners in physical therapy and related modalities. Some of the injuries discussed are ankle sprains, flexor hallucis longus tendinitis, sesamoiditis (and other sesamoid injuries), and Achilles tendinitis. As noted in the text, there are many connections with chapter 13, and to a lesser extent chapter 12.

This chapter discusses five of the most common foot and ankle injuries seen in dancers: ankle sprains, flexor hallucis longus tendinitis, sesamoid injuries, Achilles tendinitis, and plantar fasciitis. In each case it describes the basic anatomy involved, typical mechanisms of injury, treatment modalities, prognosis, and rehabilitation procedures to be considered. It is hoped that this information will help dancers to understand what is involved in diagnosing and dealing effectively with injuries to this most vulnerable anatomical unit.

Ankle Sprains

Ankle sprains are prevalent in dancers (Liebler 1976). Too often treated as insignificant, these injuries can have a major impact on a dancer's life and ability to perform. It is important to understand how the ankle joint is constructed and how these injuries occur.

Anatomy and Etiology

The talus is the part of the ankle on which the tibia, or shinbone, rests. It is relatively wide in the front and narrow in the back (Inman 1976). The talus fits into the ankle mortise, which is a niche formed by the end of the fibula and tibia (figure 4.1).

The medial aspect of the ankle has three very strong ligaments, the deltoid ligaments. These are rarely sprained. There are also three major ligaments on the lateral side of the ankle. The anterior talofibular ligament (ATF) runs from the fibula to the talus in a horizontal fashion. When a dancer

is in the demi-pointe position the ATF becomes vertical instead of horizontal. This provides mechanical stability and prevents the foot from supinating (Gould, Seligson, and Gassman 1980). The ATF also gives rotational stability to the ankle (Gould, Seligson, and Gassman 1980), preventing the talus from rotating out of its mortise, especially on outside turns. Despite, or perhaps because of, its stabilizing role, the ATF ligament is most commonly involved in minor ankle sprains.

Muscles also aid in stabilizing the ankle joint. The most important of these are the peroneal muscles, which run from the top of the fibula down the outside of the lower leg. The peroneus longus then runs along the side of the ankle and inserts under the ball of the great toe, or hallux. The peroneus brevis inserts into the base of the fifth metatarsal. On the medial side of the leg, the tibialis posterior muscle originates from underneath the calf muscle and sends its tendon around the medial malleolus, inserting on the inner aspect of the midfoot. When the foot is on demi-pointe the narrow rear part of the talus is in

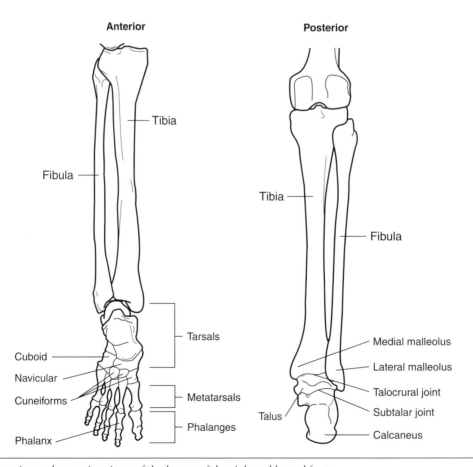

Figure 4.1 Anterior and posterior views of the bones of the right ankle and foot.

Reprinted from Behnke 2001.

Terms Describing Anatomical Location in Chapter 4

distal	away from the origin or point of attachment
lateral	farther away from the midline of the body
medial	closer to the midline of the body
posterior	behind or toward the back of the body
proximal	close to or nearest the origin or point of attachment
superficial	situated on or near the surface
superior	situated above or higher than another structure

the mortise, and thus there is little or no mechanical (bony) stability in this position (Sammarco 1982). In high demi-pointe there is some stability gained from the locking of the calcaneus against the posterior aspect of the tibia. When the ankle is dropped even a few degrees out of a very high demi-pointe, the responsibility for stabilizing the ankle falls predominantly on the ATF ligament and the peroneal and posterior tibial muscles, which form a yoke around the ankle.

Perhaps the most important cause of ankle sprains is inadequate rehabilitation of previous ankle sprains, since these injuries are often taken too lightly. Another is poor technique in landing from jumps, particularly with the foot supinated (Hardaker et al. 1988). Certain dance steps seem to carry a higher risk for ankle sprains, such as the entrechat six (Hamilton 1982). At the end of a long day, when fatigue is a factor, rehearsing new, unfamiliar, or advanced steps can also be a very real threat. Dancers must stay attuned to the workings of their bodies to know what their limits are and when those limits are reached. Other disorders, such as hallux rigidus (arthritis of the great toe joint) can cause a sickling in of the foot when attempting relevé, which may predispose to ankle sprains. Dance surfaces that are hard or uneven or steeply raked may be a factor as well (Seals 1983).

Grades of Injury

Ankle sprains are usually classified into three grades, grade 1 being the mildest and grade 3 the most severe (and fortunately the least common). The amount of pain experienced is not a reliable indicator in diagnosing the degree or severity of

an ankle sprain. A grade 1 sprain means there has been partial tearing of the fibers in the ligaments of the muscles, while a grade 2 involves a more severe tear. A grade 3 is a complete disruption or tearing of one or more of the ligaments. The ankle develops what is called a "talar tilt sign"; when the ankle is placed under a lateral stress the talus tilts and opens up, creating a gap laterally. This can be measured and diagnosed by means of a stress X ray in which the ankle is manipulated to simulate stress under normal movement conditions (Hamilton 1982). A talar tilt sign during this test indicates a complete rupture of the calcaneofibular ligament, which normally assists with lateral stability of the ankle. Clinically, a grade 3 sprain of the ATF ligament is confirmed when there is a positive "drawer sign": That is, when the tibia is stabilized and the heel is pulled forward, there is an anterior shifting of the talus out of the mortise joint.

Treatment

The first aid treatment for ankle sprains is rest, ice, compression, and elevation (RICE). This minimizes the bleeding and swelling that occur in and about the ankle joint following the sprain. Controlling the swelling significantly reduces recovery time. For first- and second-degree sprains an air-cast or gel-cast ankle brace is very useful. This consists of two plastic shells containing air- or gel-filled bladders, which are arranged on either side of the ankle and held in place by a flat stirrup that fits inside the shoe and by straps wrapped around the ankle. With each step and release the bladders cause a change of pressure, which helps force out some of the swelling. The construction of the brace prevents painful pronation and supination while still allowing for nearly full flexion and extension. The dancer wearing this device is able to bear weight earlier, walk more naturally, and return to activities in less time (Hamilton 1982).

Rehabilitation

Rehabilitation aims at restoring full range of motion, the normal levels of strength and endurance, and position sense, or *proprioception.* In many cases exercises are addressed to these rehabilitative principles or goals simultaneously. An attempt should always be made to rehabilitate the dancer in as functional a manner as possible (Molnar 1988). It is very important to maintain overall body flexibility and strength while the dancer is injured and recuperating. Allowing the entire body to become deconditioned due to an injury of a specific part is a common problem in any sport and one that is easily avoidable. In the case of ankle injuries, swimming is an excellent solution, or a ballet barre may be done in the water (Hardaker et al. 1988).

Stretching

Flexibility of the Achilles tendon must be restored through stretching, as the Achilles often becomes tight following an ankle sprain. Strengthening the peroneal muscles can be done most effectively by using a Theraband, which is a broad elastic or rubber band in varying resistance degrees, each color coded. The band can be wrapped around the balls of both feet so that when the feet are opened up to a V shape, keeping the heels together, the band applies the desired resistance. This should be done with the feet pointed as well as flexed, because the peroneal muscles come into play primarily when the foot is up on demi-pointe and must be rehabilitated in that position.

The yoke muscles, that is, the peroneal and posterior tibialis muscles, can also be strengthened effectively using manual resistance. Holding the foot, the therapist (or the dancer himself or herself) will resist movement in two different diagonals, referred to by physical therapists as "close pack" and "loose pack" (Molnar 1988). The diagonals are from dorsiflexion with supination (up and in) to plantarflexion with pronation (down and out), and the opposite, dorsiflexion with eversion or pronation (up and out) to

plantarflexion with supination (down and in). Resisting these movements in a smooth but progressively intense fashion has an advantage over the Theraband in that it rehabilitates the muscles in more directional planes.

Restoring Proprioception

Within the substance of the ankle ligaments and joint capsule lie sensory nerve endings called *proprioceptive endings.* These nerve endings transmit position information to the brain, directing muscle control about the ankle to maintain stability. When the ankle is sprained, these pathways are often disrupted and must be restored through functional rehabilitation. The wobble-type board is an excellent means of doing this; one can construct this device by simply affixing a half round dowel or half of a hard wooden ball to the underside of a piece of plywood about a foot and a half square (0.14 m²). It can be used initially in a seated position with no weight bearing and then with progressive weight bearing. A more sophisticated version of this device is called the BAPS, or biomechanical ankle platform system, manufactured by Camp International. The BAPS has five different-sized hemispheres that screw to the underside of the board. The board is designed to accommodate the difference in range of motion between pronation and supination. There are mechanisms for adding weights in different positions around the foot and ankle to provide progressive resistive exercises in addition to proprioceptive rehabilitation (Molnar 1988). The BAPS board is also useful for rehabilitation of knee injuries.

Molnar, in her article "Rehabilitation of the Injured Ankle" (1988), outlines a number of ankle rehabilitation exercises (with photographs), as does Micheli in *The Sports Medicine Bible* (1995). The reader may wish to consult these references for more detailed information.

Rehabilitation Program

A sensible plan for rehabilitation is essential to full recovery. The following 7- to 10-day program is designed primarily for mild ankle sprains. More serious grades would use a similar progression but with greater length between the stages.

> **Day 1:** Apply ice with elevation and compression; no weight bearing; air cast or gel cast.

Day 2: Do active exercises for ankle and foot two to three times a day; ice after each period; conditioning exercises for entire body, and walking when necessary with air cast.

See chapter 13, pages 176-177, figure 13.6*a-d*.

Day 3: Massage elevated lower leg, stroking upward toward heart; swimming and pool exercises; resistive exercises for ankle two to three times a day; walking with air cast.

See chapter 13, page 178, figures 13.9*a-c* and 13.10.

Day 4: Stretch to normal range of motion; increase resistance exercises; use balance board; continue use of ice after exercise.

Day 5: Warm up foot and ankle; contrast baths (alternating immersion of the leg to just below knee level in warm or hot and then cold water, for 20 minutes each); barre work, slowly with foot in tape; strength and flexibility exercises, then ice.

Day 6: Continue body conditioning exercises; resistance exercises for ankle; full barre, all speeds; walk in pointe shoes, but no work on pointe.

Days 7-10: Begin small jumps and turns; resisted balance positions; rehearsals and slow pointe work (Hamilton and Molnar 1983).

Open Versus Closed Management

One further comment about third-degree (complete) sprains: There is some controversy among dance orthopedists as to how these injuries are to be managed. Some feel that conservative or "closed" management is adequate (Norris 1988a, 1988b), whereas others favor "open" or surgical repair (Hamilton 1982). It is, however, agreed that if a reconstructive procedure is necessary to stabilize a joint, the peroneal tendons should not be sacrificed to serve as a reinforcement. The peroneal tendons are too important for stability en pointe to be sacrificed (Gould, Seligson, and Gassman 1980).

Flexor Hallucis Longus Tendinitis

The flexor hallucis longus (FHL) tendon runs behind the medial malleolus of the ankle, along with the tendons of the posterior tibialis and flexor digitorum longus. This muscle and tendon can be thought of as the Achilles tendon of the great toe, since it does for the toe what the Achilles does for the foot—that is, completes push-off during striding or jumping. When a dancer is experiencing tendinitis about the inner side of the ankle, this is the tendon that is usually involved (rather than the posterior tibialis tendon).

Anatomy and Etiology

The FHL tendon is unique among the three tendons behind the medial malleolus in that it passes through a fibro-osseous tunnel behind the malleolus (figure 4.2). This is one of the anatomical reasons why this tendon is often involved in tendinitis. In the dancer who has an abnormally low insertion of the muscle belly on the tendon, the muscle belly tends to be jammed down into the mouth of the fibro-osseous tunnel when the foot and great toe are dorsiflexed, as in doing grand pliés in fifth position. This causes irritation, often resulting in inflammation and adhesions. Interestingly, the condition seems to arise more often in the left foot than the right, perhaps due to the predominance of right turns (pirouettes, fouettés) in ballet choreography (Hamilton 1977). If adhesions do occur they can mimic an arthritic condition of the metatarsophalangeal (MTP) joint of the great toe (pseudo hallux rigidus) by not allowing for dorsiflexion of the great toe. Even without adhesions, dorsiflexion of the great toe and ankle may be limited; but when the ankle is plantarflexed the great toe can be dorsiflexed, as plantarflexion of the ankle releases the tension on the FHL tendon (Thomasen 1982).

Another common cause of FHL tendinitis is pronation, a result of a natural malalignment or of faulty technique (dancers with inadequate turnout at the hips will often "cheat" by turning out from the knee down, encouraging a pronated alignment of foot and ankle, especially in fifth position). Pronation in relevé (sickling out) also predisposes to FHL tendinitis in combination with a short first toe, the so-called Morton's foot, or lack of strength about the ankle.

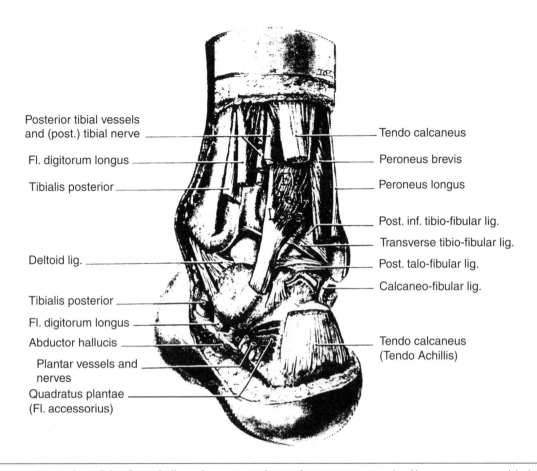

Posterior tibial vessels
and (post.) tibial nerve

Fl. digitorum longus

Tibialis posterior

Deltoid lig.

Tibialis posterior

Fl. digitorum longus

Abductor hallucis

Plantar vessels and
nerves

Quadratus plantae
(Fl. accessorius)

Tendo calcaneus

Peroneus brevis

Peroneus longus

Post. inf. tibio-fibular lig.

Transverse tibio-fibular lig.

Post. talo-fibular lig.

Calcaneo-fibular lig.

Tendo calcaneus
(Tendo Achillis)

Figure 4.2 The tendon of the flexor hallucis longus muscle can be seen entering the fibro-osseous tunnel behind the medial malleolus.

Illustration by Barry LaPoint.

Occasionally nodules may form in this region, resulting in triggering and snapping of the great toe (Hamilton 1982; Thomasen 1982).

Treatment

Treatment consists of anti-inflammatory medications, thermotherapy in the form of ultrasound, and ice massage. Electrical stimulation may be useful to decrease inflammation and swelling. Stretching and strengthening the FHL tendon with physical therapy techniques are also required. Orthotics used in street footwear may benefit the dancer who has a naturally pronated foot. Injection of steroid solution is favored by some, but to be effective the solution must enter the fibro-osseous tunnel, and this can weaken tendons; in the worst-case scenario it may predispose to rupture. Rupture is rare, but should it occur the treatment is surgical repair with six weeks in a cast and extensive rehabilitation. Full

recovery may take up to one year (Sammarco 1982).

Sesamoid Injuries

The sesamoids are small isolated bones in multiple locations in the foot and ankle (figure 4.3). This discussion will focus on the sesamoids on the undersurface of the first MTP joint.

Anatomy, Etiology, Diagnosis

These bones lie within the tendon of the flexor hallucis brevis, and their articular surfaces are covered with hyaline cartilage (Richardson 1987). There are generally two sesamoids. The medial or tibial sesamoid tends to be larger and longer than the sesamoid on the fibular, or lateral side. Besides the flexor hallucis brevis muscle, the adductor hallucis and abductor hallucis tendons contribute tendons to the sesamoids. The

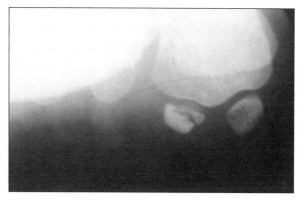

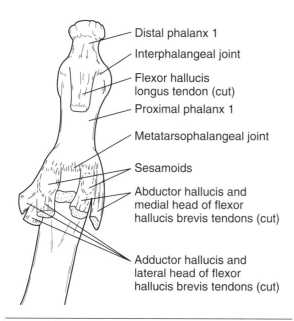

- Distal phalanx 1
- Interphalangeal joint
- Flexor hallucis longus tendon (cut)
- Proximal phalanx 1
- Metatarsophalangeal joint
- Sesamoids
- Abductor hallucis and medial head of flexor hallucis brevis tendons (cut)
- Adductor hallucis and lateral head of flexor hallucis brevis tendons (cut)

Figure 4.3 A view of the plantar aspect of the first metatarsal head, with the two heads of the flexor hallucis brevis muscle cut to reveal the sesamoids embedded in their tendons.

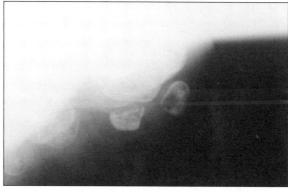

a

b

Figure 4.4 *(a)* Fracture of the lateral sesamoid in a 24-year-old dancer. *(b)* After three months of treatment with a modified shoe (figure 4.6) the fracture is nearly healed as shown by X ray, and the patient is asymptomatic.

sesamoids may be bipartite (have two parts) or multipartite. These variations may occur in approximately 10% to 33% of all feet (Hamilton 1985; Jahss 1981). Forces equal to three times the body weight have been estimated to occur beneath the sesamoids during the normal gait cycle, particularly at push-off (Drez 1982). These studies also show that the sesamoids aid push-off during gait by accentuating the flexor strength of the FHL. During weight bearing, especially in relevé, the tibial or medial sesamoid bears most of the weight, thus accounting for the higher rate of injury in this bone. Certain ethnic dances (e.g., East Indian, flamenco) may be irritating to the sesamoids because they employ slapping or stamping forefoot steps (Sammarco 1988).

Sesamoids are prone to numerous pathological processes, including fracture, stress fracture, chondromalacia, osteoarthritis, tendinitis of the flexor hallucis brevis, osteochondritis of the sesamoids, and ganglion cysts between the sesamoids (Novella 1987). One can localize problems clinically by forcibly dorsiflexing the great toe with one hand while palpating the undersurface of the head of the first metatarsal with the opposite thumb. Fracture and stress fracture must be ruled out through radiographs or bone scan,

and bipartite sesamoids should be differentiated from fractures by the same means (figures 4.4a and b). Stress fractures may not show up for several weeks, but the bone scan will confirm their presence or absence.

Treatment and Rehabilitation

Sesamoid problems must be treated vigorously, not only to relieve chronic pain and disability in the dancer, but also to avoid further injury. The dancer with pain under the head of the first metatarsal will often compensate by supinating the forefoot during relevé, leading to ankle sprains, fifth metatarsal fractures, and so on. The dancer should be examined in the relevé position, as pain in this region that was not apparent on palpation by the examiner's thumb may be evident upon weight bearing (Novella 1987).

Treatment should include physical therapy modalities such as ultrasound, deep friction massage, ice massage, and electrical stimulation. However, the cornerstone of therapy is relief of weight bearing on the sesamoids, with several considerations to be addressed. Sesamoiditis is typically treated with a sesamoid "pad" that lifts up the first metatarsal and extends far enough distally to lift up the second through fifth metatarsals when the dancer is in relevé (figure 4.5). While it is necessary to relieve weight bearing on the sesamoids, it is also important to prevent the MTP joint from flexing during normal gait, as this places increased stress on the sesamoids. The best way to accomplish this is by use of a rigid or wooden-soled shoe with a rocker bottom, which causes the foot to roll through the push-off phase of the gait cycle. A router can be used to ream out the shoe underneath the first metatarsal head, all the way to beyond the end of the great toe. This space is filled in with a soft foam (figure 4.6). Such a device relieves weight bearing on the sesamoids, prevents MTP joint flexion during push-off, and inhibits or discourages contraction of the flexor

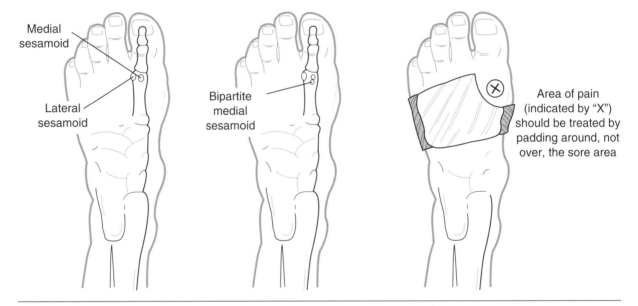

Figure 4.5 Standard padding of the sole of the foot for sesamoiditis.

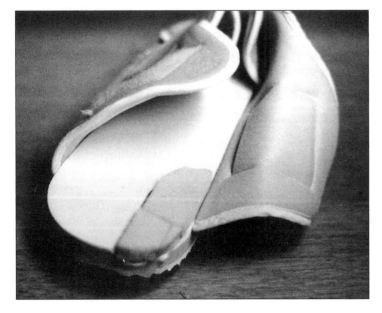

Figure 4.6 The wooden-soled, rocker-bottom shoe, modified by reaming out the sole of the shoe from behind the first metatarsal head to beyond the toe and filling the space with soft foam (Plastazote). This not only relieves weight bearing on the injured sesamoid, but prevents additional irritation by eliminating metatarsophalangeal flexion on push-off and inhibiting isometric contraction of the flexor hallucis brevis, the tendons of which contain the sesamoids.

hallucis brevis during push-off, as there is nothing substantive for the pad of the distal phalanx of the great toe to push down against. This prevents strain on the sesamoids from contraction of the flexor hallucis brevis muscle, within whose tendons the sesamoids are located.

Dancers should be told that they might need a long course of treatment with sesamoiditis, especially if there is a stress fracture or frank fracture of the sesamoids. I have, however, successfully treated several fractured sesamoids with the protocol described.

If at all possible, sesamoid problems should be treated nonsurgically, as sesamoidectomy can create imbalance, particularly with the exaggerated forces generated in the relevé position in dance. Removal of one sesamoid also places excessive force on its mate (McBryde and Anderson 1988).

When symptoms are resolved the dancer may gradually return to full activities, beginning with demi-pointe on both feet, working up to demi-pointe on one foot, then progressively to jumps on both feet, and finally one-foot jumps, such as jetés or assemblés.

Achilles Tendinitis

The Achilles tendon is the common tendon for the *triceps surae* (figure 4.7a and b). This consists of the outer calf muscle or gastrocnemius, which has two bellies, and the soleus. The gastrocnemius arises from the posterior aspect of the femoral condyles. The soleus, which is the deeper of the two calf muscles, arises from the tibia and fibula distal to the knee joint. The tendon is attached to a facet in the calcaneus where the Achilles tendon is separated from the bone by a bursa.

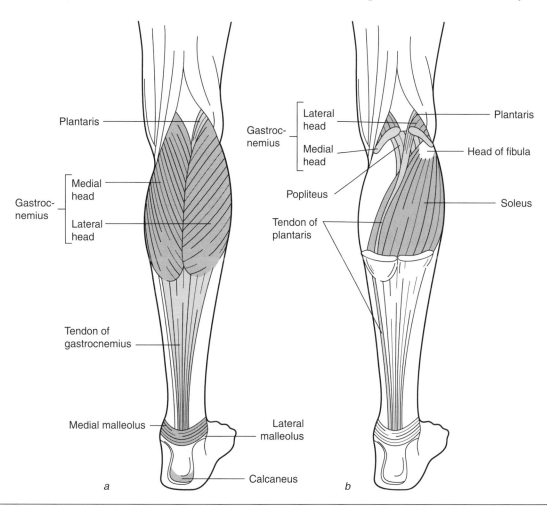

Figure 4.7 Triceps surae. *(a)* The two heads of the gastrocnemius and its tendon. *(b)* The gastrocnemius removed, revealing the soleus beneath.

Reprinted from Behnke 2001.

The tendon is shaped like an hourglass, with the narrow part 1.6 to 2.8 in. (4-7 cm) above the calcaneal insertion. There is no true synovial tendon sheath around the Achilles tendon; rather, it is covered by fascia, and a sheath, or paratenon, is formed by the fascia. The two muscle groups of the triceps surae have a different but similar function. The gastrocnemius flexes both the knee and the ankle in an open kinetic chain; the soleus plantarflexes the ankle only. The gastrocnemius is used primarily in jumps, whereas the soleus has a more static function. In relevé these muscles act together, and due to the physics involved the pull on the Achilles tendon is less in high relevé or full pointe than in low relevé (Thomasen 1982).

Etiology and Diagnosis

Numerous factors contribute to Achilles tendinitis in the dancer: (1) tightness of the heel cords, which is common in dancers, as they do most of their work in plantarflexion; (2) anatomic variation of the Achilles, smaller and thinner Achilles tendons being more susceptible to strain; (3) supination or pronation of the foot; and (4) a low relevé that places more stress on the Achilles than a high relevé because of the physics involved. A prominence of the posterior superior portion of the calcaneus may cause mechanical irritation and tendinitis of the Achilles or the retrocalcaneal bursa (or both) in plié (Hamilton 1988). Anecdotally, the neoclassical en pointe position, with its exaggerated plantarflexion, may cause toe shoe ribbons to bite tightly into the back of the Achilles in the most vulnerable area.

Achilles tendinitis occurs in various degrees, from mild irritation or fraying of the fibers to intratendinous tears or fusiform swellings. Chronic tendinitis may result in nodule formation or adhesions between the tendon and paratenon (Hamilton 1988).

Magnetic resonance imaging has been used increasingly in the diagnosis of Achilles tendinitis, and is most useful in differentiating a simple tendinitis from intratendinous tears. These latter must be treated more aggressively, as they may herald impending Achilles rupture.

Treatment

Nonsurgical management includes anti-inflammatory medications, ice massage, ultrasound with electrical stimulation to reduce edema,

and contrast baths. Range of motion should be worked only to the point of mild discomfort, not pain. There is no place in the conservative management of Achilles tendinitis for steroid injections, due to the risk of weakening the tendon and predisposing toward rupture. A heel lift in the shoe takes tension off the Achilles, while the dancer with mild Achilles tendinitis may use a character or jazz shoe with a small heel to reduce strain during plié. For more severe cases of Achilles tendinitis, this author uses an air-cast walking brace with an added heel lift (figure 4.8). This immobilizes the ankle, and the rocker-type sole

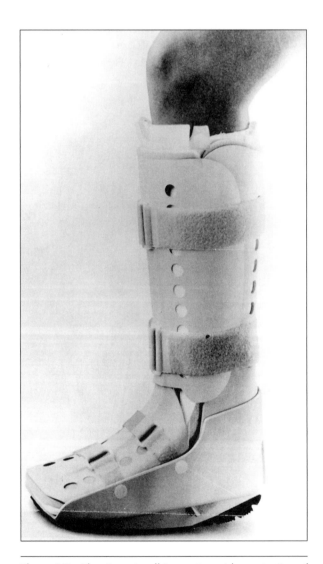

Figure 4.8 The air-cast walking cast provides protection of the inflamed Achilles tendon by eliminating ankle motion during ambulation and by placing the foot-ankle complex in slight plantarflexion. The advantage over a traditional cast is easy removal for gentle range of motion exercises to prevent joint stiffness and muscle atrophy.

prevents stretching of the Achilles just before push-off. The walking brace should be removed every 3 to 4 hours and active, pain-free range of motion exercises performed to prevent stiffness of the ankle joint. See chapter 13, pages 176-178 and 180, figures 13.6*a-d,* 13.7, 13.9*a-c,* 13.10, and 13.11*a-b.*

Rehabilitation

Once pain has diminished, full range of motion, strength, and endurance must be gradually restored. Pilates equipment, which allows for horizontal jumps on a spring-loaded board, or doing jumps in a swimming pool, can be used for this purpose. Dancers should be encouraged to do adequate heel cord stretching in and out of class in an effort to prevent this injury.

Plantar Fasciitis

Plantar fasciitis is an inflammation of the plantar fascia (PF), the thick connective tissue in the sole of the foot, superficial to the intrinsic muscles of the foot. The site of pain is frequently located at the medial calcaneal border, where the fascia originates. The inflammation is a result of the body's attempt to heal microscopic tears or avulsions of the fascia, usually from repetitive microtrauma (overuse). Excessive pronation of the foot (as found with forced turnout) is a major contributing factor (Kwong et al. 1988). The distal insertion of the PF is the base of the proximal phalanges (the first toe bone). When the toes go into dorsiflexion during demi-pointe or during the push-off phase of walking the PF tightens via a "windlass" effect (figure 4.9), thus pulling on the origin of the PF at the medial aspect of the heel (Cailliet 1980).

Diagnosis

Diagnosis can easily be made by firm palpation at the medial aspect of the heel, just where the arch starts. Pain is pronounced if palpation is done with the toes forced back into dorsiflexion to tighten the PF, and lessened if palpation is done with the toes in neutral or slight plantarflexion, which relaxes the PF.

Treatment and Rehabilitation

In the past, treatment has focused on controlling pronation by the use of various orthotics. However, this approach fails to take into consideration

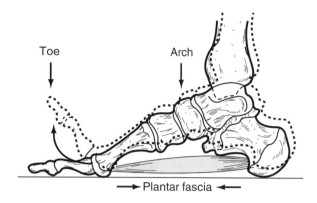

Figure 4.9 The plantar fascia has its origin from the medial calcaneus and inserts on the proximal phalanges of the toes. When the toes are in dorsiflexion as in the push-off phase of the gait cycle or in demi-pointe, the plantar fascia becomes taut, supporting the arch. This pulls on the origin, which is the usual site of microtears in plantar fasciitis. By blocking dorsiflexion of the toes, the carbon fiber footplate effectively puts the plantar fascia at rest, facilitating healing.

the "windlass" effect of pulling on the injured portion of the PF with every step one takes or with demi-pointe. In order to minimize the constant pull of the PF it is essential to immobilize the MTP joint (where the toes join the foot). This can be most effectively accomplished by the insertion of a Springlite carbon footplate beneath the insole of a running shoe. This ultra-thin, ultra-lightweight device is available at specialty foot stores, and by virtue of being fairly rigid it minimizes MTP dorsiflexion at push-off. This in turn effectively puts the PF at rest. The Springlite footplate is available with a molded arch support, which can complement or replace the normally good support already available in most running shoes. The "rocker" sole found on running shoes allows one to roll through the shoe, compensating for the lack of MTP flexion at push-off.

Dancers may dance en pointe with PF, but must avoid the demi-pointe position. Recreational walking or jogging must be kept to a minimum. Physical therapy modalities, such as ice, ultrasound, electrical stimulation, and deep friction massage, can be useful in reducing inflammation. Cortisone injections are to be avoided, as they are excruciatingly painful, can cause atrophy of the heel fat pad, and have been associated with PF ruptures. They are also unnecessary if the regimen described is adhered to. Oral anti-inflammatories are of minimal value, as delivery to the target tissue is poor due to the scant blood supply of the PF, and they may also cause gastric upset. Bone spurs, which on occasion are seen in conjunction with PF, are not the cause of the symptoms but the result of traction on the calcaneus from the tight PF (Kwong et al. 1988). Surgical removal of the spurs should rarely be considered.

Conclusion

Foot and ankle injuries, because they are so common and potentially disabling, are of the utmost importance to those concerned with dance medicine. Understanding the role of certain muscles should encourage preventive strengthening programs. Early and aggressive rehabilitation, stressing functional activities, full restoration of strength, range of motion, proprioception and endurance, and gradual return to dance activities, will serve to minimize disability. Maintaining good physical condition during the rehabilitation process cannot be overemphasized. Finally, appreciating that inadequate treatment often leads to recurrence of injury should cause us to give these injuries our full attention.

References

Cailliet, R. 1980. *Foot and ankle pain.* Philadelphia: Davis, 34.

Drez, D. 1982. Forefoot problems in runners. In *Symposium on the foot and leg in running sports,* edited by R.P. Mack. St. Louis: Mosby, 73-75.

Gould, N., D. Seligson, and J. Gassman. 1980. Early and late repair of the lateral ligament of the ankle. *Foot and Ankle* 1(2): 84-89.

Hamilton, W.G. 1977. Tendinitis about the ankle joint in classical ballet dancers. *American Journal of Sports Medicine* 5(2): 84-88.

Hamilton, W.G. 1982. Sprained ankles in ballet dancers. *Foot and Ankle* 3(2): 99-102.

Hamilton, W.G. 1985. *Surgical anatomy of the foot and ankle.* CIBA Clinical Symposia Annual 37(3). New Jersey: CIBA-Geigy.

Hamilton, W.G. 1988. Foot and ankle injuries in dancers. *Clinics in Sports Medicine* 7(1): 143-173.

Hamilton, W.G., and M. Molnar. 1983. Back to dancing after injury. *Dance Magazine* 57(4): 88-90.

Hardaker, W.T., J.C. Angelo, T.R. Malone, and M. Myers. 1988. Ankle sprains in theatrical dancers. *Medical Problems of Performing Artists* 3(4): 146-150.

Inman, V.T. 1976. *The joints of the ankle.* Baltimore: Williams & Wilkins.

Jahss, M.H. 1981. The sesamoids of the hallux. *Clinical Orthopaedics and Related Research* 157: 88-97.

Kwong, P.K., D. Kay, R.T. Voner, and M.W. White. 1988. Plantar fasciitis. Mechanics and pathomechanics of treatment. *Clinics in Sports Medicine* 7(1): 119-126.

Liebler, W.A. 1976. Injuries of the foot in dancers. In *Foot science,* edited by J.E. Bateman. Philadelphia: Saunders, 284-287.

McBryde, A.M., and R.B. Anderson. 1988. Sesamoid foot problems in the athlete. *Clinics in Sports Medicine* 7(1): 51-60.

Micheli, L.J. 1995. *The sports medicine bible.* New York: HarperPerennial.

Molnar, M.E. 1988. Rehabilitation of the injured ankle. *Clinics in Sports Medicine* 7(1): 193-204.

Norris, R. 1988a. Personal communication with John Bergfeld, MD, orthopedic surgeon, Cleveland Clinic.

Norris, R. 1988b. Personal communication with Lyle Micheli, MD, Director, Division of Sports Medicine, Children's Hospital, Boston.

Novella, T.M. 1987. Dancers shoes and foot care. In *Dance medicine: A comprehensive guide,* edited by A. Ryan and R.E. Stephens. Chicago and Minneapolis: Pluribus Press/Physician and Sportsmedicine, 139-176.

Richardson, E.G. 1987. Injuries to the hallucal sesamoids in the athlete. *Foot and Ankle* 7(4): 229-244.

Sammarco, G.J. 1982. The foot and ankle in classical ballet and modern dance. In *Disorders of the foot,* edited by M.H. Jahss. Philadelphia: Saunders, 1626-1659.

Sammarco, G.J. 1988. The dancer's foot and ankle. In *Postgraduate advances in sports medicine.* University of Pennsylvania School of Medicine. Berryville, VA: Forum Medicum.

Seals, J.G. 1983. A study of dance surfaces. *Clinics in Sports Medicine* 2(3): 557-561.

Thomasen, E. 1982. *Diseases and injuries of ballet dancers.* Denmark: Universitetsforlaget I. Arhus.

Recommended Readings (Editors)

Conti, S.F., and Y.S. Wong. 2001. Foot and ankle injuries in the dancer. *Journal of Dance Medicine & Science* 5(2): 43-50.

Denton, J. 1997. Overuse foot and ankle injuries in ballet. *Clinics in Podiatric Medicine and Surgery* 14(3): 525-532.

Kravitz, S.R., and C.J. Murgia. 1999. The mechanics of dance and dance-related injuries. In *Sports medicine of the lower extremity: Edition 2,* edited by S.I. Subotnick. New York: Churchill Livingstone, 645-655.

Liederbach, M. 2000. General considerations for guiding dance injury rehabilitation. *Journal of Dance Medicine & Science* 4(2): 54-65.

Macintyre, J., and E. Joy. 2000. Foot and ankle injuries in dance. *Clinics in Sports Medicine* 19(2): 351-368.

Malone, T.R., and W.T. Hardaker. 1990. Rehabilitation of foot and ankle injuries in ballet dancers. *Journal of Orthopaedic and Sports Physical Therapy* 11(8): 355-361.

Molnar, M. 1995. Assessment of the dancer's foot and ankle for rehabilitation. In *Rehabilitation of the foot and ankle,* edited by G.J. Sammarco. St. Louis: Mosby, 311-324.

Novella, T.M. 2001. Shim set therapy for the dancer's foot. *Journal of Dance Medicine & Science* 5(3): 87-93.

Omey, M.L., and L.J. Micheli. 1999. Foot and ankle problems in the young athlete. *Medicine and Science in Sports and Exercise* 31(7 Suppl.): S470-S485.

Stretanski, M.F., and G.J. Weber. 2002. Medical and rehabilitation issues in classical ballet. *American Journal of Physical Medicine and Rehabilitation* 81(5): 383-391.

Chapter 5

Knee Problems in Dancers

Carol C. Teitz, MD

This chapter provides an inclusive introduction to the most common knee injuries in dancers, making it a "must read" for anyone involved in training or treating dancers, and the dancers themselves. Specific injuries discussed include medial knee strain, patellofemoral pain, patellar subluxation and dislocation, patellar tendinitis, meniscal tears, and ligament injuries.

Lower extremity injuries account for 57% to 88% of all dancers' injuries (Bowling 1989; Garrick, Gillien, and Whiteside 1986; Garrick and Requa 1983; Rothenberger, Chang, and Cable 1988; Rovere et al. 1983; Washington 1978). The rate of knee injuries ranges from 9% to 17% (table 5.1). Quirk found that patellofemoral problems and patellar tendinitis accounted for approximately 16% of the knee injuries seen in professional ballet dancers, patellar subluxation (partial dislocation of the kneecap) for 0.3%, and meniscal (cartilage) problems for 16% (Quirk 1983). Patellar tendinitis is also often seen in aerobic dancers. Torn menisci are more common in male than in female dancers, particularly in folk dancers, for whom percussive squatting activities put the meniscus at risk during rapid flexion and extension of the knee (Nilsson et al. 2001; Teitz 1988a; Washington 1978). The following discussion describes the anatomy and pertinent biomechanics of the knee, followed by typical causes, clinical presentations, and recommended treatment for common knee problems.

Table 5.1 Percentage of Dancers' Injuries by Injury Site As Reported in Previous Studies

Location	Theatrical dance (Washington 1978)	Ballet and modern (Rovere et al. 1983)	Ballet (Quirk 1983)	Aerobic dance (Rothenberger et al. 1988)
Knee	14	15	17	9
Foot and ankle	23	37	42	18
Other lower extremity	21	19	21	36
Back and other	42	29	20	13

Anatomy, Biomechanics, and Kinesiology

The knee is a complex joint with no inherent bony stability (figure 5.1). It is made up of articulations (joints) between the femur and tibia, and the patella and femur, and is surrounded by a layer of synovial tissue that produces fluid, and by a tough fibrous capsule. Within the synovial tissue are folds called plicae. A plica is a synovial band that is a remnant of an embryologic partition in the knee. The medial plica is present in approximately 60% of adults and rarely produces any symptoms. However, when knee irritation results in synovial thickening, this band can harden to the point that it rubs back and forth on the undersurface of the patella, producing wear and pain (Hardaker, Whipple, and Bassett 1980; Harty and Joyce 1977). Knee joint motion is complex; it includes flexion and extension, rotation, rolling, and gliding.

Ligaments

Ligaments are collagenous structures that lend support to the connective tissue capsule around the knee and act to restrain the knee joint. Fibers in the ligaments run in the direction necessary to control loading. There are four major ligaments

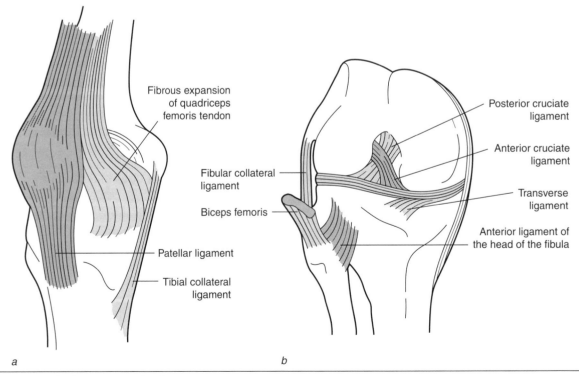

Figure 5.1 The knee joint and its ligaments, anterior views.
Reprinted from Behnke 2001.

Terms Describing Anatomical Location in Chapter 5

anterior	nearer to or toward the front of the body
extrinsic	coming from or originating outside
intrinsic	situated entirely within or pertaining exclusively to a part
lateral	farther away from the midline of the body
medial	closer to the midline of the body
posterior	behind or toward the back of the body
proximal	close to or nearest the origin or point of attachment

supporting the knee joints: two collateral ligaments (medial [MCL] and lateral [LCL]) and two cruciate ligaments (anterior [ACL] and posterior [PCL]). The collateral ligaments are located on either side of the knee and resist medial and lateral forces. The MCL has a superficial and a deep component, both running from the medial femoral condyle onto the proximal portion of the tibia. The deep portion of the MCL is attached to the capsule of the knee joint and the medial meniscus; hence, injuries that tear both the MCL and the medial meniscus can occur. The LCL is outside the capsule of the knee. The cruciate ligaments cross each other in the center of the knee and form an axis about which the knee rotates. The ACL originates on the lateral femoral condyle and inserts on the anterior aspect of the tibia. The PCL originates on the medial femoral condyle and inserts on the posterior-most margin of the tibia. The designation of these ligaments as anterior or posterior is derived from the site of insertion on the tibia (figure 5.2). The cruciate ligaments resist anterior and posterior translation (gliding movement) of the tibia on the femur and rotational stresses. Due to the differences in radius of curvature between the medial and lateral femoral condyles, tension in the cruciate ligaments changes during flexion and extension, and also during internal and external rotation of the knee (Dienst, Burks, and Greis 2002). These changes in tension are due to the twisting of the ligaments around each other, and to the twist of the fibers within the ligaments themselves (Ryman and Jackson 1987). Because collagen is viscoelastic, rate of stretch is an important factor in ligament failure. Other factors include age, ligament strength, and axis of loading. Ligament strength increases with

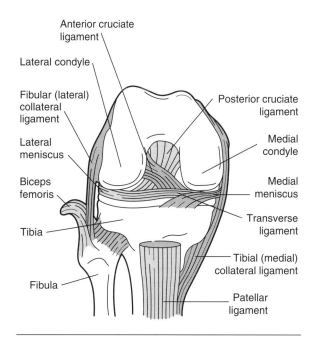

Figure 5.2 The ligaments of the knee, anterior view.
Reprinted from Behnke 2001.

exercise and decreases following immobilization (Laros, Tipton, and Cooper 1971). There is a fine line between stability brought about by ligaments and the freedom of movement necessary as the knee moves through a range of motion.

Patellofemoral Joint

The patella is a triangular-shaped bone, with the apex pointing toward the foot. On its posterior surface (the surface making contact with the femur) the patella has facets that are designed to articulate with the trochlear groove of the femur. The patella lies within the quadriceps tendon and

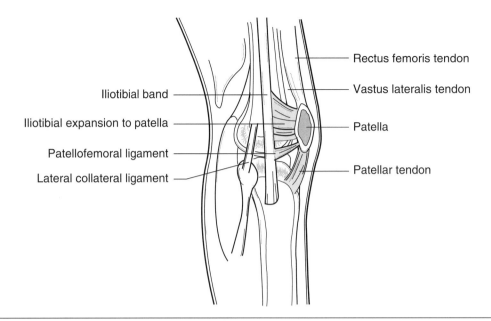

Figure 5.3 Lateral view of patellar retinacular attachments.

is held in position by connective tissue bands from the quadriceps muscle, the medial patellofemoral ligament, the iliotibial expansion, and the patellar tendon (Tuxoe et al. 2002). As illustrated in figure 5.3, the mobility and stability of the patella are determined by the patellar position in the trochlear groove, the depth of the groove, the length of the patellar tendon, and the relative flexibility or tightness of the soft-tissue attachments (Goodfellow, Hungerford, and Zindel 1976). Articulation of the patella with the femur varies as a function of knee flexion. When the knee is in full extension the patella rests on a fat pad just above the trochlear groove. As the knee begins to flex, the patella moves downward and engages the trochlear groove (Kaufer 1971).

Compressive forces between the patella and the femur are generated predominantly by the pull of the quadriceps muscle and the patellar tendon. (Although the patellar tendon is the anatomic termination of the quadriceps muscle, for purposes of biomechanical analysis the two are considered as separate structures.) These forces can be considered in two planes. When looking at the knee from the front, one can draw a line along the axis of the quadriceps muscle and tendon and a second line along the axis of the patellar tendon. The acute angle formed between these two lines makes up what is known as the Q (quadriceps)-angle. The larger this Q-angle (figure 5.4), the larger will be the "lateral vector"

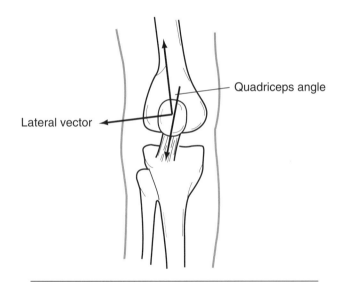

Figure 5.4 Quadriceps angle.

tending to pull the patella laterally in the trochlear groove (Nagamine et al. 1995; van Kampen and Huiskes 1990). When the knee is viewed from the side, forces generated by the quadriceps muscle can be analyzed using vectors. The resultant of the quadriceps vector and the patellar tendon vector produces compressive forces between the patella and the femur (figure 5.5). As knee flexion increases, this force increases (Huberti and Hayes 1984). The magnitude of quadriceps force has been found to increase 6% per degree of

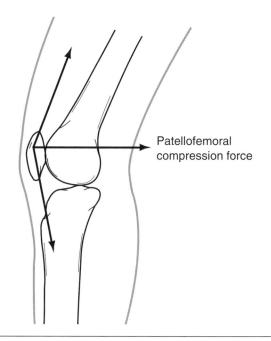

Patellofemoral
compression force

Figure 5.5 Patellofemoral compression force.

flexion. Reilly and Martens found that the patellofemoral force was half body weight during level walking, three times body weight going up and down stairs, and 7.6 times body weight during a deep knee bend (Reilly and Martens 1972). Perry, Antonelli, and Ford (1975) found that the amount of quadriceps force required to stabilize the knee when it is flexed to 30° equaled 50% of maximum quadriceps strength.

Muscles and Tendons

Collagen (mostly type I) and elastin account for 65% to 75% and 2%, respectively, of the dry weight of tendon. These two substances are embedded in a proteoglycan-water matrix (Jozsa and Kannus 1997). Whereas collagen is predominantly responsible for the structural integrity of tendon and for resisting deformation, elastin contributes to its flexibility. Scar tissue contains almost no elastin, which accounts for its relatively stiff behavior. Exercise improves the mechanical and structural properties of tendon through changes in the synthesis of the collagen and proteoglycan matrix, collagen cross-links, and the deposition and arrangement of collagen fibers (Woo et al. 1975).

The behavior of tendon under load is a function of the structural orientation of the fibers and the properties and proportions of collagen and elastin. Range of motion of a musculotendinous unit and the force applied to the tendon are in part a function of the orientation of the muscle fibers relative to the axis of the tendon. The greater the longitudinal array of muscle fibers, the greater the range of motion of the muscle and tendon. The greater the obliquity of muscle fibers, the more force is dissipated laterally relative to the axis of the tendon. A fusiform muscle (spindle shaped, tapering at the ends) exerts greater tensile force on its tendon than does a pennate (feather shaped) muscle because all of the force in a fusiform muscle is applied in series with the longitudinal axis of the tendon.

The ability of tendon to deform without suffering structural damage is due in part to its viscoelastic properties. A viscoelastic material exhibits solid and fluid properties, and the rate at which forces are applied determines the amount of force that the tendon can withstand prior to rupture. Tendon is most vulnerable to injury when tension is applied quickly or obliquely, when the tendon is tense before trauma, or when the attached muscle is maximally innervated (Barfred 1971). Eccentric muscle contraction is associated with a higher incidence of tendinitis than is concentric contraction (Newham et al. 1983). During an eccentric contraction the muscle fibers lengthen (i.e., are stretched) while the sarcomeres (contractile units) contract to produce force. This occurs, for example, when the quadriceps muscle is used to decelerate the descent of the body when landing from a jump. Concentric contraction occurs when the muscle shortens while producing force. This occurs in the quadriceps muscle, for example, during final straightening of the knee in développé. The force production during eccentric contraction is greater than during concentric contraction.

To appreciate the functional stability of the knee one must consider the dynamic stability brought about by muscle use (Czerniecki, Lippert, and Olerud 1988). Stabilization provided by the muscles is important in the normal knee and in the previously injured knee (Markolf, Graff-Redford, and Amstutz 1978). When a sudden force is applied, muscle contraction usually does not occur rapidly enough to prevent damage. When forces are applied more slowly, proprioceptive input from the ligaments and capsule is relayed to the neighboring muscles, which then contract to resist the force. Although hip muscles contribute to control of knee motion, the muscles directly affecting flexion and extension of the knee are the quadriceps and the hamstring muscles. The quadriceps straightens the knee via the patellar tendon, which transmits force from the quadriceps muscle to the anterior tibia, causing the knee to straighten. The hamstring tendons transmit forces from their respective muscles (semimembranosus, semitendinosus, biceps femoris) to the posterior tibia, causing the knee to bend. At their insertions into bone, tendon fibers become incorporated into relatively avascular fibrocartilage. The blood supply to tendons is variable, with contributions from the synovial sheaths, paratenon, and the musculotendinous and bone tendon junctions. Tendon vasculature is compromised at sites of friction, torsion, or compression. Proprioceptive information is obtained through nerve endings near the musculotendinous junction (Jozsa and Kannus 1997). Muscle function also alters knee kinematics. Quadriceps forces produce anterior tibial translation, increased strain in the ACL, and decreased strain in the PCL, whereas hamstrings produce posterior tibial translation, decreased strain in the ACL, and increased strain in the PCL (Bach and Hull 1998; Fleming et al. 2001; Takai et al. 1993).

Menisci

The menisci are small, wedge-shaped semilunar cartilages in the knee, with their thickest portion at the periphery and a paper-thin portion at their innermost margin. Collagen within the meniscus is aligned like barrel hoops to withstand centrifugal stress. In the most superficial layer of the meniscus the fibers are predominantly oriented radially (diverging from the center). In deeper layers collagen is circumferentially oriented (around the perimeter), with random branching fibers that may link the circumferentially oriented bundles. Loading of the meniscus causes radial displacement that must be resisted by the radially oriented collagen fibers. Meniscal tears usually result from compression, shear forces, or both. Due to the differences in collagen orientation between the superficial and deeper layers, the biomechanical behavior of the meniscus is not homogeneous in its response to various stresses (Arnoczky et al. 1988).

The menisci function in a number of ways. They increase the congruity between the femur and tibia, distributing weight evenly and preventing excessive wear in any one area. The lateral meniscus absorbs most of the weight applied to the lateral aspect of the knee, whereas the weight

applied on the medial side is shared equally between the medial meniscus and the articular surface. Obviously, when menisci are removed there is a considerable loss of energy-absorbing function, and increased load is transmitted to the articular cartilage (Krause et al. 1976; Walker and Erkman 1975).

By pushing synovial fluid around, the menisci contribute to the lubrication of the knee and to the nourishment of the articular cartilage. They also act as shock absorbers and provide some stability to the knee joint by acting as spacers. The medial meniscus is attached to the capsule along its peripheral margin, and is also attached to the deep MCL. The capsular attachment of the lateral meniscus is interrupted in its mid to posterior third by the passage of the popliteus tendon from the tibia to the lateral femoral condyle. The inner margins of the menisci are free (figure 5.6). Their peripheral attachments provide the outer 20% to 30% of the meniscus with a blood supply (Arnoczky and Warren 1982). When a tear occurs in the periphery—that is, the vascular area—the meniscus is capable of healing. However, the vast majority of tears occur in the nonvascular area and therefore have no potential for healing.

Knee Problems

Some of the most common medical problems encountered at the knee by dancers are described in this section.

Medial Knee Strain

The word "strain," by standard definition, refers to a change in length, and often is used to describe a microscopic tear in connective tissue. In dancers medial knee strain is seen predominantly in those who are poorly trained, either children or adult beginners. It is rare in the accomplished dancer. The strain occurs in the capsule on the medial aspect of the knee (Teitz 1983).

Etiology

During plié an imaginary plumb line dropped from the knee should land over the second toe. When the plumb line falls medial to the foot during plié, the medial capsule and collateral ligament are strained. Particularly in ballet, emphasis is placed on turnout, or external rotation of the lower extremities. In the ideal turned-out position the weight should fall from the body to the

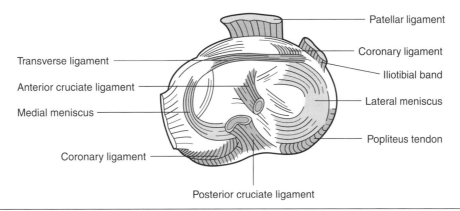

Patellar ligament

Coronary ligament

Iliotibial band

Lateral meniscus

Popliteus tendon

Posterior cruciate ligament

Transverse ligament

Anterior cruciate ligament

Medial meniscus

Coronary ligament

Figure 5.6 Section through the knee joint, superior view.
Reprinted from Behnke 2001.

thigh, and directly through the center of the knee and ankle (figure 5.7; see also chapter 11, figures 11.1, p. 136, and 11.10*a*, p. 144). This distribution of weight can be achieved if the external rotation of the lower extremities occurs at the hip. When external rotation of the hip is lacking, or as a result of poor instruction, a dancer may attempt to gain more rotation by doing a demi-plié, "turning out" the feet, and then straightening the knees. Weight will then fall medial to the knee and ankle, pro-

ducing tensile stresses on the medial side of the knee and first metatarsophalangeal joint (figure 5.8), as well as pronation of the foot. In the usual ballet class approximately one-half to two-thirds of class time is spent in barre exercises, many of which include pliés in various positions. In addition, pliés are fundamental to initiating and landing jumps. Hence, if one's plié technique is incorrect, musculoskeletal problems are likely to occur.

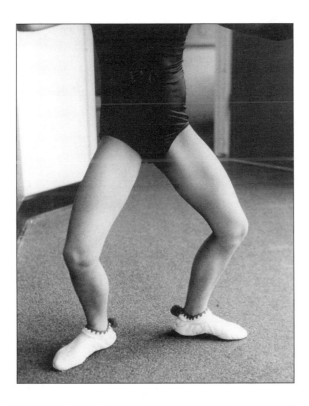

Figure 5.7 Ideally, weight should fall through the center of the knee and ankle.
Reprinted from Teitz 1982.

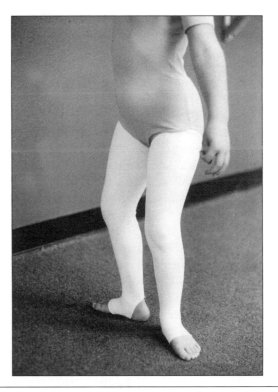

Figure 5.8 Turnout attained from the floor upward places abnormal stresses on the medial knee, ankle, and foot structures.
Reprinted from Teitz 1982.

Symptoms and Signs

Medial knee strain presents as pain along the medial side of the knee, with no history of specific injury. Pain is usually worse after class, and gradually decreases if there is a day or two hiatus between ballet classes. There is no knee swelling or locking. Physical examination often reveals some tenderness along the medial aspect of the knee, but not specifically over the joint line. No effusion (excessive fluid in the joint) is present. Ligamentous laxity, meniscal signs, and patellar tenderness are lacking. Radiographs are not usually required in this situation. One can confirm the suspicion of medial knee strain by asking the dancer to do a plié. If the positioning is inappropriate (as in figure 5.8) rather than appropriate (as in figure 5.7), technique is quite likely the culprit.

Treatment

This problem requires no specific medical care, but rather correct technical training. The best way for finding a dancer's proper position when in external rotation of the hip is to have him or her stand with legs and feet together. Then, instruct the dancer to move his or her legs from parallel to a position of comfortable external rotation, keeping the back straight and head up (figure 5.9). (Keeping the back straight is important because students may increase their lumbar lordosis to achieve increased external rotation of the lower extremity. Increasing lordosis decreases the tension on the iliofemoral ligament, allowing increased external rotation of the hip. However, it will strain the lumbar spine.) The "turnout" achieved by starting in parallel and then turning out while the knees are kept straight will be a function of the dancer's femoral neck–shaft angle (figure 5.10). Keeping the knees straight ensures that the rotation will occur at the hips. (See also chapter 11, figure 11.14, p. 148.) Once in this position the dancer can be instructed to keep the feet at this angle when assuming the various ballet positions. When this technique is used the feet may not be externally rotated to full parallel in third, fourth, and fifth positions. Nonetheless, during performance of pliés in these positions the knees should fall directly over the feet (figures 5.7 and 5.9). Ballet instructors who are concerned with the well-being of their students will accept this variation in foot positioning, realizing that most of them cannot achieve a 180° angle with their feet. In addition, good instructors will teach

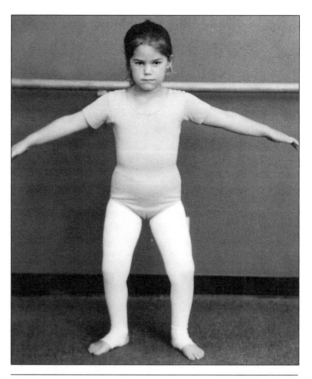

Figure 5.9 This child's natural turnout allows second position with the feet at a 145° angle at most.
Reprinted from Teitz 1982.

their students to obtain more external rotation by using the short external rotators of the hip rather than "cheating" through excessive lordosis of the lumbar spine or twisting the knee (see "Torn Cartilage"). (Turnout is discussed frequently throughout the chapters that follow. See especially chapters 6 and 11, and consult the index for other references.)

Patellofemoral Pain

Patellofemoral pain is responsible for a large percentage of knee complaints in dancers. When one has a good grasp of the basic biomechanics of the patellofemoral joint, it is not difficult to understand why abnormalities in lower extremity alignment, overuse, and faulty dance technique can lead to pain originating in the patellofemoral joint.

Etiology

Small variations in anatomic alignment of the lower extremities can produce patellar problems in dancers due to the requirement for frequent knee flexion and for turnout. The most common form of lower extremity malalignment seen is a triad consisting of excessive femoral anteversion, external tibial torsion, and pronated feet. Femoral anteversion describes the angle of the femoral neck at the hip relative to the plane of the femoral condyles at the knee. In most individuals this angle is 10°. In individuals with excessive femoral anteversion the angle between the neck of the femur and its shaft may equal as much as 20° (figure 5.10). This is reflected clinically by an excessive amount of internal rotation of the hip. The tibia compensates for this excessive internal rotation by rotating externally with relation to the femur. Finally, in order to get the foot flat on the ground, it must pronate at the subtalar joint. As femoral anteversion and tibial torsion increase, so do the Q-angle and the forces, tending to pull the patella laterally (Hvid and Andersen 1982). Subsequent abnormal patellar tracking results in wear of the articular surfaces, patellar subluxation, or excessive pressure on the lateral facet of the patella. The first of these conditions has been called chondromalacia of the patella, whereas the last is known as excessive lateral pressure syndrome (Arendt and Teitz 1997; Fulkerson 1994; Teitz, Hu, and Arendt 1997). The two conditions produce similar symptoms.

Overuse and poor technique also create abnormal pressure in the patellofemoral joint. Excessive compressive loading of the patella occurs due to the frequency of knee flexion and to improper use of the quadriceps muscle. Many students contract their quadriceps muscles tightly during an entire plié, producing constantly high patellofemoral compression forces that theoretically will wear patellar and femoral surfaces. In addition, quadriceps strains may result from chronic eccentric use.

Additional minor aberrations in plié technique, repeated over time, may produce clinical problems. In the dancer with excessive femoral

anteversion, particularly the dancer attempting ballet, knee pain is frequently produced due to the lack of turnout at the hips and compensatory faulty technique. The dancer who attempts to achieve turnout from the floor upward uses the iliotibial band to gain further external rotation of the tibia. This is called "screwing the knee" because of the torque applied. Simultaneously, the patellar attachments of the iliotibial band pull the patella into an abnormal lateral position while it is being subjected to the large compressive forces generated during a plié. Functionally, because ballet dancers rarely work their lower limbs in adduction, their iliotibial bands tighten and pull the patella laterally (Reid et al. 1987). Tight iliotibial bands are also associated with patellofemoral pain in dancers (Winslow and Yoder 1995).

Determining the exact source of anterior knee pain in a dancer—for example, malalignment, thickened plica, or faulty technique—demands a thorough history and physical exam by someone versed in dance technique as well as in anatomy, pathophysiology, and clinical musculoskeletal problems.

Symptoms and Signs

Dancers with patellofemoral problems generally complain of poorly localized anterior knee pain that is exacerbated by dance activities, particularly those incorporating plié. This pain is also aggravated by stair climbing, knee bends, or running, particularly when pronated feet are present. Sitting with the knee flexed for any length of time will produce discomfort. "Giving way" is common, due to reflex quadriceps inhibition. A crackling sound is frequently described but is also present in many people without patellofemoral problems. Also, one may find relatively weak external rotator muscles of the hip, tightness in the iliotibial band and quadriceps, and pronated feet.

Treatment

For most dancers with patellofemoral pain, improving the position of the patella with regard to the femur and correcting faulty technique and training schedules will solve the problem and prevent recurrence. In some cases assistive bracing, and rarely surgery, are required to relieve the pain and return the dancer to full activity. In attempting to gain optimal position of the patella

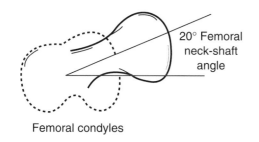

Figure 5.10 Viewed from above, the angle of the femoral neck in relation to the shaft of the femur.

in the trochlear groove, one must balance the forces of the vastus medialis obliquus (VMO) and the iliotibial band, both of which insert on the patella (Steinkamp et al. 1993). Usually the iliotibial band is tight, and stretches (especially those in which the knee crosses the midline) are recommended. For the VMO component of the quadriceps, muscle strengthening is recommended (Teitz, Hu, and Arendt 1997). Although in the past isometric contractions and straight-leg raises with the leg externally rotated were used, the most effective way to strengthen the VMO in isolation is with closed kinetic chain short arc exercises (any exercise in which the distal aspect of the extremity remains in contact throughout with a support surface such as the floor). The VMO is electrically active in the last 15° before complete extension (Steinkamp et al. 1993). The closed kinetic chain decreases the forces on the joint (Kibler and Livingston 2001). When even this mini-plié produces pain, moving the center of gravity back—so that the knee lines up over the ankle—will decrease the forces at the patellofemoral joint. To decrease patellofemoral forces, quadriceps flexibility is also important both at the knee and in the rectus femoris component at the hip. Full arc isotonic exercises are generally discouraged due to the high patellofemoral compression forces produced. In dancers who have difficulty contracting the vastus medialis muscle, or who have pain during isometric exercise, electrogalvanic muscle stimulation will produce a vastus medialis contraction with less force across the knee joint than a voluntary quadriceps contraction (Laughman et al. 1983).

Close assessment of technique and correction thereof are often necessary. Again, dancers should be taught to position their feet to correspond to their hip rotation. Additional turnout can be achieved by working the short external rotators at the hip and stretching the iliofemoral ligaments anteriorly (Hvid and Andersen 1982). Hamstring strengthening and working on centering body weight, especially during demi-pointe and pointe, will decrease the tendency toward hyperextension of the knee. Learning proper control of one's core muscles is facilitated by Pilates exercises. When excessive quadriceps use is noted, the dancer must be taught to initiate plié using the short external rotators of the hip and to end plié using adductors of the thigh. Technique can be modified in several ways. Some teachers

use terms such as "pull up the thigh" and "don't sit in your knees." Other professionals dealing with dancers, including physical therapists, kinesiologists, and movement analysts, have varying approaches to help the dancer find a healthier and more appropriate way of moving. Some utilize imagery techniques or proprioceptive neuromuscular facilitation. Many dancers have a keen awareness of muscle usage and are able to change quickly once they are made to realize what they are doing incorrectly.

Some cases of patellofemoral knee pain will require a knee sleeve that incorporates a lateral pad to hold the patella in position. In approximately 10% of patients with pain due to malalignment, arthroscopic surgery will be indicated to release the lateral retinacular structures pulling the patella laterally. Dancers with extremely anteverted hips should be directed toward types of dance (e.g., tap) that do not demand external rotation.

Subluxating and Dislocating Patellae

Patellar subluxation (partial dislocation) and dislocation usually are due to abnormal rotatory stresses at the knee when the feet are planted. This may occur, for example, when initiating a pirouette. Jumps, particularly those associated with turns in midair, are likely to produce abnormal lateral patellar movement, as the torque necessary to produce the lift and rotation comes from the foot pushing against the ground as the body begins to rotate prior to becoming airborne (Laws 1984).

Etiology

These injuries are most common in people who have increased femoral anteversion. Whereas we are unlikely to find this malalignment in the professional dancer, it is certainly rampant in the adolescent dancer. In dancers with shallow trochlear grooves, abnormal Q-angles, or excessive ligamentous laxity, abnormal lateral patellar movement is common. In addition, faulty technique, particularly screwing the knee, produces excessive pull by the iliotibial band on the patella and increases the likelihood of patellar subluxation. Dancers whose knees hyperextend may also have subluxing patellae. Hyperextension may be due to excessive ligamentous laxity, or may be a compensation for limited plantarflexion at the ankle or for poor trunk stability. Hyperextension of the knee moves the patella away from the trochlear groove and increases its potential mobility.

Symptoms and Signs

When patellar subluxation occurs the dancer feels an unpleasant sense of the knee coming apart and the supporting musculature turning to jelly. This is more dramatic during dislocation, which is usually associated with severe pain. The flatter the trochlear groove and the looser the medial retinacular structures, the less trauma is suffered during lateral patellar dislocation, because nothing has to tear to allow the patella to dislocate. In most cases, however, for dislocation to occur the patella must ride up and over the lateral trochlear facet. Once the patella is out of its normal position the quadriceps mechanism in which it resides is useless, as its fulcrum has been displaced. Hence, the dancer usually falls to the ground. During the fall, or often as a reflex, the leg straightens and the quadriceps muscles pull the patella back into position. In some cases a chip of cartilage, with or without bone, is knocked off the underside of the patella on its way out of or back into the trochlear groove. When this occurs, or when the medial patellofemoral ligament or retinaculum tears, the torn soft tissue or fractured bone ends will bleed into the joint. The dancer then presents with a tensely swollen knee filled with blood. The presence of fat droplets in the blood suggests communication with the fatty bone marrow, that is, a fracture. The dancer's knee will be tender at the site of damage. In the dancer with marked laxity or a very shallow trochlea, in whom patellar mobility is great, dislocation can occur readily without any damage. These dancers will report a similar history but will not have much, if any, swelling or tenderness.

Treatment

Immediate care should include rest, ice, compression, and elevation (RICE). Rapid application of ice and compressive wrapping of the injured area will minimize hemorrhage and swelling. Elevation of the leg, preferably above heart level, will markedly decrease the amount of swelling after injury. If one can minimize swelling and bleeding immediately following an injury the body will need to do less "cleanup" before the healing process begins. The injured area should be rested to avoid further trauma and a diagnosis should be made as soon as possible so that treatment can proceed quickly.

In the dancer whose knee joint is filled with blood, magnetic resonance imaging (MRI) will identify fracture fragments, and tears of the medial patellofemoral ligament or retinaculum (Elias, White, and Fithian 2002). Patellar fracture, chondral injury, patellofemoral ligament tears, or complete medial retinaculum tears will require surgical procedures. These might include removal or replacement and fixation of a fragment, drilling or "microfracturing" the base of a chondral defect to stimulate new cartilage growth, or suture of the ligament or retinaculum. When none of these injuries is found, the patient's knee is placed in a knee immobilizer for about one week to allow resolution of swelling. Rehabilitation is then initiated and emphasizes strengthening of the VMO, which is the key to patellar control (Teitz, Hu, and Arendt 1997). Electrical stimulation is especially useful in these patients to initiate quadriceps contractions. Again we begin with isometric contractions of the quadriceps muscle (quad sets) and straight-leg raises in external rotation to strengthen the adductors. Closed kinetic chain short arc exercises are then added to the program. We never recommend full arc isotonic exercises to patients with patellar injury, as these exercises produce additional patellar damage and are poorly tolerated.

Dancers who have suffered patellar dislocation are often found to have tight lateral retinacular structures, particularly the iliotibial band attachment to the patella. Hence, iliotibial band stretching should be added to the quadriceps rehabilitation program. Since hyperextension of the knee can also lead to patellar subluxation or dislocation, hamstring strengthening is recommended to prevent hyperextension. Because of the frequent finding of technical faults, we often recommend the supine barre and learning to use hip short external rotators and thigh adductors. Well-trained movement analysts can be extremely helpful in assessing and correcting poor mechanics that contributed to the injury. Patellar restraining braces, though useful in providing additional support to the returning athlete, can be used by the dancer during class or rehearsal but usually are not worn in performance.

Tendinitis

Inflammation of the patellar tendon is a common problem in the dancer's knee. Patellar tendinitis is often called "jumper's knee," because it is frequently seen in hurdlers and in basketball and volleyball players. Hamstring tendinitis is also common, but is usually located more proximally in the thigh rather than near the muscles' insertions at the knee.

Etiology

Tendinitis represents an overuse injury. By definition, overuse injuries are those that occur from trying to do too much too quickly—that is, being poorly conditioned. They imply that the musculoskeletal tissues involved may not be strong enough, warm enough, or in the case of soft tissues, flexible enough to withstand the stresses imposed. Generally the tissues of the musculoskeletal system have a capacity for functionally adapting to loads that are gradually increased. Overuse injuries are caused by relatively low loads that are applied too frequently for normal adaptive and reparative processes to occur (Teitz et al. 1997).

Recognized causes of overuse injuries include poor training, technique, equipment, and environment. Poor training is probably the most common of these. Training considerations include frequency of participation, intensity of that participation, and duration of each burst of activity. Obviously the more intense the activity, the shorter the duration needs to be to stress the musculoskeletal system. High-intensity activity produces the type of loads seen in traumatic injuries. Duration of activity will be limited by the vascular supply to the involved tissues and by utilization of glucose and glycogen by these tissues, both of which are affected by previous conditioning. Frequency of participation is often the critical factor producing an overuse injury. Practicing new jumps during every class for a week, or adding rehearsals and performances to routine classes, often leads to patellar tendinitis. Many dancers have experienced sore muscles 48 hours after undertaking more activity than usual. This muscle ache is a sign that the metabolic and load-bearing capacities of the involved muscles have been exceeded. By 72 hours, however, recovery generally occurs and return to activity is possible. Trying to return to the same activity within the first 48 hours, often prior to the appearance of clinical symptoms of overuse, is likely to potentiate the inflammatory response to the initial stress and thereby produce a clinically significant overuse injury with symptoms described in the subsequent section.

Technique is often a factor in overuse injuries as well. Although there are "natural" dancers, one of the important aspects of training is developing efficient technique. For the recreational dancer in particular, or for the dancer who has been poorly trained, inefficient use of various musculotendinous units will cause unnecessary stress (Solomon and Micheli 1986). For example, a dancer who uses her rectus femoris muscle to raise her leg to the front is using a muscle that does not have much mechanical advantage across the hip joint, and she may ultimately develop rectus femoris tendinitis. Hypothetically, if she can be taught to use her iliopsoas muscle, a much stronger hip flexor, achieving this particular movement will be much more efficient, will be less likely to produce tendinitis, and will be aesthetically more desirable as there will not be an obvious contraction of thigh muscle. In addition, a dancer can often raise the leg higher using the iliopsoas because the rectus femoris tendon at the hip joint will be more relaxed and therefore can fold into the groin crease without blocking the ability to fold the leg up onto the torso. Similarly, constant use of the quadriceps muscle during plié, instead of short external rotator and adductor use, may lead to tendinitis and to the patellar problems previously described. Pilates training often helps the dancer to gain the core strength required to re-pattern muscle use.

Equipment and the environment in which a dancer practices or performs often play a role in overuse injuries. Dancers generally work barefooted or in shoes with no shock absorption capability. Hence, the lower extremity muscles must act (usually eccentrically) to decelerate the legs and cushion impact with the floor. Although aerobic dancers wear more shock absorbent shoes, they frequently dance on cement floors or on linoleum or carpeting covering cement. Professional dancers, whenever possible, dance on sprung wood floors that are more shock absorbent.

Symptoms and Signs

Tendinitis is the inflammatory response to a microscopic tear in the tendon and usually presents as pain during use of the involved musculotendinous unit. One often finds tenderness to palpation of the involved tendon and pain when the dancer is asked to use the musculotendinous unit against resistance. Stretching the tendon also may produce pain. In the case of patellar tendinitis, straightening the knee against resistance or flexing it beyond 120° produces pain in the patellar tendon. These symptoms are brought about by the components of the inflammatory response to a microscopic tear, which include the migration of white blood cells to the area with the intent of digesting the damaged tissue. In the process, these cells also contribute to tissue destruction by releasing enzymes and other substances called prostaglandins. The E family of prostaglandins is capable of producing redness, swelling, and pain. The inflammatory response is regulated at the cellular level, and if mild may last only 48 hours (Jozsa and Kannus 1997). Continued excessive physical activity during this period is likely to induce further microscopic damage to the tendon in its already weakened state. During the second week following injury the tendon feels better, but only low levels of activity are tolerated without further injury. Early mobilization of the area, without placing it under resistance, appears to improve tendon tensile strength and excursion (Houghum 1992). Although there is still a small amount of remodeling that occurs up to one year after injury, most tendons are able to withstand normal stresses by six weeks after injury. One is at risk for injury recurrence during that six-week period, so submaximal activity is preferred.

Treatment

Initially the inflammatory process should be kept under control with ice and rest, but not totally eliminated, as it is the inflammatory process which brings to the injured area the cells that will make new collagen. Ice is especially useful in the first few days after injury as it decreases the swelling and reduces the rate of chemical activity, thereby minimizing the inflammatory response. In addition, cold is effective for relieving pain. Two commonly discussed medications in the treatment of tendinitis are nonsteroidal anti-inflammatory drugs (NSAIDs) such as aspirin and ibuprofen, and steroids such as cortisone. The nonsteroidal drugs inhibit the synthesis of prostaglandins, thereby reducing some of the components of the inflammatory response. However, whether the use of NSAIDs in the immediate post-injury period is harmful or helpful is debated (Almekinders 1988). Injecting corticosteroids into

inflamed tendons is frowned on. Evidence indicates that steroid injection decreases the tensile strength of tendon and inhibits the production of collagen and the matrix between collagen fibers, potentially leading to tendon rupture (Halpern, Horowitz, and Nagel 1977; Kennedy and Willis 1976). Ice-friction massage improves circulation to the injured tissue and encourages functional alignment of the newly forming collagen fibers (Chamberlain 1982).

Because eccentric loading elicits greater force production, increased stress on the tendon is produced during this type of activity and is often associated with tendinitis. However, jumping requires eccentric quadriceps work and therefore treatment should also include eccentric training. For the quadriceps muscle emphasis should be placed during isotonic short arc exercises on lowering the weight just as slowly as it is raised. Lifting weights and then dropping them produces only concentric strength and may actually damage the tendon further. Plyometrics (exercises involving eccentric and rapid concentric muscular contractions, such as jumping) should also be incorporated into rehabilitation. In a situation in which the injured dancer is unable to progress with muscle strengthening after an episode of tendinitis, transcutaneous electrical muscle stimulation provides pain relief and the ability to strengthen the muscle without the risk of overloading it. A jumper's knee brace can also decrease the symptoms of patellar tendinitis and allow earlier return to jumping activity.

Torn Cartilage

The medial meniscus is more commonly injured than the lateral meniscus. Many believe that this is due to its shape and attachments. Others believe that the lateral capsular ligaments attached to the lateral meniscus help to pull it out of harm's way during flexion of the knee.

Etiology

Medial meniscal tears are commonly due to twisting the knee while the foot is planted, whereas lateral meniscal injuries are commonly due to hyperflexion of the knee. Previous ACL injury can also contribute to tears of the meniscus by increasing rotatory instability in the knee. In dancers the most common mechanism for tearing the medial meniscus is screwing the knee to increase turnout. The lateral meniscus is at risk during plié, particularly when landing from jumps and, for example, in certain forms of Russian folk dancing, where the forced hyperflexion movement in a squatting position puts a great deal of radial stress on the meniscus.

Symptoms and Signs

The patient with a torn meniscus will usually present with knee pain well localized to either the medial or lateral joint line. Swelling often occurs one or two days after the injury. The patient may report inability to flex or extend the knee completely. In addition, the patient may report that the knee has "given out." This does not reflect any ligamentous instability, but rather reflex inhibition of the quadriceps muscle secondary to pain.

Physical examination often reveals quadriceps atrophy when the injury is more than a week old. Effusion and tenderness are usually present at the site of meniscal tear. Typically, range of motion is decreased and pain may be produced by forced flexion or extension of the knee and by twisting maneuvers. Movements that are likely to cause symptoms in a dancer with a torn meniscus might include pliés, jumps, or développé. True locking occurs when the knee is mechanically limited from full extension or flexion, and when varying amounts of rotation in combination with flexion are required to unlock it. This scenario is different from the ratchety feeling often found in dancers after sitting (which is relieved by straightening the knee). Persistent pain and swelling in the knee suggests that the torn meniscus is irritating the knee and may produce damage to the articular cartilage if not removed.

Treatment

Initially, the general rules of first aid pertain. The patient should rest the knee by wrapping it with an Ace bandage and decreasing activity for a few days. During this period, frequent applications of ice will decrease the swelling. Quadriceps setting exercises (e.g., straight-leg isometric contractions, straight-leg raises, or leg presses) are recommended to avoid atrophy. As the effusion resolves, the patient should attempt to regain range of motion, continue quadriceps strengthening, and gradually return to activity (Teitz 1986). Injured dancers can try to return to full activity when full range of motion and normal strength are achieved, and when limited participation has resulted in no aggravation of knee pain or swelling. This often takes four to six weeks. If pain or effusion persists or recurs, or if the knee locks, further diagnostic evaluation is indicated. The diagnosis can be confirmed using MRI or arthroscopy (looking in the joint with a fiber optic telescope). Arthroscopic excision of the torn part of the meniscus is then recommended, unless the tear is peripheral, in which case the meniscus can be repaired rather than partially excised (Belzer and Cannon 1993). The amount of meniscal tissue removed is determined by the pattern and size of the tear. The part left behind must still resemble the original horseshoe shape in order to retain the normal biomechanical properties of resisting centrifugal stress.

Following surgery the knee must once again be rehabilitated, including range of motion exercises, strengthening, and gradual return to dance, initially omitting activities that torque the knee. When a technical fault such as screwing the knee contributed to the meniscal injury, this fault must be corrected prior to the return to dance. Practicing barre exercises while lying on the floor is useful in learning to use the lower limbs correctly. Exercises to encourage using the hip short external rotators for obtaining turnout, and abdominal muscle strengthening and stretching of the hip flexors to control the pelvis, are useful to decrease torque on the knee.

- For exercises to encourage using the hip short external rotators for obtaining turnout, see chapter 11, page 140, figure 11.7.

- Chapter 9 features exercises to help strengthen abdominal muscles; see especially pages 118 to 127, figures 9.8 through 9.20.

- Appropriate hip flexor stretches may be found in chapter 11, page 139, figures 11.5 and 11.6.

Torn Ligaments

Ligament injuries are traumatic in nature; they occur when a sudden deforming force exceeds the tensile strength of the ligament. The ligaments most commonly injured about the knee are the MCL and ACL. Fortunately, these injuries are uncommon among dancers because most dance movements are choreographed and therefore predictable.

Etiology

When it does occur, ligament injury in dancers is usually caused by hyperextension of the knee or improper landing of a jump. The LCL can be injured in a dancer who lands a jump on one leg with his or her body weight to the outside of center, thereby putting greater stress on the LCL. The MCL can be injured, as can the ACL, from planting the foot and then changing direction, as in initiating a pirouette or other turns during which torsional stresses are placed between the leg and the floor. Anterior cruciate ligament tears may also result from hyperextension of the knee, landing jumps with the center of gravity behind the knee (Griffin et al. 2000), or maximal quadriceps contraction (Kirkendall and Garrett 2001). To my knowledge a PCL injury has not been reported in a dancer.

Symptoms and Signs

Knee ligament injuries present as knee pain following a specific painful incident. It is helpful to know the position of the knee at the time of injury, whether there was an outside force, and whether any sound was heard (an audible pop is often associated with a ligamentous rather than a meniscal injury). Swelling that occurs within 12 hours after injury represents blood in the joint. Seventy percent of the time, blood in the joint is associated with injury of the ACL, whereas in 20% of cases it is associated with fractures, often related to patellar dislocation (DeHaven 1980; Noyes et al. 1980). A collateral ligament tear does not always cause bleeding inside the joint, because only the deep part of the MCL is intracapsular. Patients with collateral ligament injuries usually note swelling and bruising a day or two after injury, and often are able to bear weight on the injured leg.

The patient with chronic ligament insufficiency often will present with a history of knee injury producing pain and rapid swelling followed by subsequent episodes of instability in the knee. This type of instability takes the form of feeling the femur dissociate from the tibia during rotational maneuvers. Instability in a straight-ahead direction is rare because the knee is well controlled by the quadriceps and the hamstring muscles in extension and flexion, respectively. Dancers with a torn ACL have a difficult time turning, as well as landing from jumps. In addition, such jumps as tour jeté and saut de basque are particularly difficult as they require torque to be developed prior to leaving the ground (Laws 1984).

Findings on physical examination of a patient with an acute ligament injury will depend on whether the ligament is a collateral or cruciate ligament. In the case of a collateral ligament injury, the knee is often swollen and may well have bruising either medially or laterally (figure 5.11).

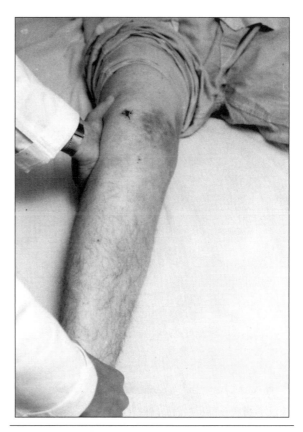

Figure 5.11 Valgus stress testing in a patient with a medial collateral ligament injury.
Reprinted from Teitz 1983.

Tenderness will be present either at the origin or the insertion or along the course of the ligament. Applying varus and valgus stress to the knee will often reproduce pain as the injured ligament is stretched. Occasionally, stressing a completely torn collateral ligament is painless; however, the examiner will feel abnormal angular joint motion. Applying angular stresses to the fully extended knee tests the integrity of the PCL, whereas stressing the knee at 20° of flexion tests for collateral ligament damage. A grade 1 injury is characterized by tenderness but no abnormal opening of the joint. When stress testing produces an abnormal opening of between 0.2 and 0.4 in. (5 mm and 1 cm), the ligament injury is called a grade 2. Grades 1 and 2 imply a partial ligament tear. Grade 3 is defined by an opening equal to or greater than 1 cm, or by no palpable end point, and implies a complete ligament rupture.

In the patient with an acute cruciate ligament tear, one usually finds tense swelling in the knee caused by intra-articular bleeding. Tests of stability will demonstrate abnormal anterior and posterior movement of the tibia on the femur (figure 5.12*a* and *b*), and provocative rotatory tests will demonstrate abnormal rotational movement of the tibia on the femur.

Treatment

The treatment of collateral ligament injuries is a function of the injury grade. Grade 1 injuries can usually be treated symptomatically using immo-

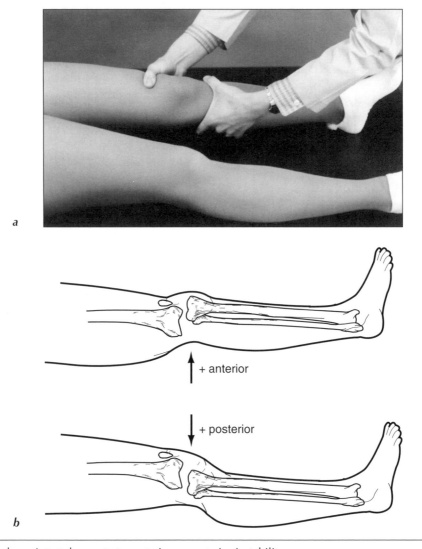

Figure 5.12 Lachman's test demonstrates anterior or posterior instability.

Photo: Reprinted from Teitz 1983.

Art: Reprinted from Teitz 1988.

bilization and ice in the first three to four days, with quadriceps exercises and weight bearing as tolerated. Generally, full flexion of the knee is not possible for four to six weeks because it creates increased tension on the ligament and is painful. Grade 2 and grade 3 ligament injuries are treated using a knee brace with bilateral metal hinged stays. These stays allow flexion and extension, but protect the knee from abnormal angulatory forces medially and laterally. The ligaments are thus shielded from abnormal strains that would stretch the newly forming collagen and make the knee permanently lax. At the same time, mobilization provides a better environment for creating stronger new collagen tissue (Frank 1996). A patient with a grade 2 injury is weaned from the brace gradually over a two- to three-week period. Patients with a grade 3 injury use these braces for six weeks. Quite often the dancer can be kept in class doing barre exercises within a pain-free range, but should avoid jumping and turning.

The situation with cruciate ligaments is entirely different. Torn cruciate ligaments do not heal, because once they have ruptured they untwist and are bathed inside the joint in synovial fluid, which prevents healing of collagenous tissue. Because direct repair yields poor functional results, ACL reconstruction has become the procedure of choice. In the past, debates between surgeons advocating immediate reconstruction and those advocating a trial of rehabilitation and bracing were based on factors such as the movement demands of the patient, the chance of future degenerative arthritis, and the likelihood of functional instability and future meniscal tears (Satku, Kumar, and Ngoi 1986). Athletes in many sports wear functional knee braces that restrict motion of the knee and allow for continued performance. Unfortunately for dancers, although a brace can be worn during rehearsal, the dancer is still at risk during performance, when costuming usually does not allow wearing a brace. The dancer also requires full extension of the knee for stability on pointe and demi-pointe and for aesthetic reasons, and reconstructive procedures often are associated with a loss of 5° to 10° of knee extension (Petsche and Hutchinson 1999). Hence, most orthopedic surgeons who take care of dancers agree that reconstruction, particularly of the ACL, should be undertaken only after the conservative approach to rehabilitation using hamstring strengthening and proprioceptive training has failed (Larson and Tailon 1994).

Anterior cruciate ligament reconstruction may also result in subsequent anterior knee pain. Debates about the origin of this pain center on the graft used and scarring. Those advocating use of the patellar tendon argue that it is stronger in vitro than hamstring tendon (Jansson et al. 2003). Concern about potential hamstring weakness after using semitendinosus as graft has led others to propose using allograft (Peterson, Shelton, and Bomboy 2001).

The principal goal of rehabilitating a patient with a cruciate ligament injury is to produce a stable knee. In the case of an ACL injury, hamstring strengthening is utilized because the hamstrings insert on the back of the tibia and will restrict it from abnormal forward sliding motion. Dancers' hamstring muscles often can benefit markedly from rehabilitation because they are lax due to frequent knee extension, and should be strengthened using isotonic exercises as well as isokinetic exercises (e.g., prone leg curls or leg presses). Before return to full activity, the strength of the injured knee should be at least equal to that of the uninjured knee, or preferably exceed it by approximately 10%. Despite muscular strengthening and reconstruction of a torn ligament, the knee is occasionally perceived to be less stable than before injury. This perception may be due to the lack of proprioceptive input in the scar or reconstructed ligament. When proprioceptive fibers have been torn with the ligament, the recruitment of muscles is often too late to be protective (Schultz et al. 1984; deAndrade, Grant, and Dickson 1965). Training dancers in proprioceptive exercises during which they practice turning and changing direction may help prevent further episodes of knee instability.

An example of a proprioceptive exercise to practice turning and changing direction may be found in chapter 4, page 42.

Conclusion

The discussion in this chapter has dealt with knee problems seen in dancers. Fortunately, the most common problems are those of patellofemoral pain and tendinitis, and for the most part, following proper diagnosis, they can be dealt with utilizing proper principles of rehabilitation. These must include analysis of any predisposing factors such as weakness, tightness, or poor technique, so that those problems can be corrected and recurrence of injury avoided.

References

Almekinders, L.C. 1988. Tendinitis and other chronic tendinopathies. *Journal of the American Academy of Orthopaedic Surgeons* 6(3): 157-164.

Arendt, E.A., and C.C. Teitz. 1997. The lower extremities. In *The female athlete.* Rosemont, IL: American Academy of Orthopaedic Surgeons.

Arnoczky, S., M. Adams, K. DeHaven, D. Eyre, and V. Mow. 1988. Meniscus. In *Injury and repair of the musculoskeletal soft tissue,* edited by S.L.-Y. Woo and J.A. Buckwalter. Parkridge, IL: American Academy of Orthopaedic Surgeons, 489-537.

Arnoczky, S.P., and R.F. Warren. 1982. Microvasculature of the human meniscus. *American Journal of Sports Medicine* 10(2): 90-95.

Bach, J.M., and M.L. Hull. 1998. Strain inhomogeneity in the anterior cruciate ligament under application of external and muscular loads. *Journal of Biomechanical Engineering* 120: 497-503.

Barfred, T. 1971. Experimental rupture of the Achilles tendon: Comparison of various types of experimental rupture in rats. *Acta Orthopaedica Scandinavica* 42(6): 528-543.

Belzer, J.P., and W.D. Cannon. 1993. Meniscal tears. Treatment in the stable and unstable knee. *Journal of the American Academy of Orthopaedic Surgeons* 1(1): 41-47.

Bowling, A. 1989. Injuries to dancers; prevalence, treatment, and perceptions of causes. *British Medical Journal* 298(6675): 731-734.

Chamberlain, G.J. 1982. Cyriax's friction massage: A review. *Journal of Orthopaedic and Sports Physical Therapy* 4: 16-22.

Czerniecki, J.M., F. Lippert, and J.E. Olerud. 1988. A biomechanical evaluation of tibiofemoral rotation in anterior cruciate deficient knees during walking and running. *American Journal of Sports Medicine* 16(4): 327-331.

deAndrade, J.R., C. Grant, and A.S. Dickson. 1965. Joint distension and reflex muscle inhibition in the knee. *Journal of Bone and Joint Surgery* 47A: 313-322.

DeHaven, K.E. 1980. Diagnosis of acute knee injuries with hemarthrosis. *American Journal of Sports Medicine* 8(1): 9-14.

Dienst, M., R.T. Burks, and P.E. Greis. 2002. Anatomy and biomechanics of the anterior cruciate ligament. *Orthopedic Clinics of North America* 33(4): 605-620.

Elias, D.A., L.M. White, and D.D. Fithian. 2002. Acute lateral patellar dislocation and MR imaging injury patterns of medial patellar soft-tissue restraints and osteochondral injuries of the inferomedial patella. *Radiology* 225(3): 736-743.

Fleming, B.C., P.A. Renstrom, B.D. Beynnon, B. Engstrom, G.D. Peura, C.J. Badger, and R.J. Johnson. 2001. The effect of weightbearing and external loading on anterior cruciate ligament strain. *Journal of Biomechanical Engineering* 34(2): 163-170.

Frank, C.B. 1996. Ligament healing: Current knowledge and clinical applications. *Journal of the American Academy of Orthopaedic Surgeons* 4(1): 74-83.

Fulkerson, J.P. 1994. Patellofemoral pain disorders: Evaluation and management. *Journal of the American Academy of Orthopaedic Surgeons* 2(2): 124-132.

Garrick, J.G., D.M. Gillien, and P. Whiteside. 1986. The epidemiology of aerobic dance injuries. *American Journal of Sports Medicine* 14(1): 67-72.

Garrick, J.G., and R.K. Requa. 1993. Ballet injuries. An analysis of epidemiology and financial outcome. *American Journal of Sports Medicine* 21(4): 586-590.

Goodfellow, J., D.S. Hungerford, and M. Zindel. 1976. Patellofemoral mechanics and pathology. 1. Functional anatomy of the patellofemoral joint. *Journal of Bone and Joint Surgery* 58B(3): 287-290.

Griffin, L.Y., J. Agel, M.J. Albohm, E.A. Arendt, R.W. Dick, W.E. Garrett, J.G. Garrick, T.E. Hewett, L. Huston, M.L. Ireland, R.J. Johnson, W.B. Kibler, S. Lephart, J.L. Lewis, T.N. Lindenfeld, B.R. Mandelbaum, P. Marchak, C.C. Teitz, and E.M. Wojtys. 2000. Noncontact anterior cruciate ligament injuries: Risk factors and prevention strategies. *Journal of the American Academy of Orthopaedic Surgeons* 8(3): 141-150.

Halpern, A.A., B.C. Horowitz, and D.A. Nagel. 1977. Tendon ruptures associated with corticosteroid therapy. *Western Journal of Medicine* 127(5): 378-382.

Hardaker, W.T., T.L. Whipple, and F.H. Bassett. 1980. Diagnosis and treatment of the plica syndrome of the knee. *Journal of Bone and Joint Surgery* 62A(2): 221-225.

Harty, M., and J.J. Joyce. 1977. Synovial folds in the knee joint. *Orthopaedic Review* 6: 91-92.

Houghum, P.A. 1992. Soft tissue healing and its impact on rehabilitation. *Journal of Sports Rehabilitation* 1: 19-39.

Huberti, H.H., and W.C. Hayes. 1984. Patellofemoral contact pressures. *Journal of Bone and Joint Surgery* 66A(5): 715-724.

Hvid, I., and L.I. Andersen. 1982. The quadriceps angle and its relation to femoral torsion. *Acta Orthopaedica Scandinavica* 53(4): 577-579.

Jansson, K.A., E. Linko, J. Sandelin, and A. Harilainen. 2003. A prospective randomized study of patellar versus hamstring tendon autografts for anterior cruciate ligament reconstruction. *American Journal of Sports Medicine* 31(1): 12-18.

Jozsa, L.G., and P. Kannus. 1997. Structure and metabolism of normal tendons. In *Human tendons, anatomy, physiology, and pathology.* Champaign IL: Human Kinetics.

Kaufer, H. 1971. Mechanical function of the patella. *Journal of Bone and Joint Surgery* 53A(8): 1551-1560.

Kennedy, J.C., and R.B. Willis. 1976. The effects of local steroid injections on tendons: A biochemical and microscopic correlative study. *American Journal of Sports Medicine* 4(1): 11-21.

Kibler, W.B., and B. Livingston. 2001. Closed-chain rehabilitation for upper and lower extremities. *Journal of the American Academy of Orthopaedic Surgeons* 9(6): 412-421.

Kirkendall, D.T., and W.E. Garrett Jr. 2001. Biomechanical considerations. In *Prevention of noncontact ACL injuries*, edited by L.Y. Griffin. Rosemont, IL: American Academy of Orthopaedic Surgeons.

Krause, W.R., M.H. Pope, R.J. Johnson, and D.G. Wilder. 1976. Mechanical changes in the knee after meniscectomy. *Journal of Bone and Joint Surgery* 58A(5): 599-604.

Laros, G.S., C.M. Tipton, and R.R. Cooper. 1971. Influence of physical activity on ligament insertions in the knees of dogs. *Journal of Bone and Joint Surgery* 53A(2): 275-286.

Larson, R., and M. Tailon. 1994. Anterior cruciate ligament insufficiency: Principles of treatment. *Journal of the American Academy of Orthopaedic Surgeons* 2(1): 26-35.

Laughman, R.K., J.W. Youdas, T.R. Garrett, and E.Y.S. Chao. 1983. Strength changes in the normal quadriceps femoris muscle as a result of electrical stimulation. *Physical Therapy* 63(4): 494-499.

Laws, K. 1984. *The physics of dance.* New York: Schirmer Books.

Markolf, K.L., A. Graff-Radford, and H.C. Amstutz. 1978. In vivo knee stability: A quantitative assessment using an instrumented clinical testing apparatus. *Journal of Bone and Joint Surgery* 60A(5): 664-674.

Nagamine, R., T. Otani, S.E. White, D.S. Carthy, and L.A. Whiteside. 1995. Patellar tracking measurement in the normal knee. *Journal of Orthopaedic Research* 13(1): 115-122.

Newham, D.J., K.R. Mills, B.M. Quigley, and R.H.T. Edwards. 1983. Pain and fatigue after concentric and eccentric muscle contractions. *Clinical Science* 64(1): 55-62.

Nilsson, C., J. Leanderson, A. Wykman, and L.E. Strender. 2001. The injury panorama in a Swedish professional ballet company. *Knee Surgery, Sports Traumatology, Arthroscopy* 9(4): 242-246.

Noyes, F.R., R.W. Bassett, E.S. Grood, and D.L. Butler. 1980. Arthroscopy in acute traumatic hemarthrosis of the knee. *Journal of Bone and Joint Surgery* 62A(5): 687-695.

Perry, J., D. Antonelli, and W. Ford. 1975. Analysis of knee-joint forces during flexed-knee stance. *Journal of Bone and Joint Surgery* 57A(7): 961-967.

Peterson, R.K., W.R. Shelton, and L.A. Bomboy. 2001. Allograft versus autograft patellar tendon anterior cruciate ligament reconstruction: A 5-year follow-up. *Arthroscopy* 17(1): 9-13.

Petsche, T.S., and M.R. Hutchinson. 1999. Loss of extension after reconstruction of the anterior cruciate ligament. *Journal of the American Academy of Orthopaedic Surgeons* 7(2): 119-127.

Quirk, R. 1983. Ballet injuries: The Australian experience. *Clinics in Sports Medicine* 2(3): 507-514.

Reid, D.C., R.S. Burnham, L.A. Saboe, and S.F. Kushner. 1987. Lower extremity flexibility patterns in classical ballet dancers and their correlation to lateral hip and knee injuries. *American Journal of Sports Medicine* 15(4): 347-352.

Reilly, D.T., and M. Martens. 1972. Experimental analysis of the quadriceps muscle force and patellofemoral joint reaction force for various activities. *Acta Orthopaedica Scandinavica* 43(2): 126-137.

Rothenberger, L.A., J.I. Chang, and T.A. Cable. 1988. Prevalence and types of injuries in aerobic dancers. *American Journal of Sports Medicine* 16(4): 403-407.

Rovere, G.D., L.X. Webb, A.G. Gristina, and J.M. Vogel. 1983. Musculoskeletal injuries in theatrical dance students. *American Journal of Sports Medicine* 11(4): 195-198.

Ryman, P.R., and D.W. Jackson. 1987. Anatomy of the anterior cruciate ligament. In *The anterior cruciate deficient knee*, edited by D.W. Jackson and D. Drez. St. Louis: Mosby.

Satku, K., V.P. Kumar, and S.S. Ngoi. 1986. Anterior cruciate ligament injuries: To counsel or to operate? *Journal of Bone and Joint Surgery* 68B(3): 458-461.

Schultz, R.A., D.C. Miller, C.S. Kerr, and L.J. Micheli. 1984. Mechanoreceptors in human cruciate ligaments: A histological study. *Journal of Bone and Joint Surgery* 66A(7): 1072-1076.

Solomon, R.L., and L.J. Micheli. 1986. Technique as a consideration in modern dance injuries. *Physician and Sportsmedicine* 14(8): 83-92.

Steinkamp, L.A., M.F. Dillingham, M.D. Markel, J.A. Hill, and K.R. Kaufman. 1993. Biomechanical considerations in patellofemoral joint rehabilitation. *American Journal of Sports Medicine* 21(3): 438-444.

Takai, S., SL-Y. Woo, G.A. Livesay, D.J. Adams, and F.H. Fu. 1993. Determination of the in situ loads on the human anterior cruciate ligament. *Journal of Orthopaedic Research* 11(5): 686-695.

Teitz, C.C. 1982. Sports medicine concerns in dance and gymnastics. *Pediatric Clinics in North America* 29(6): 1399-1421.

Teitz, C.C. 1983. Office management of common knee problems. *Current Concepts in Pain* 1(4): 13-14.

Teitz, C.C. 1983. Sports medicine concerns in dance and gymnastics. *Clinics in Sports Medicine* 2(3): 571-593.

Teitz, C.C. 1986. First aid, immediate care and rehabilitation of knee and ankle injuries in dancers and athletes. In *The *dancer as athlete,* edited by C.G. Shell. Champaign, IL: Human Kinetics.

Teitz, C.C. 1988a. Gymnastics and dance athletes. In *The sports medicine team and athletic injury prevention,* edited by F.E. Mueller and A. Ryan. Philadelphia: Davis.

Teitz, C.C. 1988b. Ultrasonography in the knee: Clinical aspects. *Radiographic Clinics in North America* 26(1): 55.

Teitz, C.C., W.E. Garrett, A. Miniaci, M.H. Lee, and R.A. Mann. 1997. Tendon problems in athletic individuals. *Journal of Bone and Joint Surgery* 79A: 138-152.

Teitz, C.C., S.S. Hu, and E.A. Arendt. 1997. The female athlete: Evaluation and treatment of sports-related injuries. *Journal of the American Academy of Orthopaedic Surgeons* 5(2): 87-96.

Tuxoe, J.I., M. Teir, S. Winge, and P.L. Nielsen. 2002. The medial patellofemoral ligament; a dissection study. *Knee Surgery, Sports Traumatology, Arthroscopy* 10(3): 138-140.

van Kampen, A., and R. Huiskes. 1990. The three-dimensional tracking pattern of the human patella. *Journal of Orthopaedic Research* 8(3): 372-382.

Walker, P.S., and M.J. Erkman. 1975. The role of the menisci in force transmission across the knee. *Clinical Orthopaedics and Related Research* 109: 184-192.

Washington, E.L. 1978. Musculoskeletal injuries in theatrical dancers: Site, frequency, and severity. *American Journal of Sports Medicine* 6(2): 75-98.

Winslow, J., and E. Yoder. 1995. Patellofemoral pain in female ballet dancers: Correlation with ilio-tibial band tightness and tibial external rotation. *Journal of Orthopaedic and Sports Physical Therapy* 22(1): 18-21.

Woo, S.L., J.V. Matthews, W.J. Akeson, D. Amiel, and F.R. Convery. 1975. Connective tissue response to immobility. *Arthritis and Rheumatism* 18(3): 257-264.

Recommended Readings (Editors)

Barnes, M.S., D. Krasnow, S.J. Tupling, and M. Thomas. 2000. Knee rotation in classical dancers during the grand-plié. *Medical Problems of Performing Artists* 15(4): 140-147.

Credico, M., and A. Davis. 1999. Knee injury in ballet dancers: Incidence and the effect of preventive exercises. *Sports Chiropractic and Rehabilitation* 13(2): 43-49.

Ireland, M.L., and M.R. Hutchinson. 1995. Women. In *Rehabilitation of the injured knee,* edited by L.Y. Griffin. St. Louis: Mosby, 297-312.

Jenkinson, D.M., and D.J. Bolin. 2001. Knee overuse injuries in dance. *Journal of Dance Medicine & Science* 5(1): 16-20.

Scoscia, T.N., J.R. Griffin, and F.H. Fu. 2001. Knee ligaments and meniscal injuries in dancers. *Journal of Dance Medicine & Science* 5(1): 11-15.

Teitz, C.C. 1995. Dance. In *Rehabilitation of the injured knee,* edited by L.Y. Griffin. St. Louis: Mosby, 274-282.

Chapter 6

Iliopsoas Tendinitis in Dancers

Ruth Solomon, Professor Emerita; Lyle J. Micheli, MD

As with the anatomic sites discussed in the two preceding chapters (and the one that follows), dancers are, of course, vulnerable to a variety of injuries at the hip. Several surveys of these injuries are available in the periodical literature: See especially Stone in the Recommended Readings at the end of the chapter. This chapter highlights one such injury because it is (a) uniquely common in dancers, (b) still not well understood in the dance community, and (c) easily prevented if its warning signs are promptly and properly addressed. Chapter 11 provides additional information on how the biomechanics of dance movement can contribute to hip injuries.

History and Etiology

Clicking and popping about the hip in athletes and dancers is a common phenomenon, and generally remains asymptomatic. Early reports of "snapping hip" treated the condition as a single entity involving movement of the tensor fascia lata or iliotibial band over the greater trochanter on the external aspect of the hip (Binne 1913; Dickinson 1929; Jones 1920; Mayer 1919; Parsons 1930). With Moreira (1940) and especially Nunziata and Blumenfeld (1951), however, a distinction came to be made between this variety and an "internal" snapping hip experienced in the groin area on the anterior aspect of the hip. Initially some observers suggested that this medial snapping was due to a tear of the labrum, and in some instances surgical exploration of these hips was carried out.

Chapter adapted by permission, from L.J. Micheli and R. Solomon, 1997, "Treatment of recalcitrant iliopsoas tendinitis in athletes and dancers with corticosteroid injection under fluoroscopy," *Journal of Dance Medicine & Science* 1(1): 7-11.

Terms Describing Anatomical Location in Chapter 6

medial	closer to the midline of the body
abducted	moved away from the midline of the body
anterior	nearer to or toward the front of the body

However, subsequent investigative studies, spearheaded by Schaberg et al. (1984, 1985), demonstrated that medial snapping results from movement of the iliopsoas tendon over the neck of the femur (figure 6.1*a* and *b*). This finding was subsequently replicated by several other investigators (Harper, Schaberg, and Allen 1987; Silver, Connell, and Duncan 1989; Staple, Jung, and Mork 1988).

In certain circumstances, especially when the spine is in hyperextension and the femur is moving into external rotation, the same condition that produces these sounds (the "snapping" tendon) may also cause pain in that area severe enough to restrict or prohibit activity, and therefore requires medical attention. Internal snapping hip poses a greater problem for dancers and other athletes than the external variety as the pain associated with it tends to be more intense and

therefore more debilitating. We were apparently the first to propose that this pain is the result of a stenosing tenosynovitis of the iliopsoas tendon near its insertion on the femur—essentially an iliopsoas tendinitis (Micheli 1983). Repeated loading of the iliopsoas with many ballet movements (editors' note: for examples, see "Diagnosis" below) results in a progressively stronger, but also tighter iliopsoas muscle–tendon unit (the iliopsoas is sometimes called "the dancer's muscle"). This tightening may be further enhanced by lumbar lordosis, since the iliopsoas takes its origin from the front of the lumbar spine (T12, L1-L4). A third factor is that stretching of this muscle–tendon is very difficult to do on one's own, and even with professional supervision and assistance is not easily accomplished. The end result is a tightened muscle–tendon complex in which the tendon begins to snap over the femur

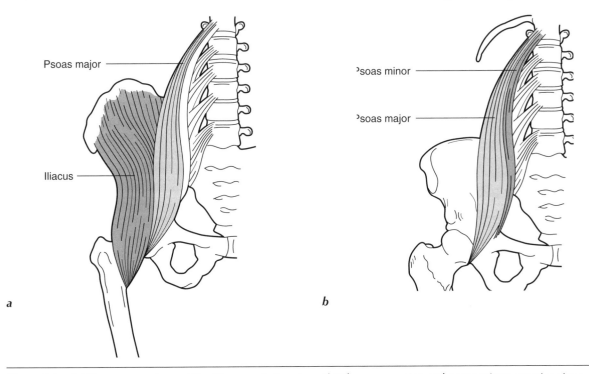

Figure 6.1 *(a)* The psoas major and the iliacus, anterior view. *(b)* The psoas major and psoas minor, anterior view.
Reprinted from Donnelly 1990.

head as the leg is flexed at the hip, sometimes causing inflammation of the iliopectineal bursa. A number of early observers have implicated this bursa as the primary source of pain (Lyons and Peterson 1984; Staple 1972).

Diagnosis

The differential diagnosis of iliopsoas tendinitis must take into account, and ultimately eliminate, a number of other clinical entities commonly associated with hip pain, namely anterior labral tears, hip arthritis, adductor tendinitis, and referred pain to the hip from the spine and pelvis. Nonetheless, in most cases the diagnosis of iliopsoas tendinitis can be strongly suspected from the history provided by the dancer or athlete. Dancers will often describe a slow progressive onset of an initially painless snap as they perform the maneuver of développé à la seconde. In particular, this snap occurs as the gesturing leg is brought down from the elevated, abducted, and externally rotated position of the hip and aligned with the standing leg. Rond de jambe en l'air also presents a problem for those with this condition, especially at the moment of transition from en avant or à la seconde to en ayer. The snap occurs when the leg passes through the front or back diagonal. Eventually there is pain accompanying the snap, which progresses to the point where dancing must be discontinued.

See chapter 11, pages 144 to 146, for more detailed explanation and illustration of développé à la seconde.

In addition to this characteristic history we have found three simple diagnostic tests useful for confirming the presence of iliopsoas tendinitis. The first is a provocative hyperflexion test. With the patient supine upon the examination table and the hip in neutral rotation and neutral abduction, the hip is slowly, progressively, and passively flexed by the examiner (figure 6.2). In all of the cases of iliopsoas tendinitis we have encountered, this action results in pain, while the same test on the uninvolved hip is painless. In the second test the knee is placed in a "frog" position. The patient is then asked to flex and adduct the extremity against the hand of the examiner placed at the knee (figure 6.3). This maneuver elicits pain when tendinitis is present. In the third test the limb is placed in a posi-

tion of hyperextension and abduction with the leg hanging over the side of the examining table and the knee flexed at 90° (figure 6.4). The hip is then slowly, provocatively rotated internally, which again appears to put stress upon the iliopsoas unit and the associated bursa and results in pain.

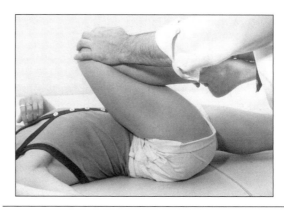

Figure 6.2 Provocative hyperflexion test: The hip is slowly, progressively, and passively flexed by the examiner.
Photo courtesy of Dr. Lyle Micheli.

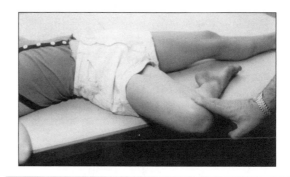

Figure 6.3 "Frog" position test: The patient flexes and adducts the extremity against the examiner's resistance.
Photo courtesy of Dr. Lyle Micheli.

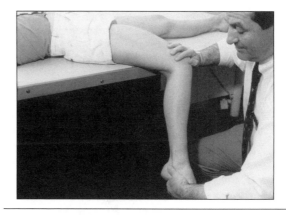

Figure 6.4 With the leg hanging over the table the hip is slowly, provocatively rotated internally.
Photo courtesy of Dr. Lyle Micheli.

Treatment

Whether the injury we are attempting to manage is strictly defined as a tendinitis or a bursitis, the preferred initial treatment involves

- "relative rest";
- the use of anti-inflammatory medication and therapeutic modalities such as deep heat or ultrasound; and
- anti-lordotic exercises. Most important, peripelvic stretching and strengthening exercises, particularly of the iliopsoas, should be initiated both for immediate relief and to correct the biomechanical conditions that caused the problem in the first place.

> The exercises in chapter 9 are excellent for stretching and strengthening the peri-pelvic area and the iliopsoas.

These "conservative" measures have generally been found to be quite efficacious, particularly if diagnosis is made early and intervention begun immediately thereafter (Micheli 1988; Paletta and Andrish 1995; Reid 1988; Quirk 1983; Sammarco 1983, 1987; Taunton, McKenzie, and Clement 1988). Unfortunately, many dancers and athletes, and their teachers and coaches, tend to dismiss snapping hip in its early stages as a minor mechanical problem. In other cases ineffectual treatment that simply approaches it as an inflammatory condition, without attempting to correct the excessive tightness and muscle imbalances about the hip, can result in persistence of this syndrome to the point where chronic inflammation of the tendon sheath and bursa occurs.

At this point surgery becomes an option. Successful surgical release of the contracted iliopsoas tendon was first described by Schaberg, Harper, and Allen (1984). Subsequently, Jacobson and Allen (1990) and Rotini, Spinozzi, and Ferrari (1991) also reported successful treatment of internal snapping hip with surgical lengthening of the muscle–tendon unit. Our own experience with this intervention has also been favorable, but more recently we have preferred a trial of up to three corticosteroid injections before proceeding to surgery, as suggested by a number of other physicians (Howse 1972; Sammarco 1987; Schaberg, Harper, and Allen 1984; Silver, Connell, and Duncan 1989). While initially we attempted the injections in an office setting using palpation and anatomic landmarks for guidance, we subsequently found that the success rate could be increased with fluoroscopy, using a dye infusion prior to injection of the steroid itself to ensure the exact site of injection into the tendon sheath and associated bursa at the femoral head. The results achieved with this procedure are summarized in a scientific study, utilizing data gathered by way of a postoperative questionnaire administered in telephone interviews with ex-patients, that appeared in the literature several years ago (Micheli and Solomon 1997).

"If It Doesn't Hurt, Don't Worry About It"

Whatever treatment modality is used, once it has achieved its goal of returning these dancers to full activity the concern of those who oversee their medical well-being, and especially those who teach them, should turn to preventing recurrence of the injury. This requires an accurate understanding of what initially precipitated the problem. As indicated previously, in its early stages medial snapping hip is usually painless, and therefore seemingly benign. It is only with repetition over time that the tendon becomes irritated and inflamed enough to get stuck in its sheath and sustain the tearing and scarring that characterize tendinitis. This no doubt explains in part why many dance teachers advise that snapping hip is really nothing to worry about unless it is painful. Such advice may also mask a lack of information regarding how to correct dance technique to eliminate the snapping. At any rate, it is widely known that dancers are prone to snapping hip, and one might well wonder why more of them do not progress to iliopsoas tendinitis.

Our theory is that when many dancers say their hips "snap" or "click" or "pop" they mean occasionally—that this is something they have experienced and taught themselves to avoid by subtly altering their technique when performing hip abducting movements (many dancers can intentionally snap their hips; hence, it is to some extent a controllable phenomenon). The unfortunate few who present for medical attention with full-blown iliopsoas tendinitis are those who have taken too much to heart the injunction not to worry about the snapping until there is pain.

Rehabilitation

What we attempt to do in treating this condition is to reduce the inflammation, restore the excursion of the tendon in its sheath, and relieve the bursal impingement. These corrections are not, however, necessarily permanent. Our findings with regard to the pattern of response in the weeks and months immediately following treatment and resumption of dance activities indicate that there is only a brief window of opportunity for the dancer to learn to work in a less injurious manner; those who simply continue the practices that have precipitated the injury run a high risk of recurrence. With careful management the risk can be dramatically reduced.

The basic components of rehabilitative management are therapeutic exercises to increase flexibility of the iliopsoas as well as the hip external rotators, and strengthening exercises for the external rotators, adductors, and internal rotators. This should be combined with anti-lordotic exercises, since a tightened iliopsoas muscle, as already indicated, is inevitably associated with hyperlordosis. Most physical therapists—at least those with some experience in dealing with athletes—will have such exercises at their disposal. The main responsibility, however, may be thought to rest with the patient's ballet teacher(s), who can be assumed to have a trained eye for detecting such alignment problems as excessive anterior pelvic tilt. This corrective work in the dance studio can be accomplished in a number of ways, seldom requiring more than a slight adjustment or augmentation of one's standard teaching practices. Our own methods, dictated by a strong background in modern dance, utilize mainly floor work, and are briefly described in chapter 9 (see especially pages 118-121), but the same therapeutic effects can be achieved by a thoughtful application of ballet technique.

> Figures 9.8 through 9.13 are good examples of anti-lordotic exercises.

Conclusion

This chapter highlights what has become one of the major issues in dance medicine and science: how to bridge the gap between the findings of researchers and the practices of dancers and those people who are directly responsible for their well-being. In this case medical science has made it known that the traditional tendency in the dance field to ignore "snapping hip" is misconstrued; if not acknowledged and dealt with early on, this condition can result in serious medical complications. Hence, we owe it to young dancers to help them effect the changes initially required to prevent a truly unnecessary injury, or at least to avoid its recurrence. Hopefully publications of this sort help to disseminate that information.

References

Binne, J.F. 1913. Snapping hip (hanche a ressort; Schnellend Hefte). *Annals of Surgery* 58: 59-66.

Dickinson, A.M. 1929. Case reports by Dr. Arthur M. Dickinson. Bilateral snapping hip. *American Journal of Surgery* 6: 97-101.

Harper, M.C., J.E. Schaberg, and W.C. Allen. 1987. Primary iliopsoas bursography in the diagnosis of disorders of the hip. *Clinical Orthopaedics and Related Research* 221: 238-241.

Howse, A.J.G. 1972. Orthopaedists aid ballet. *Clinical Orthopaedics and Related Research* 89: 52-63.

Jacobson, T., and W.C. Allen. 1990. Surgical correction of the snapping iliopsoas tendon. *American Journal of Sports Medicine* 18(5): 470-474.

Jones, F.W. 1920. The anatomy of snapping hip. *Journal of Orthopaedic Surgery* 2: 1-3.

Lyons, J.C., and L.F.A. Peterson. 1984. The snapping iliopsoas tendon. *Mayo Clinic Proceedings* 59(5): 327-329.

Mayer, L. 1919. Snapping hip. *Surgery Gynecology and Obstetrics* 29: 425-428.

Micheli, L.J. 1983. Overuse injuries in children's sports: The growth factor. *Orthopedic Clinics of North America* 14(2): 337-360.

Micheli, L.J. 1988. Dance injuries: The back, hip, and pelvis. In *Science of dance training,* edited by P.M. Clarkson and M. Skrinar. Champaign, IL: Human Kinetics, 193-207.

Micheli, L.J., and R. Solomon. 1997. Treatment of recalcitrant iliopsoas tendinitis in athletes and dancers with corticosteroid injection under fluoroscopy. *Journal of Dance Medicine & Science* 1(1): 7-11.

Moreira, F.E.G. 1940. Anca a scatto (snapping hip). *Journal of Bone and Joint Surgery* 22A: 506.

Nunziata, A., and I. Blumenfeld. 1951. Cadeva a resorte. A proposito de una variedad. *Prensa Medica Argentina* 38: 1997-2001.

Paletta, G.A., and J.T. Andrish. 1995. Injuries about the hip and pelvis in the young athlete. *Clinics in Sports Medicine* 14(3): 591-628.

Parsons, E.B. 1930. The snapping hip. *Texas State Medical Journal* 26: 361-362.

Quirk, R. 1983. Ballet injuries: The Australian experience. *Clinics in Sports Medicine* 2(3): 507-514.

Reid, D.C. 1988. Prevention of hip and knee injuries in ballet dancers. *Sports Medicine* 6(5): 295-307.

Rotini, R., C. Spinozzi, and A. Ferrari. 1991. Snapping hip: A rare form with internal etiology. *Italian Journal of Orthopaedics and Traumatology* 17(2): 283-288.

Sammarco, G.J. 1983. The dancer's hip. *Clinics in Sports Medicine* 2(3): 485-498.

Sammarco, G.J. 1987. The hip in dancers. *Medical Problems of Performing Artists* 2(1): 5-14.

Schaberg, J.E., M.C. Harper, and W.C. Allen. 1984. The snapping hip syndrome. *American Journal of Sports Medicine* 12(5): 361-365.

Schaberg, J.E., M.C. Harper, and W.C. Allen. 1985. Snapping hip syndrome. *Advances in Orthopaedic Surgery* 12: 340-342.

Silver, S.F., D.G. Connell, and C.P. Duncan. 1989. Case report 550. *Skeletal Radiology* 18: 327-328.

Staple, T.W. 1972. Arthrographic demonstration of iliopsoas bursa extension of the hip joint. *Diagnostic Radiology* 102: 515-516.

Staple, T.W., D. Jung, and A. Mork. 1988. Snapping tendon syndrome: Hip tenography with fluoroscopic monitoring. *Radiology* 166(3): 873-874.

Taunton, J.E., D.C. McKenzie, and D.B. Clement. 1988. The role of biomechanics in the epidemiology of injuries. *Sports Medicine* 6(2): 107-120.

Recommended Readings (Editors)

Anderson, K., S.M. Strickland, and R. Warren. 2001. Hip and groin injuries in athletes. *American Journal of Sports Medicine* 29(4): 521-533.

Janzen, D.L., E. Partridge, P.M. Logan, D.G. Connell, and C.P. Duncan. 1996. The snapping hip: Clinical imaging findings in transient subluxation of the iliopsoas tendon. *Canadian Association of Radiologists Journal* 47(3): 202-208.

Johnston, C.A., J.P. Wiley, D.M. Lindsay, and D.A. Wiseman. 1998. Iliopsoas bursitis and tendinitis: A review. *Sports Medicine* 25(4): 271-283.

Morelli, V., and V. Smith. 2001. Groin injuries in athletes. *American Family Physician* 64(8): 1405-1414.

Stone, D. 2001. Hip problems in dancers. *Journal of Dance Medicine & Science* 5(1): 7-10.

Stretanski, M.F., and G.J. Weber. 2002. Medical and rehabilitation issues in classical ballet. *American Journal of Physical Medicine and Rehabilitation* 81(5): 383-391.

Chapter 7

Spinal Problems in Dancers

Elly Trepman, MD; Arleen Walaszek, PT; Lyle J. Micheli, MD

This chapter presents an anatomical and biomechanical description of the spine, followed by discussion of the etiology, diagnosis, and treatment of common dance injuries at that site. Emphasized are lumbar hyperlordosis (as a cause of injury), spondylolysis, scoliosis, facet arthrosis, disc herniation, mechanical low back pain, and upper back and neck injuries.

Injury to the spine accounts for 7% to 18% of all dance injuries (Francis, Francis, and Welshons-Smith 1985; Garrick, Gillien, and Whiteside 1986; Rovere et al. 1983; Solomon, Trepman, and Micheli 1989; Washington 1978). The percentage of dancers who have a history of back injury ranges from 8% to 11% of aerobic dancers (Garrick, Gillien, and Whiteside 1986) to 60% to 80% of ballet and modern dancers (Solomon, Trepman, and Micheli 1989). The majority of spinal injuries in dancers involve the lumbar region, but cervical and thoracic injury is not uncommon (Rovere et al. 1983). Other spinal conditions such as scoliosis are prevalent in dancers (Warren et al. 1986). Furthermore, poor spinal posture and technique can contribute to pelvic and lower extremity malalignment and injury (Gelabert 1986). Therefore, attention to the anatomy and biomechanics of the spine during dance training should be a top priority for both student and teacher. Such attention should decrease the incidence and severity of spinal and lower extremity dance injuries.

Authors' note: This chapter is dedicated to Elaine Bauer, principal dancer for the Boston Ballet Company, in honor of her retirement from the stage.

Terms Describing Anatomical Location in Chapter 7

bilateral	occurring or appearing on two sides
contralateral	associated with a particular part on an opposite side
inferior	situated below another structure
ipsilateral	pertaining to the same side of the body
lateral	farther away from the midline of the body
posterior	behind or toward the back of the body
posteromedial	situated behind and to the inner side
proximal	close to or nearest the origin or point of attachment
superior	situated above or higher than another structure

For additional information regarding the epidemiology of dance injuries in general, or spinal injuries in particular, see chapter 1.

Anatomy and Biomechanics of the Spine

The skeletal framework of the spine consists of an undulated arrangement of 7 cervical, 12 thoracic, and 5 lumbar vertebrae perched on the sacrum (figure 7.1). The vertebrae are separated by intervertebral discs, which absorb impact and allow for motion between the vertebrae. The normal spinal column is curved into lordosis (concave posterior) in the cervical and lumbar regions and into kyphosis (convex posterior) in the thoracic region (figure 7.1). The magnitudes of the lumbar lordosis and pelvic tilt are inter-related: A greater degree of lumbar lordosis is associated with more pelvic extension relative to the spine, with the coccyx tipped backward and upward.

The spinal curves themselves are determined by a balance of the action of the supporting muscles of the spine and allow for impact absorption. However, when the curves are exaggerated in magnitude, as with excessive lumbar lordosis ("swayback"), undue stresses are placed on the spinal elements (as described further on), which may lead to injury. The development of excessive lumbar lordosis and thoracic kyphosis may be a result of muscle imbalance, which in dancers can often be traced to errors in posture and technique.

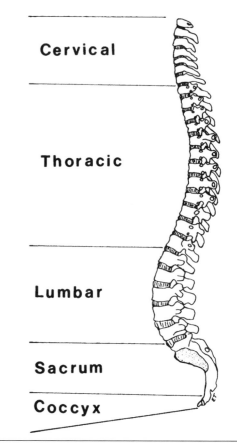

Figure 7.1 The spinal column viewed from the side. The cervical and lumbar regions are curved into lordosis (concave posterior), balancing the kyphosis (convex posterior) of the thoracic spine.

Illustration by Elly Trepman, M.D.

The Vertebrae

Each vertebra is a complex bone, analogous in basic structure to a padlock, consisting of an anterior cylindrical body and a posterior bony arch (figure 7.2a). The vertebrae surround and protect the dural sac containing the spinal cord, which sends branches (nerve roots) to the trunk and extremities for control of motion and other bodily functions (figure 7.2b). The vertebral arch consists of the laminae and pedicles, which connect the arch to the body. Each arch has seven bony projections: two transverse processes and one posterior spinous process, which provide attachments for ligaments and muscles; and two superior and two inferior facets, which articulate with facets of the adjacent vertebrae above and below to form the facet (apophyseal) joints (figure 7.2a and b). These are true synovial joints, consisting of articular cartilage, joint fluid, and a surrounding capsule. Motion between adjacent

vertebrae occurs at the intervertebral disc and the two facet joints. The superior and inferior facet on each side of the vertebral arch is separated by a supporting bar of bone known as the pars interarticularis (figure 7.2a). A foramen formed between the pedicles, disc and facet joint of two adjacent vertebrae allows passage of the nerve root from the spine; and injury to any of these structures can result in nerve root irritation, as in certain types of sciatica (figure 7.2a).

The regional differences in vertebral structure partially account for the differences in motion characteristics of the regions (figure 7.3). The plane of orientation of facet joints in the cervical spine is more horizontal than in the other regions and allows for more rotation of the neck

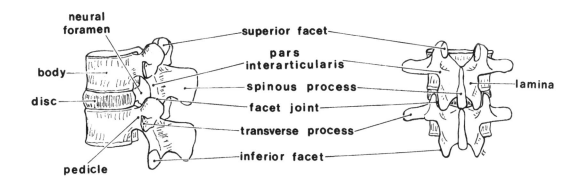

ANTERIOR

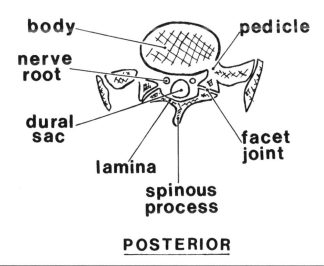

POSTERIOR

Figure 7.2 *(a)* Normal anatomy of the lumbar spine. Lateral (left) and posterior (right) views of two adjacent lumbar vertebrae and intervertebral disc. The detailed anatomy is clarified in *(b)*. (One pedicle is not seen because the cross section is slightly oblique from the horizontal plane.)

Illustration by Elly Trepman, M.D.

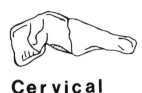

Cervical

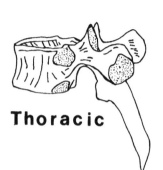

Thoracic

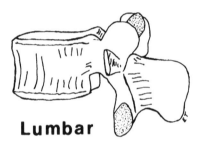

Lumbar

Figure 7.3 Structural differences between cervical, thoracic, and lumbar vertebrae partially account for the different ranges of motion of the neck, upper back, and lower back.

Illustration by Elly Trepman, M.D.

in the horizontal plane. The lumbar facet joints are more vertical, thus limiting rotation while allowing flexion and extension of the lumbar spine. The thoracic spine is restricted by rib attachments and longer, more vertical posterior spinous processes, and this partly explains the relatively smaller range of motion in this region (White and Panjabi 1978).

Excessive lumbar lordosis or repetitive hyperextension of the lumbar spine results in increased stresses on the facet joints and the pars interarticularis and may lead to facet arthritis or stress fracture of the pars. Sudden flexion of the spine results in compressive stress on the vertebral bodies and may cause compression fracture and loss of body height.

The Intervertebral Discs

The bodies of adjacent vertebrae are separated by intervertebral discs, which consist of a fibrous ring (annulus fibrosus) enclosing a pulpy center (nucleus pulposus), analogous in cross section to a jelly donut (figure 7.4). The discs act as cushions that absorb impact and allow for motion between adjacent vertebrae. Flexion of the spine, in either the sitting or standing position, results in an increase in load on the disc (Nachemson 1966). This may explain the contribution of flexion injury to disc herniation, as discussed later. Tightness associated with excessive lumbar lordosis may also increase the risk of injury to the disc.

Muscular and Ligamentous Support

The ligaments of the spine connect and stabilize the vertebral bodies, transverse processes, posterior spinous processes, laminae, and facet joint capsule. They allow for normal motion in the

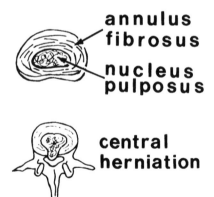

annulus fibrosus

nucleus pulposus

central herniation

lateral herniation

Figure 7.4 The normal intervertebral disc (top) consists of a fibrous annulus that encloses a pulpy central nucleus. Central disc herniation (middle) may result in pressure on the dural sac, whereas lateral herniation (bottom) may compress a nerve root as it exits the neural foramen.

Illustration by Elly Trepman, M.D.

physiological range and provide a static, protective constraint to abnormal motion (White and Panjabi 1978).

The spine is extremely unstable in the absence of active muscular control (White and Panjabi 1978). The many muscles that provide stability and control movement can be grouped into categories based on anatomic location and function.

Paraspinal Muscles

The paraspinal muscles (erector spinae) are long muscles located posterior and lateral to the vertebrae (figure 7.5). They arise from the sacrum and attach to the posterior spinous processes and ligaments of the lumbar and lower thoracic vertebrae. They then branch into three major muscle groups—the iliocostalis, longissimus, and spinalis muscles—that insert on vertebrae, ribs, and the skull. These muscles extend the spine when right and left sides are working in synchrony, and laterally flex the spine when acting unilaterally.

Deep Back Muscles

The deep back muscles connect the posterior elements of vertebrae (for example, transverse process of one vertebra to spinous process of another)

over shorter distances than the erector spinae. The main function of the deep muscles, such as the multifidus, semispinalis, and rotatores, includes spinal extension, rotation, and stabilization.

Abdominal Muscles

The abdominal muscles, consisting of the rectus abdominis, external oblique, internal oblique, and transversus abdominis, join the rib cage to the pelvis (figure 7.6). This muscle group assists in flexion of the lumbar spine, and when acting unilaterally causes lateral flexion or rotation of the trunk. Furthermore, by increasing intra-abdominal (hydrostatic) pressure, the abdominal muscles facilitate the support of the erect body, thereby decreasing the supportive work required of the erector spinae muscles. Weakness of the abdominal muscles may result in excessive lumbar lordosis and therefore may contribute to spinal and lower extremity dance injury.

The quadratus lumborum, which originates from the posterior iliac crest and inserts on the 12th rib and the transverse processes of the lumbar vertebrae, is classified as an abdominal muscle (figure 7.5). It laterally flexes the lumbar spine when working unilaterally.

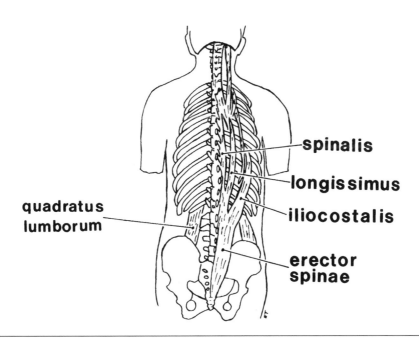

Figure 7.5   The paraspinal muscles and quadratus lumborum. The erector spinae arise from the sacrum and branch into the iliocostalis, longissimus, and spinalis groups. The quadratus lumborum is an abdominal muscle that originates from the posterior iliac crest and inserts on the 12th rib and transverse processes of the lumbar vertebrae.

Illustration by Elly Trepman, M.D.

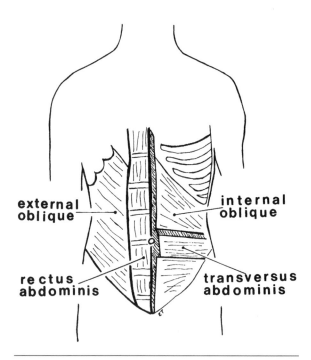

Figure 7.6 The abdominal muscles originate from the ribs and insert on the pelvis. The rectus abdominis is located adjacent to the midline. The external oblique, internal oblique, and transversus abdominis muscles are arranged as three layers, with muscle fibers of each oriented in a different direction.

Illustration by Elly Trepman, M.D.

Iliopsoas

The iliopsoas, one of the most powerful muscles of the body, is the only muscle that attaches to the spine, pelvis, and femur (Michele 1960). The two components of the iliopsoas are the iliacus, which originates from the inside of the iliac crest, and the psoas, which takes origin from the vertebrae between the 12th thoracic (T12) and fifth lumbar (L5) vertebrae (figure 7.7). The iliacus and psoas are joined in the common iliopsoas tendon, which inserts on the lesser trochanter of the femur. This insertion is on the posteromedial aspect of the proximal femur (figure 7.7). Therefore, iliopsoas contraction with shortening of the muscle (concentric contraction) would appear primarily to cause hip flexion, with possibly some associated adduction and external rotation (McKibbin 1968; Michele 1960). There is controversy regarding the effect of the iliopsoas on hip rotation (Williams and Warwick 1980).

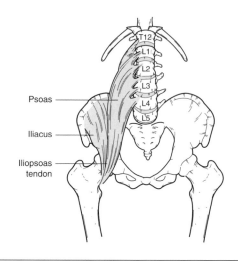

Figure 7.7 The iliopsoas consists of the iliacus and psoas muscles. The iliopsoas tendon inserts on the lesser trochanter of the femur.

Illustration by Mary Consenza.

Some authors believe that in certain circumstances it may act as an internal rotator of the hip (Bachrach 1987; Ranney 1979). Nevertheless, the effect of the iliopsoas on hip rotation is probably small in comparison with other hip rotators. Bilateral concentric iliopsoas contraction results in flexion (forward bending) of the lumbar spine and pelvis. Unilateral concentric iliopsoas contraction results in lateral bending (scoliosis) of the lumbar spine (Michele 1960).

The iliopsoas is important in stabilizing the lumbar spine and pelvis and is a major determinant of posture and movement (Michele 1962). The psoas has been shown by electromyography to be active in the upright sitting and standing positions, thereby contributing to the stability of the lumbar spine (Nachemson 1968).

Stabilization of the lumbar spine by bilateral eccentric (lengthening) or isometric (constant length) iliopsoas contraction may decrease lumbar lordosis (Solomon 1988). Weakness of the psoas and peripheral abdominal muscles is associated with hyperlordosis (Micheli and Solomon 1987). An exercise program that improves iliopsoas strength and flexibility may reduce lumbar hyperlordosis and associated technical errors that can lead to dance injury (Micheli and Solomon 1987; Solomon 1988). A further benefit of such a program is an increase in postural stability centrally, which may free peripheral muscles for finer control of extremity movement (Micheli and Solomon 1987; Solomon 1988).

> The exercises in chapter 9 are excellent for improving iliopsoas strength and flexibility.

Anatomic and Technical Factors Contributing to Lumbar Hyperlordosis

Lumbar hyperlordosis may contribute to many dance injuries because of the associated increased stresses on the posterior elements and discs (figure 7.8*a* and *b*). Therefore, it is important to determine the etiology of this posture in the individual dancer (table 7.1) (Gelabert 1986; Howse and Hancock 1988). With appropriate attention to technical errors and rehabilitation, hyperlordosis can often be corrected and this may prevent injury and prolong the career of the dancer. The young dancer is especially at risk for the development of lumbar hyperlordosis because of the tightening of the lumbar fascia and hamstrings that occurs during the adolescent growth spurt (Gurewitsch and O'Neill 1944).

Dynamics of the Spine and Muscular Control in Dance Movement

There are no available electromyographic studies of spinal muscle function in dance movement. Furthermore, quantitative estimates of individual muscle strength, such as those available for the muscles about the knee (Minkoff and Sherman 1987), are difficult to obtain for the musculature of the spine. Therefore, the current understanding of the muscular control of the spine in dance is based on the astute clinical observations of dance instructors, therapists, physicians, and dancers themselves.

Concentric muscle contraction, in which the muscle shortens as it contracts, is only one of several mechanisms by which muscles control the dynamics of spinal movement. Isometric

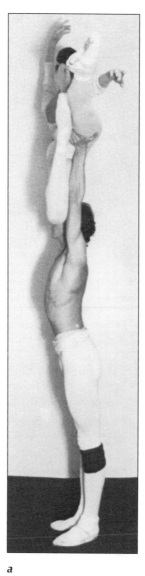 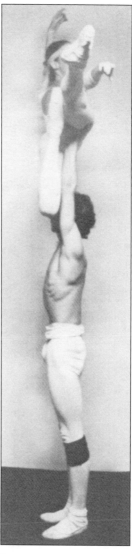

a   *b*

Figure 7.8 *(a)* Incorrect lifting posture, with excessive lumbar lordosis, may contribute to disc herniation. *(b)* Proper lifting posture, with stabilization of the lumbar spine, is promoted by an anti-lordotic strengthening and flexibility program and postural awareness.

contraction, in which the length of the muscle remains constant during contraction, is important for the stability of the spine. The concept of eccentric muscle contraction, in which the muscle contracts as it lengthens ("controlled letting go"), has resulted in an improved understanding of the importance of antagonist muscle function and strength in movement.

Table 7.1 Factors Associated With Lumbar Hyperlordosis

Anatomic factors	Technical errors	Other factors
Thoracic hyperkyphosis	Compensation for limited hip turn-out (i.e., flexing the pelvis on the hip to allow for greater turnout in the flexed hip)	Decreased flexibility during the growth spurt
Weak psoas	Arabesque or attitude with extension from the lumbar spine instead of the hip	
Tight hip flexors (e.g., ilio-psoas)	Poor lifting posture	
Hip flexion contracture	Lack of postural awareness	
Femoral anteversion		
Weak abdominal muscles		
Tight lumbar fascia		
Tight hamstrings		
Genu recurvatum ("sway-back knees")		

A specific muscle may work in any of these varied manners during different dance movements. For example, a powerful concentric contraction of the abdominal muscles provides the impulse for movement in a Graham contraction or return from a back arch; in contrast, during a back arch, control is accompanied by eccentric contraction of the abdominal muscles (Ryman 1979b). Isometric contraction of the abdominal muscles provides stability to the lumbar spine during a lift. Therefore, it may be important to strengthen the abdominal muscles in these three different modes in order to optimize function and minimize risk of injury.

Differences in flexibility of the cervical, thoracic, and lumbar regions may also affect the dynamics of spinal movement in dance. The thoracic spine is intrinsically less flexible because of the orientation of the facet joints and posterior spinous processes, as well as rib attachments (Ryman 1979a; White and Panjabi 1978). Therefore, the long graceful arch of the classical arabesque may be difficult to achieve, and a compensatory exaggeration of the cervical and lumbar lordosis may occur, resulting in increased stress and risk of injury (Ryman 1979b). This problem may be corrected by the use of a program directed at increasing thoracic extension flexibility and cervical and lumbar strength (Ryman 1979b; Dowd 1984).

Spinal motion and stability are also influenced by the muscles of the extremities. The hip extensors, including the gluteus maximus and hamstrings, may stabilize the hip in extension and assist in reducing lumbar lordosis (Ryman 1979b). However, as noted previously, use of the iliopsoas for stabilization of the lordosis may be more advantageous, as the extensors can then be used primarily for movement (Solomon 1988).

Overuse Injuries of the Spine

Although single-impact trauma is the cause of some injuries to the spine in dancers, many others result from overuse (Stanish 1987). The stresses and strains of repetitive dance training may lead to microscopic injury; if the rate of occurrence of this microtrauma exceeds that of tissue healing, then macroscopic overuse injury will occur (Hunter-Griffin 1987; Trepman and Micheli 1988).

Risk Factors

Several risk factors have been identified as contributors to overuse injury of the spine in dancers (table 7.2) (Micheli 1983). Abrupt increases in dance intensity or changes in choreographic technique may not allow musculoskeletal adaptation

Table 7.2   Risk Factors for Overuse Injuries of the Spine

Abrupt changes	Training style
	Intensity
	Duration
	Frequency
Technical errors	Excessive dynamic lumbar hypertension (lordosis) in movements such as *attitude and arabesque*
	Lifting a partner incorrectly
	Increasing hip flexion to force turnout
Anatomic malalignment	Lumbar hyperlordosis
	Femoral anteversion
	Limb length discrepancy
	Other
Footwear	Spike heels
Dance surface	Poor impact absorption
Growth factors	Decreased flexibility with growth spurt
	Growth cartilage
Hormonal factors	Delayed menarche
	Amenorrhea
	Hypoestrogenism

to the increased rate or altered pattern of stresses on the bones, discs, ligaments, and muscles of the back. This may occur when a dancer returns from a layoff period or begins intensive training in an unfamiliar style of dance. Overuse injuries are also seen in students who suddenly increase classes from 2 hours per day during the school year to 6 or 8 hours per day at a summer program.

As noted earlier, excessive lumbar lordosis resulting from anatomic causes or technical errors may result in increased stresses on the discs, pars interarticularis, and facet joints. Therefore, hyperlordosis is a major risk factor for overuse injury to the spine, such as stress fracture or ligament sprain. Muscle imbalance, weak abdominal muscles, or femoral anteversion may contribute to lumbar hyperlordosis and overuse injury.

The use of high spike heels in jazz dance may increase lumbar lordosis and strain (Micheli 1983). Poor impact absorption by the dance surface may result in increased stress on the lower extremities and lumbar spine (Seals 1983).

Adolescents have growth-dependent risk factors that may contribute to overuse injury. The decrease in flexibility during the adolescent growth spurt

(Gurewitsch and O'Neill 1944) may result in tight lumbodorsal fascia and increased lumbar lordosis. Traction injury to growth cartilage may also cause back or pelvic pain, as with ischial apophysitis associated with tight hamstrings (Micheli 1987). Furthermore, delayed menarche may predispose the young female dancer to stress fractures and scoliosis (Warren et al. 1986).

Treatment

The treatment of overuse injuries begins with an accurate diagnosis and removal of contributing risk factors. The dancer is prescribed alternate activities that do not exacerbate the injury in order to maintain aerobic and musculoskeletal fitness during the recovery period. Inflammatory conditions such as tendinitis may respond to a short course (one to two weeks) of oral anti-inflammatory medication. Physical therapeutic modalities, such as ice, heat, ultrasound, and electrical stimulation, may also accelerate healing (Gieck and Saliba 1987). Braces may be useful in specific situations such as disc herniation or spondylolysis (as discussed later).

The cornerstone of any good therapeutic program for overuse injuries of the spine is a directed, progressive, strengthening and flexibility exercise program. A program of exercises to improve iliopsoas strength and flexibility may be especially useful in the overall rehabilitation of overuse injuries of the spine (Solomon 1988). The use of floor work may minimize stresses on the lower back during the gradual return to dance activity after overuse injury (Solomon 1988).

> The exercises offered in chapter 9 would be useful in a therapeutic program for overuse injuries of the spine.

Specific Problems

Some common medical problems encountered at the spine by dancers are described in this section.

Spondylolysis

Spondylolysis is a defect in the normal bony structure of the pars interarticularis that is present in 6% of adults (Fredrickson et al. 1984). This condition usually occurs at L4 or L5, unilaterally or bilaterally, and is believed to have a hereditary predisposition (Fredrickson et al. 1984; Pizzutillo 1985). When separation at a bilateral defect occurs, spondylolisthesis may result, in which the upper vertebra slips forward over the lower one. If the amount of slippage is severe, spinal instability may result, requiring surgical fusion of the two levels. Fortunately, the degree of spondylolisthesis is usually mild and progression is unusual (Fredrickson et al. 1984).

Spondylolysis may be more common in the dancer than in the general population. Repetitive hyperextension of the lumbar spine in arabesque or attitude can result in stress at the pars interarticularis, and this may be exacerbated by excessive lumbar lordosis or poor technique (table 7.1). The dancer with this condition may notice a gradual onset of localized low back pain, which is often in a discrete location on the side of the involved pars. The pain is increased by lumbar hyperextension, particularly during standing on the leg of the affected side. The physical examination may be notable for paraspinous muscle spasm, hyperlordosis, and limitation of forward bending due to tightness of the hamstrings and

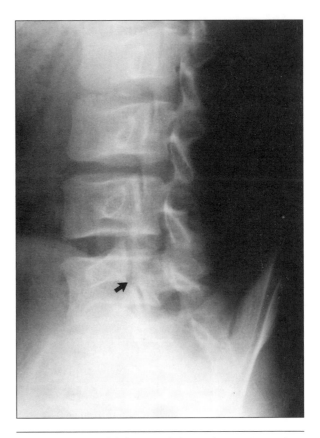

Figure 7.9   Spondylolysis is a defect in the pars interarticularis (arrow) that may be seen on the oblique radiograph of the lumbar spine.

lumbar fascia. Radiographs of the lumbar spine may reveal a frank bony pars defect that has the appearance of a stress fracture (figure 7.9). A technetium pyrophosphate radionuclide bone scan, which is more sensitive than radiography, may show increased activity at the involved pars, even if no pars defect is detected on radiographs (Jackson et al. 1981). An occasional dancer with this condition will nonetheless have normal radiographs and bone scan.

Treatment of spondylolysis includes the discontinuation of dance activity and immobilization of the low back with an anti-lordotic brace for six months (figure 7.10, *a-c*). This must be supplemented with a program of abdominal and pelvic strengthening exercises and a stretching program for the hamstrings and lumbodorsal fascia, to prevent atrophy, weakness, and tightness that may otherwise be associated with immobilization.

> The exercises offered in chapter 9 are excellent for abdominal and pelvic strengthening.

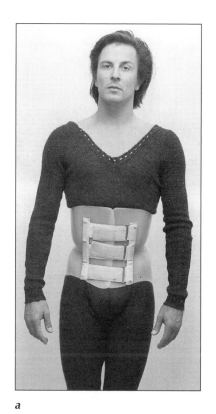 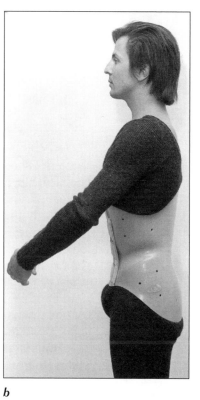 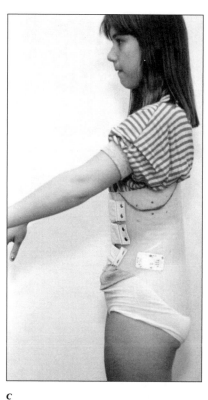

a b c

Figure 7.10 (a) The Boston brace is a plastic anterior-opening orthosis that may be useful in the treatment of back problems in dancers. (b) The brace can be constructed with a mild amount (15°) of lordosis to minimize stresses on the discs, as in the treatment of disc herniation. (c) Alternatively, the anti-lordotic (0° lordosis) version is used to treat posterior element conditions such as spondylolysis or facet arthrosis.

Such a treatment regimen may result in bony and radiographic healing of the pars stress fracture (Steiner and Micheli 1985). However, failure to heal radiographically does not preclude return to dance activity. In this situation, fibrous healing may have occurred, or the symptoms may have been due to mechanical back pain or strain with a coincident old spondylolysis. Frequently, avoiding painful technique and instituting the anti-lordotic rehabilitation program without bracing may eliminate pain and allow return to full dance activity. Spinal fusion is only rarely required for treatment of painful spondylolysis that interferes with dance activity despite bracing and exercises (Micheli 1983).

The older dancer with intermittent episodes of low back pain associated with spondylolysis may be helped by a short period of full-time bracing, followed by part-time use of the brace, thus enabling dance activity to be continued. Healing of the spondylolytic defect is not expected in this instance, but use of the brace appears to speed clinical recovery.

Injury to the lumbar pedicle is rare in the dancer. Stress fracture of the pedicle, resulting from repetitive flexion and hyperextension of the lumbar spine, has been reported in only one dancer (Ireland and Micheli 1987). Occasionally, stress fracture of the pars is associated with reactive hypertrophy of the contralateral pedicle and lamina, which may be difficult to differentiate from benign bone conditions such as osteoid osteoma (Sherman, Wilkinson, and Hall 1977).

Scoliosis

Scoliosis is a spinal deformity that consists of a structural curvature of the spine sideways, with an associated rotational deformity of the vertebrae (figure 7.11). The curvature of scoliosis is usually associated with a flexible compensatory curve in the opposite direction (figure 7.11) in order to maintain trunk balance. The rotational component is manifested by the characteristic unilateral thoracic rib hump or

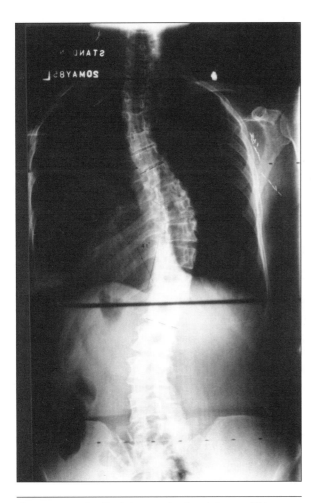

Figure 7.11 Scoliosis in a professional dancer. This curve (41°) is balanced, with the head, shoulders, and torso centered over the pelvis. It has not interfered with her 30-year career of modern dance performance, choreography, and teaching.

lumbar asymmetry observed when the affected individual bends forward to touch the floor.

Scoliosis is significantly more common in dancers than in the general population (Warren et al. 1986). Most commonly this is the adolescent idiopathic type, which may progress from a small to a large curve during growth. This may be a result of a relative decrease in rate of bone growth on the concavity of the curve because of the greater pressure on the growth cartilage on this side of the spine. Adolescent idiopathic scoliosis occurs in up to 10% to 16% of the general population (Brooks et al. 1975; Bunnell 1988; Edmonson 1987). In most cases specific treatment is not required other than observation until growth is completed, after which progression of curve

magnitude is unlikely for small curves. Above the age of 10 to 11 years, scoliosis is more common in females (Edmonson 1987) and risk of progression is greater prior to menarche (Bunnell 1988). The higher prevalence of scoliosis in ballet dancers (24%) has been attributed to hypoestrogenism secondary to delayed menarche and prolonged intervals of amenorrhea (Warren et al. 1986).

Screening children for scoliosis, which can be accomplished by a school nurse, physical education teacher, or dance instructor, can lead to early detection and nonoperative treatment of mild curves that may otherwise progress in severity and require spinal fusion (Renshaw 1988). In the screening examination, the child is observed as he or she bends forward to 90° at the hips with the knees straight, arms dangling, and the feet and hands together. An asymmetric prominence of one side of the thoracic or lumbar region compared with the other side, resulting from vertebral rotation, is an early sign of scoliosis (Renshaw 1988). In the upright standing position, asymmetry of shoulder height or scapular prominence, unequal arm height, pelvic obliquity, unequal waistline, and lower limb length inequality should be noted and are indications for orthopedic referral (Renshaw 1988).

The most accurate determination of magnitude of scoliosis is from a standing radiograph of the spine (figure 7.11). Individuals with small curves (less than 20°) who do not show signs of radiographic progression are followed until growth is completed. If progression by 10° to 15° does occur, or if the curve is larger than 20°, then a plastic brace, similar to that used for spondylolysis, may prevent further progression. The brace may be removed for dance activities, and is worn the rest of the day and night (Micheli and Marotta 1989). We do not use electrical stimulation or exercise alone for progressive scoliosis. If the severity of the curve progresses despite bracing or if it is greater than 40°, spinal fusion may be required.

A well-balanced curve, even if large, does not necessarily preclude a successful dance career (figure 7.11). Problems such as diminished pulmonary function, back pain, neurological compromise, or loss of self-esteem, which may occur with very large curves, are not generally observed with curves of up to 40° to 50° (Winter 1987). Therefore, low back pain in the dancer should not be attributed to scoliosis and a thorough investigation of other potential causes should be performed.

Facet Arthrosis

The repetitive lumbar hyperextension in dance technique places enormous stresses on the facet joints as well as the pars. After many years of dance these stresses may result in degenerative changes of the facet joints characteristic of osteoarthritis, including erosion of the cartilage surface of the facets and secondary joint space narrowing and irregularity, with osteophyte formation ("bone spurs") at the edges of the joints.

Although the degenerative changes of facet arthrosis may develop over many months or years, the symptoms can appear in a relatively short period of time. During a vigorous schedule, a fracture of an osteophyte at the edge of the facet, or of the facet itself, may occur with hyperextension of the lumbar spine in attitude or arabesque. The pain may be localized to the low back on the side of the lumbar facet involved, or may radiate down the lower extremity because of irritation of the nerve root adjacent to the facet. The pain may be exacerbated by lateral bending toward the involved side, or by hyperextension of the lumbar spine during standing on the ipsilateral lower extremity.

Radiographs may reveal irregularity of the facet joint, and a bone scan may show an area of increased activity if a fracture has occurred (figure 7.12a and b). A computed tomography (CT) scan may demonstrate the facet joint irregularity in better detail (figure 7.12c).

Initial treatment consists of rest, anti-inflammatory medication, and anti-lordotic exercises. If the pain continues, immobilization of the facet joint with an anti-lordotic brace (figure 7.10c) may encourage healing of the injury. In rare instances, surgical exploration of the facet joint and excision of the osteophyte may be considered if nonoperative treatment fails. As a last resort, limited spinal fusion may provide relief.

The dancer with this condition usually has been performing for many years and is often among the older members of the company. Depending on the severity of the pain, he or she may be faced with the difficult decision of whether to dance in pain, undergo surgery that may yield limited improvement, accept technical limitations secondary to the arthrosis, or retire from professional performance.

Disc Herniation

Discogenic back pain may result from inflammation of a disc, disc protrusion, or frank disc herniation or rupture ("slipped disc"). These problems are more common in male than in female dancers because of the stresses imposed by lifting. Forward flexion of the lumbar spine results in a major increase in the load on the lumbar discs compared with that during neutral

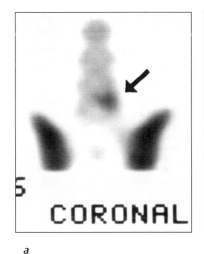
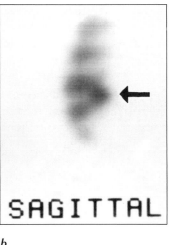
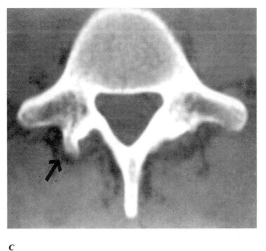

a   b   c

Figure 7.12 Facet arthrosis in a 36-year-old professional ballet dancer. Bone scans *(a* and *b)* showed increased activity of the posterior elements of the left L4-5 region. A computed tomography (CT) scan *(c)* demonstrated left L4-5 facet arthrosis, with osteophyte ("bone spur") and fracture of the inferior L4 facet.

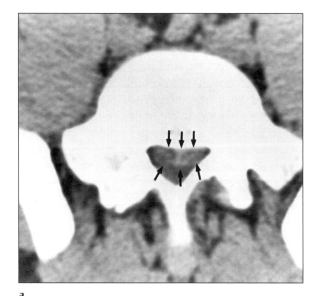

a

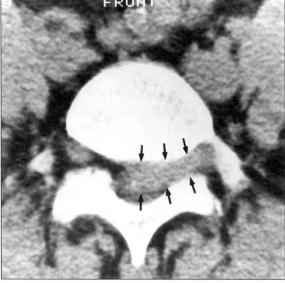

b

Figure 7.13 *(a)* A computed tomography (CT) scan demonstrating disc herniation at L5-S1 (arrows). *(b)* CT scan of a large central and lateral L5-S1 disc herniation (arrows), with compression of the dural sac and left S1 nerve root.

(Andersson, Ortengren, and Nachemson 1976). Lifting with hyperlordosis of the lumbar spine may place extensive stress on the discs and cause herniation (figure 7.8*a*).

With herniation, the pulpy disc center (nucleus) extrudes through a tear in the fibrous annulus and causes pain because of pressure on the neural elements of the spine (figures 7.4 and 7.13*a*). If the herniation is in the midline, the extruded nucleus presses on the central neural sac, and the pain is felt in the low back; if the nucleus herniates more laterally, it may press on the nerve roots that run to the lower extremity on that side and pain may radiate down this extremity (figures 7.4, 7.13*b*).

Discogenic back pain is exacerbated by forward bending, sitting, coughing, sneezing, or straining, because these activities increase disc pressure. In addition to pain, disc herniation may result in numbness or paresthesia ("pins and needles") radiating down the lower extremities as a result of pressure on specific nerve roots. Passively flexing the hip with the knee extended may cause pain and spasm because of stretch on an irritated nerve root. A detailed neurological examination is important because pressure on the nerve roots may result in muscle weakness or loss of a reflex. Sometimes, though rarely, pressure on the nerves to the bladder or bowel may result in incontinence, which requires emergency attention.

Most disc herniations resolve over several weeks or months, possibly because the extruded nucleus fragment shrinks as its water content is resorbed. Therefore, treatment usually consists of rest, analgesics, anti-inflammatory medication, and muscle relaxants, followed by a progressive anti-lordotic strengthening and flexibility rehabilitation program. A plastic brace or corset (figure 7.10, *a-c*) in conjunction with the exercise program may immobilize the lumbar spine, prevent further lordosis, and improve comfort during the first four to six months after injury (Micheli 1985b). The dancer may be able to continue limited dance classes, perform character roles, and maintain fitness with swimming and gentle, directed exercises.

Every attempt is made to manage disc herniation nonoperatively. Surgical excision of a herniated disc is indicated if bowel or bladder symptoms or signs are present. If pain and spasm are severe, and are associated with specific neurological loss such as muscle weakness or loss of

upright stance, and this load is further increased when a weight is held in the arms or when the flexed spine is rotated (Nachemson 1966, 1981). This may be exacerbated by the presence or accentuation of lumbar hyperlordosis. Poor lifting technique, with outstretched arms away from the body, may increase disc pressure and hence disc-related pain, or even result in herniation a reflex, disc excision can be considered if there is no improvement with nonoperative treatment. However, the dancer may not be able to perform for a full year following discectomy, and extensive rehabilitation is required. Further professional dancing may not be possible, depending on the extent of recovery.

Mechanical Low Back Pain

Mechanical low back pain is a syndrome in which localized aching low back pain is exacerbated by motion, turns, lifts, or prolonged standing or sitting but no definite anatomic cause can be defined. The dancer with mechanical low back pain usually has lumbar hyperlordosis; and the pain may be a reflection of facet joint stress, muscular strain, or ligament sprain secondary to the lordotic posture. The pain may be reproduced by motion of the lumbar spine, possibly in more than one direction. The hamstrings and lumbodorsal fascia may be tight, but neurological examination is normal. The diagnosis of mechanical low back pain can be made only after other specific causes of low back pain, such as spondylolysis, disc herniation, infection, or tumor, have been excluded by appropriate studies such as radiography, bone scans, and CT scans (Micheli 1979; Micheli, Hall, and Miller 1980).

Management of mechanical low back pain begins with attention to technical errors that contribute to hyperlordosis. A directed anti-lordotic rehabilitation program may result in improvement of pain and hyperlordosis. In cases refractory to an exercise program alone, anti-lordotic bracing has been helpful in accelerating pain relief and improving a tight hyperlordosis (Micheli, Hall, and Miller 1980). When used for mechanical back pain, the brace is worn full-time initially except during dance activity, and pain is often relieved after 6 to 12 weeks of bracing. The dancer is then tapered from the brace over the next three to four months, with emphasis on the exercise program throughout the entire period of bracing. Recurrence rate after bracing is low if anti-lordotic strengthening and flexibility are maintained.

Sciatica

The term sciatica does not refer to a specific diagnosis, but rather to the symptom of pain along the course of the sciatic nerve, the largest peripheral nerve in the body. The pain of sciatica may radiate from the back to the buttock and down the posterior aspect of the lower extremity.

Any condition that causes mechanical or inflammatory irritation of the nerve roots that join to form the sciatic nerve, or of the sciatic nerve itself, may cause sciatic pain. The possible causes of sciatica are manifold, including disc herniation, facet arthrosis, low back strain, spondylolisthesis, or pressure on the nerve by muscles at the back of the hip (piriformis syndrome). The treatment of these problems may differ. Therefore, it is important to define the etiology of the pain, rather than to simply attribute the pain to "sciatica."

Upper Back Injuries

Upper back and periscapular injuries in dancers usually consist of muscle strains or ligament sprains. They may occur during lifting of a partner, as a result of weakness or being off balance. Periscapular strains can result from repetitive elevation and rotation of the upper arm.

First aid includes ice massage or cold spray, which may enable completion of a performance. Massage may minimize muscle spasm and stiffness. Physical therapeutic modalities, including ice, heat, ultrasound, massage, and electrical stimulation, may accelerate recovery. Anti-inflammatory medications can be useful. A strengthening and flexibility exercise program may promote healing and prevent recurrence.

Injury to the bony elements and discs of the thoracic spine is unusual in the dancer. The most common problem of the thoracic vertebrae in the adolescent is a variant of Scheuermann's disease, or dorsal kyphosis ("roundback") deformity. This condition is caused by increased stress on the vertebral bodies of the thoracic spine, leading to stress fracture and wedging. Contributing factors include repetitive flexion of the thoracic spine, loss of flexibility associated with the growth spurt, and increased lumbar lordosis with compensatory thoracic kyphosis. Dorsal back pain may be present, and there is usually a tight lumbar hyperlordosis and tightness of the hamstrings. Treatment consists of dorsal extension and lumbar anti-lordotic strengthening and flexibility exercises, hamstring stretching, and, occasionally, bracing for 9 to 12 months (Micheli 1979; Micheli, Hall, and Miller 1980).

Neck Injuries

Injury to the neck and cervical spine is less common in the dancer than lumbar spine injuries. Cervical spondylolysis, brachial plexus injury, and thoracic outlet syndrome in the dancer are considered elsewhere (Nixon 1983).

Rehabilitation of the Injured Back in the Dancer

The goals of rehabilitation include return to pain-free performance and prevention of recurrent injury (Walaszek 1982). Rehabilitation begins with an accurate diagnosis of the injury and any anatomic malalignment. Specific exercise programs for different injuries, as noted earlier, are planned and modified as pain and spasm improve. The dancer's awareness of body mechanics and alignment facilitates the rehabilitation process.

In addition to rest, directed exercises, and bracing for the specific injury, it is important to prescribe a program to maintain cardiovascular and musculoskeletal fitness. Swimming is particularly useful because it minimizes stresses of gravity on the injured spine and provides water resistance for strengthening. Floor work is also useful because gravitational stresses can be minimized and dance exercises maintain interest (Solomon 1988). Progression to chair exercises (Dowd 1984) and barre work may be modified to minimize stresses on the back and preserve good technique.

The contribution of lumbar hyperlordosis to many injuries was noted previously. The mainstay of rehabilitation for this postural malalignment is a program of abdominal muscle and psoas strengthening, including gentle sit-ups, pelvic tilts, and flexibility exercises for the low back and hamstrings. Attention to concentric, eccentric, and isometric exercises may be important. Postural awareness in daily life, in and out of the classroom, is emphasized throughout rehabilitation. Vocalization is particularly useful as a means of monitoring effort and tension in movement (Solomon 1988). Breathing and relaxation techniques may be useful in rehabilitation and may help improve lumbar expansion and awareness (Walaszek 1982).

For exercises to strengthen the abdominal muscles and psoas and increase flexibility in the low back and hamstrings, see chapter 9, figures 9.8 through 9.20 on pages 118 to 127.

Therapeutic modalities such as ice, heat, ultrasound, and massage, may be useful in decreasing spasm and pain and improving passive stretch and relaxation. Postural mechanics may be improved with techniques such as those based on the work of Alexander (Jones 1979) and Feldenkrais (Feldenkrais 1972a, 1972b; Galeota-Wozny 2002). Sleeping posture with the low back maximally flexed may allow a passive anti-lordotic stretch, whereas prone positions should be discouraged because they may exacerbate tight lumbar lordosis.

The upper back muscles can be strengthened with directed weight training. This will improve upper extremity control during lifting of a partner.

An excellent upper back and shoulder strengthening program can be found in Micheli, *The Sports Medicine Bible* (p. 225).

For the purposes of rehabilitation, the standard elements of a dance class can be thought of as separate units. The importance of warm-up should be emphasized, and the dancer with back problems can progress from barre to center work as recovery proceeds.

If surgery has been necessary, the return to dance participation is individualized. Successful resumption of training and performance will depend on the nature of the injury, type of surgery, level of the spine involved, extent of spinal fusion if any, and the potential for subsequent instability or neurological injury (Micheli 1985a).

Conclusion

It is a common theme throughout this book that the prevention of dance injuries is based in an understanding of what injuries are likely to occur, and how they make their presence known.

All of the injuries discussed in this chapter, with the exception of scoliosis (which is not properly an injury, but rather a pathological condition), are of the overuse variety. That is, they develop over time as a result of repetitive stresses on the spine that it is incapable of absorbing. Hence, their symptoms tend to develop gradually. This provides an opportunity for knowledgeable and vigilant dancers, teachers, choreographers, and others to interdict their development by altering or discontinuing those dance activities that are causing problems. As spinal injuries can be especially debilitating if allowed to become full-blown, often requiring long periods of rest and rehabilitation, it obviously behooves the dance community to learn as much about them as possible.

References

Andersson, G.B.J., R. Ortengren, and A. Nachemson. 1976. Quantitative studies of back loads in lifting. *Spine* 1: 178-185.

Bachrach, R.M. 1987. Dance injuries of the low back. *Kinesiology for Dance* 9(3): 4-8.

Brooks, H.L., S.P. Azen, E. Gerberg, R. Brooks, and L. Chan. 1975. Scoliosis: A prospective epidemiological study. *Journal of Bone and Joint Surgery* 57-A(7): 968-972.

Bunnell, W.P. 1988. The natural history of idiopathic scoliosis. *Clinical Orthopaedics and Related Research* 229: 20-25.

Dowd, I. 1984. Technique and training: How to arch your back. *Dance Magazine* 58(4): 118-119.

Edmonson, A.S. 1987. Scoliosis. In *Campbell operative orthopaedics* (Vol. 4). 7th ed., edited by A.H. Crenshaw. St. Louis: Mosby, 3167-3236.

Feldenkrais, M. 1972a. *Awareness through movement.* Harper & Row.

Feldenkrais, M. 1972b. *Body and mature behavior.* Harper & Row.

Francis, L.L., P.R. Francis, and K. Welshons-Smith. 1985. Aerobic dance injuries: A survey of instructors. *Physician and Sportsmedicine* 13(2): 105-111.

Fredrickson, B.E., D. Baker, W.J. McHolick, H.A. Yuan, and J.P. Lubicky. 1984. The natural history of spondylolysis and spondylolisthesis. *Journal of Bone and Joint Surgery* 66-A(5): 699-707.

Galeota-Wozny, N. 2002. "Ouch"—dancers find a path out of pain with the Feldenkrais Method. *Dance Magazine* 76(11): 37, 70.

Garrick, J.G., D.M. Gillien, and P. Whiteside. 1986. The epidemiology of aerobic dance injuries. *American Journal of Sports Medicine* 14(1): 67-72.

Gelabert, R. 1986. Dancers spinal syndromes. *Journal of Orthopaedic and Sports Physical Therapy* 7(4): 180-191.

Gieck, J.H., and E.N. Saliba. 1987. Application of modalities in overuse syndromes. *Clinics in Sports Medicine* 6(2): 427-466.

Gurewitsch, A.D., and M.A. O'Neill. 1944. Flexibility of healthy children. *Archives of Physical Therapy* 25: 216-221.

Howse, J., and S. Hancock. 1988. *Dance technique and injury prevention.* New York: Theatre Arts Books/Routledge.

Hunter-Griffin, L.Y., ed. 1987. Overuse injuries. *Clinics in Sports Medicine* 6: 225-470.

Ireland, M.L., and L.J. Micheli. 1987. Bilateral stress fracture of the lumbar pedicles in a ballet dancer: A case report. *Journal of Bone and Joint Surgery* 69-A(1): 140-142.

Jackson, D.W., L.L. Wiltse, R.D. Dingeman, and M. Hayes. 1981. Stress reactions involving the pars interarticularis in young athletes. *American Journal of Sports Medicine* 9(5): 304-312.

Jones, F.P. 1979. *Body awareness in action: A study of the Alexander Technique.* Revised. New York: Schocken.

McKibbin, B. 1968. The action of the iliopsoas muscle in the newborn. *Journal of Bone and Joint Surgery* 50-B(1): 161-165.

Michele, A.A. 1960. The iliopsoas muscle: Its importance in disorders of the hip and spine. *CIBA Clinical Symposia* 12(3): 66-101.

Michele, A.A. 1962. *Iliopsoas: Development of anomalies in man.* Springfield, IL: Charles C Thomas.

Micheli, L.J. 1979. Low back pain in the adolescent: Differential diagnosis. *American Journal of Sports Medicine* 7(6): 362-364.

Micheli, L.J. 1983. Back injuries in dancers. *Clinics in Sports Medicine* 2(3): 473-484.

Micheli, L.J. 1985a. Sports following spinal surgery in the young athlete. *Clinical Orthopaedics and Related Research* 198: 152-157.

Micheli, L.J. 1985b. The use of the modified Boston brace system (B.O.B.) for back pain: Clinical indications. *Orthotics and Prosthetics* 39: 41-46.

Micheli, L.J. 1987. The traction apophysites. *Clinics in Sports Medicine* 6(2): 389-404.

Micheli, L.J. 1995. *The sports medicine bible.* New York: HarperPerennial.

Micheli, L.J., J.E. Hall, and M.E. Miller. 1980. Use of modified Boston brace for back injuries in athletes. *American Journal of Sports Medicine* 8(5): 351-356.

Micheli, L.J., and J.J. Marotta. 1989. Scoliosis and sports. *Your Patient and Fitness* 2: 5-11.

Micheli, L.J., and R. Solomon. 1987. Training the young dancer. In *Dance medicine: A comprehensive guide,* edited by A.J. Ryan and R.E. Stephens. Chicago and Minneapolis: Pluribus Press/Physician and Sportsmedicine, 51-72.

Minkoff, J., and O.H. Sherman. 1987. Considerations pursuant to the rehabilitation of the anterior cruciate injured knee. *Exercise and Sports Science Reviews* 15: 297-349.

Nachemson, A. 1966. The load on lumbar disks in different positions of the body. *Clinical Orthopaedics and Related Research* 45: 107-122.

Nachemson, A. 1968. The possible importance of the psoas muscle for stabilization of the lumbar spine. *Acta Orthopaedica Scandinavica* 39(1): 47-57.

Nachemson, A.L. 1981. Disc pressure measurements. *Spine* 6(1): 93-97.

Nixon, J.E. 1983. Injuries to the neck and upper extremities of dancers. *Clinics in Sports Medicine* 2(3): 459-472.

Pizzutillo, P.D. 1985. Spondylolisthesis: Etiology and natural history. In *The pediatric spine*, edited by D.S. Bradford and R.M. Hensinger. New York: Thieme, 395-402.

Ranney, D.A. 1979. The functional integration of trunk muscles and the psoas. *Kinesiology for Dance* 9: 10-12.

Renshaw, T.S. 1988. Screening school children for scoliosis. *Clinical Orthopaedics and Related Research* 229: 26-33.

Rovere, G.D., L.X. Webb, A.G. Gristina, and J.M. Vogel. 1983. Musculoskeletal injuries in theatrical dance students. *American Journal of Sports Medicine* 11(4): 195-198.

Ryman, R. 1979a. Training the dancer VIII: The spine. *Dance in Canada* 20: 19-22.

Ryman, R. 1979b. Training the dancer IX: The spine in motion. *Dance in Canada* 21: 14-18.

Seals, J.G. 1983. A study of dance surfaces. *Clinics in Sports Medicine* 2(3): 557-561.

Sherman, F.C., R.H. Wilkinson, and J.E. Hall. 1977. Reactive sclerosis of a pedicle and spondylolysis in the lumbar spine. *Journal of Bone and Joint Surgery* 59-A(1): 49-54.

Solomon, R. 1988. *Anatomy as a master image in training dancers* (videorecording). Santa Cruz, CA: 1 videocassette; 59 minutes; color; 1/2 inch, VHS or Beta; 3/4 inch, U-matic. (Available from Princeton Books, Pennington, NJ.)

Solomon, R., E. Trepman, and L.J. Micheli. 1989. Foot morphology and injury patterns in ballet and modern dancers. *Kinesiology and Medicine for Dance* 12(1): 20-40.

Stanish, W. 1987. Low back pain in athletes: An overuse syndrome. *Clinics in Sports Medicine* 6(2): 321-344.

Steiner, M.E., and L.J. Micheli. 1985. Treatment of symptomatic spondylolysis and spondylolisthesis with the modified Boston brace. *Spine* 10(10): 937-943.

Trepman, E., and L.J. Micheli. 1988. Overuse injuries in sports. *Seminars in Orthopaedics* 3(4): 217-222.

Walaszek, A. 1982. Physical therapy rehabilitation for dance injuries. In *Sports medicine, sports science: Bridging the gap*, edited by R.C. Cantu and W.J. Gillespie. Lexington, MA: Collamore Press, 151-159.

Warren, M.P., J. Brooks-Gunn, L.H. Hamilton, L.F. Warren, and W.G. Hamilton. 1986. Scoliosis and fractures in young ballet dancers: Relation to delayed menarche and secondary amenorrhea. *New England Journal of Medicine* 314(21): 1348-1353.

Washington, E.L. 1978. Musculoskeletal injuries in theatrical dancers: Site, frequency and severity. *American Journal of Sports Medicine* 6(2): 75-98.

White, A.A., and M.M. Panjabi. 1978. *Clinical biomechanics of the spine.* Philadelphia: Lippincott.

Williams, P.L., and R. Warwick, eds. 1980. *Gray's anatomy.* 36th ed. Philadelphia: Saunders.

Winter, R.B. 1987. Natural history of spinal deformity. In *Moe's textbook of scoliosis and other spinal deformities.* 2nd ed., edited by D.S. Bradford, J.E. Lonstein, J.H. Moe, J.W. Ogilvie, and R.B. Winter. Philadelphia: Saunders, 89-95.

Recommended Readings (Editors)

Fehlandt, A.F., and L.J. Micheli. 1993. Lumbar facet stress fracture in a ballet dancer. *Spine* 18(16): 2537-2539.

Gerbino, P.G., and L.J. Micheli. 1995. Back injuries in the young athlete. *Clinics in Sports Medicine* 14(3): 571-589.

Hall, H., and J. Piccinin. 1996. Dance. In *The spine in sports*, edited by R.G. Watkins. St. Louis: Mosby, 465-474.

McMeeken, J., E. Tully, C. Natrass, and B. Stillman. 2002. The effect of spinal and pelvic posture and mobility on back pain in young dancers and non-dancers. *Journal of Dance Medicine & Science* 6(3): 79-86.

Micheli, L.J., and L. Backe. 1999. Low-back injuries in young athletes. *Sport and Medicine Today* 2(1): 48-52.

Micheli, L.J., R. Solomon, and P.G. Gerbino. 1998. Ballet and dance. In *Sports neurology: Second edition*, edited by B.D. Jordan, P. Tsairis, and R.F. Warren. Philadelphia: Lippincott-Raven, 331-349.

Micheli, L.J., R. Solomon, J. Solomon, and P.G. Gerbino. 1999. Low back pain in dancers. *Medscape Orthopaedics and Sports Medicine* 3(5). [Available at www.medscape.com/viewarticle/408509]

Chapter 8

Stress Fractures in Dancers

Lyle J. Micheli, MD; Ruth Solomon, Professor Emerita

Stress fractures are so prevalent and debilitating in dancers as to justify a chapter devoted exclusively to them. While this type of injury is primarily associated with the tibia, as illustrated here with the aid of case studies, a number of other sites are also vulnerable. The risk factors that can give rise to stress fractures which have been introduced in chapter 7, pages 86-87, are discussed in greater detail.

Etiology and Diagnosis

Doctors who have incorporated dance medicine into their practice and research know that most injuries to dancers result from repetitive microtrauma and are therefore properly classified as overuse injury. The endless repetition of prescribed movements that is so basic to the discipline makes the dancer's body particularly susceptible to these injuries. There are often additional etiologic factors that contribute to the overuse injury in each dancer's case, but repetitive movement is always present.

Overuse injuries may affect different tissues, including bone, articular cartilage lining the joints, tendons, and ligaments. A stress fracture (also known as"fatigue" or "insufficiency" fracture) is the overuse injury of bone. Like an acute fracture, it involves an interruption of the continuity and structure of a bone, but it presents in different ways. When someone falls on an outstretched arm or receives a severe impact to the leg and has a frank, acute fracture of the arm bones or leg bones, there is usually pain, swelling, and obvious deformity at the site of injury. With stress fracture, however, the onset is often insidious. The fracture may present as simply a low-grade aching that is activity related. With continuation of activity the hairline crack in the bone, which is what the stress fracture is, may deepen or promulgate into additional small

Terms Describing Anatomical Location in Chapter 8

distal	away from the origin or point of attachment
dorsal	referring to the top side of a structure
lateral	farther away from the midline of the body
proximal	close to or nearest the origin or point of attachment
varus	bent or turned inward toward the midline

cracks in the same bone, resulting in more pain. Throughout this process the body is attempting to heal the stress fracture site, but is unsuccessful. A repetitive cycle of microfracture—partial healing—microfracture—partial healing, and so on, is established. Rarely, the stress fracture may suddenly develop into a frank fracture through the bone following a particular dance movement, as in one of our cases reported in this chapter. More typically the pain persists and worsens until the activity that has caused the injury becomes almost impossible. It is usually at this point that medical assistance is sought.

Diagnosis of stress fracture is seldom a simple matter. Ailments that do not involve bones per se—tendinitis, bursitis, strains, sprains, and tumors—can produce the same symptoms and need to be ruled out. In the lower leg, the most common site of stress fractures, shinsplints, a frequent precursor of stress fracture, can be confused with the real thing. A qualified medical person who has access to imaging technologies must be consulted. Specialized techniques like tomography or bone scans may allow early diagnosis before plain X rays demonstrate a problem. The earlier the diagnosis is made the sooner corrective action can be initiated, lessening the period of disability.

History

Not only dancers but anyone regularly involved in repetitive activities is at increased risk for stress fractures. The first published report of this injury type was by a German military physician named Briethaupt in 1855. He discovered a high incidence of what came to be called "march fractures" in Prussian Army soldiers experiencing painful feet after long marches. Subsequent publications have continued to associate stress fractures with military training systems. In 1975 Dr. Angus McBryde reviewed the current literature on stress fractures. "In the military," McBryde observed, "the inciting activity is standard for that particular service or installation, causing a group injury and permitting a group diagnosis. The military experience has been, by far, the primary contributor in the understanding of stress fractures" (p. 213). That is, because the military tends to subject groups of men and women to standardized physical regimens for which they have had no prior training, the physiological reactions of those groups—for example, a predisposition to stress fractures of the feet after sustained marching—provide a particularly pure measure of the effects of physical activity on the body. McBryde noted similarities between the military and typical sport training as regards susceptibility to stress fracture.

A review of sport-related stress fractures was done by Dr. Carl Stanitski (1978). "Interestingly," Stanitski observes, "in only three animals have stress fractures been documented: thoroughbred racing horses, racing greyhounds and man. These all have been systematically trained to produce maximum performance with certain types of repetitive physical exertion. Sufficient time is often not allowed for the normal reparative processes of bone to withstand the relentless forces demanded by the athlete" (p. 394). Stanitski uses case studies of subjects involved in various sport activities to speculate on the nature of stress fractures. Ultimately he theorizes that "It is the rhythmic repetitive muscle action [required in the practice of most sports] that causes subthreshold mechanical insults that summate beyond the stress-bearing capacity of the bone" (p. 394).

Risk Factors

Sports that involve running, jumping, or repetitive throwing have been particularly indicted. Our own early work on stress fractures encompassed several sports, but focused on running. In a review of stress fractures of the lower extremities in runners, we found them in every major bone of the lower extremity. We presented a checklist (table 8.1) that we believe represents risk factor categories to be considered in analyzing the etiology of these injuries (Micheli et al. 1980). In every stress fracture site studied, training error was the most frequently associated etiology, followed by muscle—tendon imbalance and so on down the list to those factors that are rarer or more difficult to assess. (For more detailed information regarding these risk factors the reader may wish to consult the Micheli et al. 1980 article.)

This list points to a close correlation between the causes of stress fractures in runners and in dancers. Not only do these two groups experience many of the same injuries in much the same ratio to the number of participants in the activity studied (dancers seem to have a slightly higher percentage of stress fractures than runners), but the mechanics that at least in part precipitate the injury are similar (Barrow and Saha 1988; Warren et al. 1986). Simply put, if you train and perform regularly in an activity that requires your lower extremities to repetitively exchange energy with a hard surface for prolonged periods of time, you are a prime candidate for stress fractures.

Since we made our original list, other probable risk factors have come to our attention:

- Dance technique training
- Gender
- Nutrition

In our study of injuries in modern dancers we found differences in the techniques studied to be of significance (Solomon and Micheli 1986). Modern dance encompasses many techniques, each of which makes unique demands on the dancer's body, thereby creating its own stress patterns. More recently, authors in this field have suggested additional factors that have to do with nutrition and gender. In female dancers and athletes a correlation between menstrual irregularities and bone disorders has been observed. Dr. Michelle Warren, for example, suggests that the very high incidence of fractures in the group of young ballet dancers she studied (46 fractures in 75 dancers, or 61%) may be related to hypoestrogenism as reflected in delayed menarche and prolonged amenorrhea (Warren et al. 1986). Similarly, a study of female

Table 8.1 Factors to Check in Overuse Syndrome

Training errors	Muscle-tendon imbalance	Anatomical malalignment of the lower extremities	Footwear	Running surface	Associated disease state of the lower extremity
Abrupt changes in intensity, duration, or frequency of training	Strength, flexibility, or bulk	Femoral anteversion	Improper fit	Concrete pavement	Osteoarthritis
		Patella alta or lateral alignment	Inadequate impact-absorbing material	Asphalt	Neuromuscular disease
		Genu valgum	Excessive stiffness of sole	Running track	Vascular insufficiency
		Tibia vara	Insufficient support of hindfoot	Dirt or grass	Old fracture
		Pes planus			
		Cavo varus			

distance runners reported in *The American Journal of Sports Medicine* indicates that "female distance runners who have a history of irregular or absent menses and who have never used oral contraceptives [i.e., artificially altered their estrogen balance] may be at an increased risk for developing a stress fracture" (Barrow and Saha 1988, p. 209). Both articles go on to draw eating disorders into an equation that might be expressed as follows: Extreme concern with physical fitness (and, perhaps, with body image) yields exercise and eating patterns that produce hypoestrogenism (and resulting menstrual irregularities), which in turn contributes to bone disorders such as stress fractures. This syndrome has subsequently been defined by the American College of Sports Medicine as the "female athlete triad. "

> The female athlete triad is discussed in detail in chapter 17.

These considerations in explaining the etiology of stress fractures can be assimilated to produce a more complete picture. To remain healthy, bones require certain nutrients that result from proper food intake and the maintenance of normal hormone balances. If bones are not receiving these nutrients—as a result of such classic eating disorders as anorexia nervosa or bulimia, or excessive dieting, or the loss of appetite that can accompany heavy physical training—they lose their normal ability to "remodel," or rebuild themselves, and are prone to injury. This condition can produce what we sometimes call (when we split stress fractures into subgroups) insufficiency fractures. If at the same time these bones are being asked to do hard, repetitive work, they may develop fatigue fractures.

Treatment

The dancer who develops a stress fracture must anticipate a fairly substantial period of time away from dancing. When a stress fracture is recognized early and diagnosed properly we normally treat it with "relative rest," by which we mean a period of approximately three weeks during which dancing is discontinued and replaced with such nonimpact activities as swimming, cycling, or floor work. Whatever alternate activity is used, it should not involve impacting on the already

fatigued site; inherent in the injury we call stress fracture is an attempt by the bone to restructure itself, and it can do this healing work only when the stress that has caused the injury is removed. Initially we may use crutches, a cane, casting, or pneumatic bracing (air cast) to augment the non-weight-bearing approach to treatment. It is important to keep the patient (dancer) functioning for both physical and psychological reasons, but unfortunately the dance activity that caused the stress fracture must be temporarily suspended.

Case Studies

We now turn to case studies from our practice that should help to exemplify the subject of stress fracture. The dancers reported in these cases are all professionals who were thoroughly involved in taking classes, rehearsing, and performing when their injuries materialized.

Case 1

A 24-year-old jazz dancer came in with persistent pain at the ball of her foot. This is a common complaint of dancers that does not necessarily raise the prospect of stress fracture; quite often it is diagnosed as a "bone bruise." In this case the X ray taken after her initial visit *did* give clear indication of stress fracture, although in an early stage, of one of the two small bones at the base of the first toe, the sesamoid bones (figure 8.1). We recommended no classes for four weeks, substituting careful stretching and strengthening

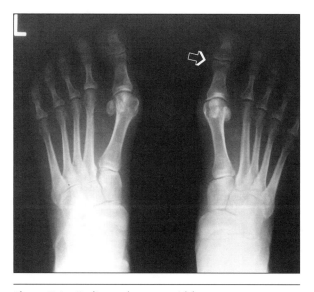

Figure 8.1 Radiograph: sesamoid fracture.

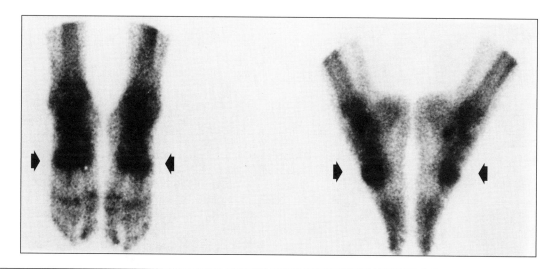

Figure 8.2   Bone scan: bilateral stress fracture second metatarsal.

exercises, and the use of a special rigid shoe insert. The injury healed. Other cases of this sort, when not treated promptly, have gone on to non-union fractures, which may then require surgical fusion or resection.

Case 2

This 29-year-old female ballet dancer presented with pain in the forefoot. She had a long history of stress fractures involving both fibulas and bilateral fractures of the first and third metatarsals. This proven predisposition increased our suspicion of stress fracture. X rays were inconclusive, showing only a cortical thickening of the second and third metatarsals; but a subsequent bone scan confirmed our diagnosis through increased uptake, or "hot spots" (unexpectedly in *both* feet), at the base of the metatarsals and adjacent tarsal bones, including the cuneiform bones (figure 8.2).

It should be noted that ballet dancers who perform on pointe are at high risk for another apparently unique stress fracture of the metatarsal bones. This involves the Lisfranc joint, at the proximal end of the second metatarsal (figure 8.3). In such cases pain usually occurs not in the forefoot, but in the middle portion of the foot, at or near the point where the second metatarsal articulates with all three cuneiforms. The mechanism of this injury is of particular interest: When the foot goes on pointe the proximal head of the second metatarsal essentially locks in place, becoming rigid in its socket and therefore

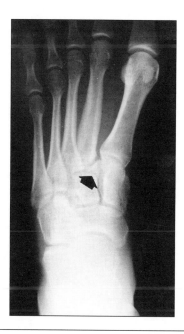

Figure 8.3   Radiograph: Lisfranc fracture proximal head of second metatarsal.

vulnerable to injury. This is not an easy injury to diagnose (it was not reported in the literature on dancers until our article of 1985), and, like the sesamoid stress fracture described earlier, it can easily develop into a non-union fracture.

Case 3

This 22-year-old male ballet dancer had been experiencing pain over the dorsum and lateral aspect of the foot for three to four weeks as

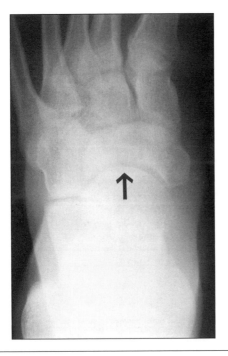

Figure 8.4 Radiograph: negative for navicular fracture.

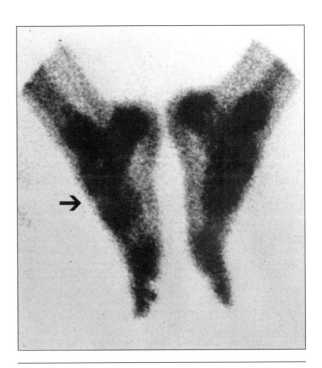

Figure 8.5 Bone scan: stress fracture of the navicular along with additional areas of increased uptake.

pressure was released from the foot, especially after plié. There was also significant tenderness over the navicular. His X ray was negative (figure 8.4), yet we remained suspicious of stress fracture and ordered both bone scan (figure 8.5) and computed tomography scan. These were positive, confirming the diagnosis. The dancer was placed in a short leg cast for four weeks, on crutches for two more weeks, and progressed to barre and center work over a one-month period.

Case 4

A 24-year-old female ballet dancer experienced generalized pain in her right foot during an intense run of *The Nutcracker*. Although the pain was persistent, she waited two months after the run had ended before seeking medical help. The X ray taken at her initial visit showed suspicious cortical thickening of her distal fibula, above the ankle (figure 8.6). A bone scan four days later confirmed increased uptake over the right fibular shaft (figure 8.7). Diagnosis of right fibular stress fracture was made and the patient was given an air cast and taken off all physical activity except swimming. Two and one-half weeks later she was allowed to do a gentle barre, and one week thereafter she resumed across-the-floor

work. However, pain over the fibula recurred. Four more weeks of total rest were prescribed, followed by a gradual, pain-free return to full dance work.

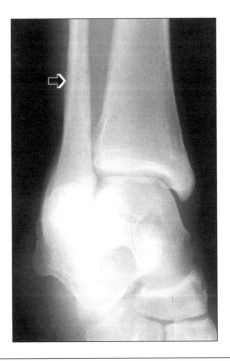

Figure 8.6 Radiograph: cortical thickening indicating fibular stress fracture.

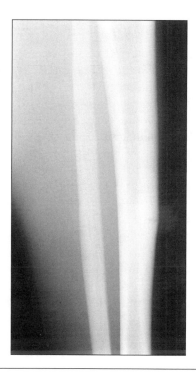

Figure 8.8   Radiograph: incomplete healing of tibial stress fracture.

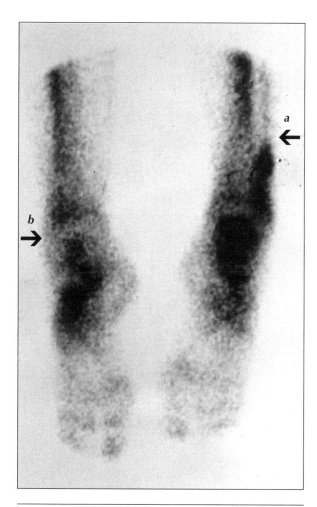

Figure 8.7   Bone scan: *(a)* confirmed stress fracture right fibular and *(b)* stress reaction over left tarsal bone.

Case 5

This 22-year-old female ballet dancer presented with pain suggestive of stress fracture in the tibia. X rays showed a clear but incomplete fracture, with a dense margin across the tibial cortex. She was removed from dancing and given electro-stimulation to encourage bone formation. Two months later there was little pain, swelling, or tenderness, and she was returned to partial dance activity. However, an X ray taken after another month showed incomplete healing, so she was not allowed to dance full out (figure 8.8). After six months there was still some pain in the area, and the X ray taken then indicated that whereas the original fracture was healed, the patient had at some point had bilateral stress fractures in the mid-third of the tibias (figure 8.9).

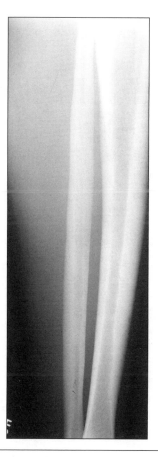

Figure 8.9   Radiograph: original tibial fracture healed, but X ray shows past stress fracture in mid-third of tibia.

Case 6

This is a case referred to in passing earlier. It involves fractures of the tibia and fibula in a male ballet dancer that occurred during a rehearsal from the sudden explosive force of jumping while in an extreme turned-out position. This was obviously a macrotrauma injury, but review of his X rays suggested multiple stress fracture sites of the tibia, doubtless of variable recurrences and duration. The spiral fracture of the midshaft of the left tibia was initially treated with closed reduction and placed in a long-leg cast. Over the next few weeks there was progressive loss of reduction (separation of the bone fragments) and an exacerbation of the varus position of the bones (figure 8.10). Hence, an open (surgical) reduction of the fracture was performed and fixation with stainless steel lag screws was accomplished. An X ray taken a month later shows the screws in place and sig-

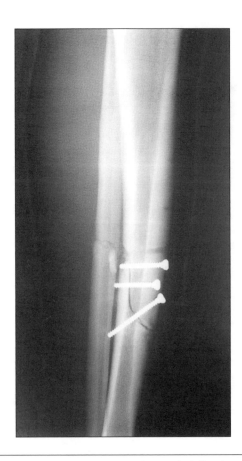

Figure 8.11 Postoperative radiograph following open reduction and internal fixation.

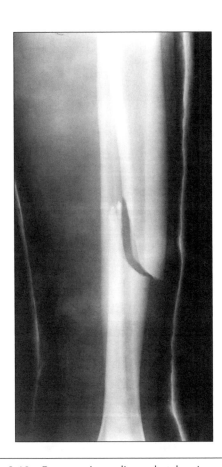

Figure 8.10 Preoperative radiograph: taken in cast, fracture showing loss of reduction and exacerbation of varus position.

nificant healing under way (figure 8.11). It goes without saying that this is an extreme example of what can happen if stress fractures are not attended to promptly.

Case 7

Finally, we turn to the case of a 35-year-old ballerina who, also during a run of *The Nutcracker*, was experiencing unrelenting pain in the area of the femur. An X ray taken at that time showed new bone formation (figure 8.12), and a bone scan supported the diagnosis of stress fracture of the femur. Three months later the pain persisted; there was a sense that the bone damage was not healing, and additional X rays confirmed this. The patient was taken off all dance activities and given a cane to limit weight bearing. Swimming was recommended and Pilates exercises were allowed. Two months later the pain was gone and she was able gradually to resume dancing.

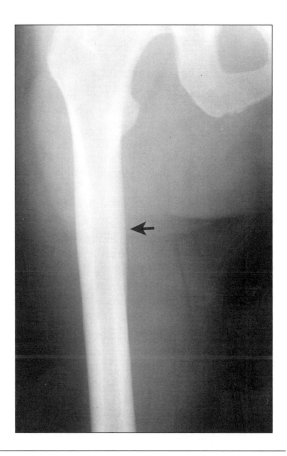

Figure 8.12 Radiograph: femur showing new bone formation.

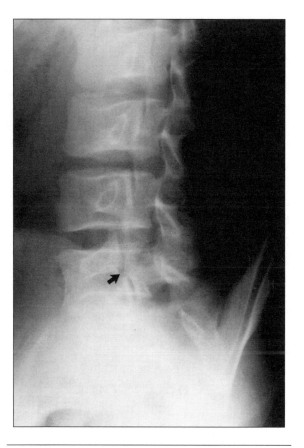

Figure 8.13 Spondylolysis: radiograph of lumbar spine, demonstrating fracture defect in the pars interarticularis of L5.

Spinal Stress Fractures

This survey of case studies has intentionally moved up the foot and leg, reflecting the pattern in which stress fractures in dancers are most frequently seen. It should be understood, however, that like active people in all walks of life, dancers might experience stress fracture in any part of the body. Stress fractures in the spine, especially, occur with increased frequency in dancers.

The majority of spinal stress fractures are called spondylolysis–tiny (sometimes not so tiny) cracks in the bone at the site of the pars interarticularis, most often in the lumbar spine (figure 8.13). If not dealt with properly the loss of continuity at the pars interarticularis can weaken the spinal structure and contribute to low back pain, particularly with movements involving extension to the rear, such as the arabesque. When a dancer—or a gymnast—presents with pain upon performing back extension, this injury must be suspected. One study of female gymnasts showed spondylolysis

in over 11% of its subjects upon X ray, whereas no more than 2.3% of the female population at large might be expected to have it (Jackson, Wiltse, and Cirincione 1976). Another study of two ballet companies showed spondylolysis in over 7% of the members X-rayed (Garrick 1986). Bracing for months, often in combination with pelvic strengthening exercises, has proven a successful method of treating this particular fracture (Steiner and Micheli 1985).

> Spondylolysis and stress fractures of the lumbar pedicles are discussed in greater detail in chapter 7, pages 88 and 89.

The pars interarticularis is clearly the most vulnerable site in the spine, but stress fractures have also been found in the lumbar pedicles (figure 8.14). This is another possibility that must be considered in diagnosing and treating lower back pain in dancers (Ireland and Micheli 1987).

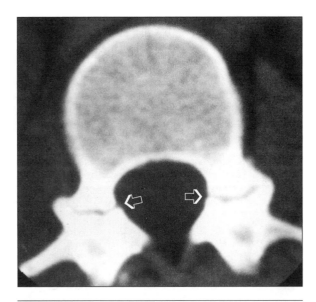

Figure 8.14 Tomogram: bilateral stress fracture of lumbar pedicles.

Conclusion

We close with a word about prevention. Virtually everything in the way dancers are trained, and much, we suspect, in the lifestyle they share as a group, predisposes them to stress fractures. To gain and maintain the skills required for their art, dancers have to subject their bodies to severe and repetitive extremes of motion. However, this regimen *can* be pursued in ways that minimize the risk. The keys to prevention of stress fractures may lie in a slow, progressive approach to training, with careful attention to avoiding rapid changes of style or technique; a reasoned attempt to match the anatomical characteristics of the individual dancer to the demands of the technique he or she is practicing; and a general awareness of body mechanics, especially as they pertain to avoiding excessive fatigue. Maintaining proper nutrition may be another important factor. Attention to these matters by dancers and those who are responsible for their training can reduce the incidence of stress fracture.

References

Barrow, G.W., and S. Saha. 1988. Menstrual irregularity and stress fractures in collegiate female distance runners. *American Journal of Sports Medicine* 16(3): 209-216.

Breithaupt, M.D. 1855. Zur Pathologie des menschlichen fusses. *Medicinische Zeitung* 24: 169-171, 175-177.

Garrick, J.G. 1986. Ballet injuries. *Medical Problems of Performing Artists* 1(4): 123-127.

Ireland, M.L., and L.J. Micheli. 1987. Bilateral stress fracture of the lumbar pedicles in a ballet dancer: A case report. *Journal of Bone and Joint Surgery* 69A(1): 140-142.

Jackson, D.W., L. Wiltse, and R.J. Cirincione. 1976. Spondylolysis in the female gymnast. *Clinical Orthopaedics and Related Research* 117: 68-73.

McBryde, A.M. 1975. Stress fractures in athletes. *Journal of Sports Medicine* 3(5): 212-217.

Micheli, L.J., F. Santopietro, P. Gerbino, and P. Crowe. 1980. Etiologic assessment of overuse stress fractures in athletes. *Nova Scotia Medical Bulletin* 59: 43-47.

Micheli, L.J., R.S. Sohn, and R. Solomon. 1985. Stress fractures of the second metatarsal involving Lisfranc's joint in ballet dancers: A new overuse injury of the foot. *Journal of Bone and Joint Surgery* 67A(9): 1372-1375.

Solomon, R., and L.J. Micheli. 1986. Technique as a consideration in modern dance injuries. *Physician and Sportsmedicine* 14(8): 83-92.

Stanitski, C.L., J.H. McMaster, and P.E. Scranton. 1978. On the nature of stress fractures. *American Journal of Sports Medicine* 6(6): 391-396.

Steiner, M.E., and L.J. Micheli. 1985. Treatment of symptomatic spondylolysis and spondylolisthesis with the modified Boston brace. *Spine* 10(10): 937-943.

Warren, M.P., J. Brooks-Gunn, L.H. Hamilton, L.F. Warren, and W.G. Hamilton. 1986. Scoliosis and fractures in young ballet dancers: Relation to delayed menarche and secondary amenorrhea. *New England Journal of Medicine* 314(21): 1348-1353.

Recommended Readings (Editors)

Bennell, K., and P. Brukner. 1997. Epidemiology and site specificity of stress fractures. *Clinics in Sports Medicine* 16(2): 179-196.

Bolin, D.J. 2001. Evaluation and management of stress fractures in dancers. *Journal of Dance Medicine & Science* 5(2): 37-42.

Brukner, P., C. Bradshaw, K. Khan, S. White, and K. Crossley. 1996. Stress fractures: A review of 180 cases. *Clinical Journal of Sport Medicine* 6(2): 85-89.

Coady, C.M., and L.J. Micheli. 1997. Stress fractures in the pediatric athlete. *Clinics in Sports Medicine* 16(2): 225-238.

Denton, J. 1997. Overuse foot and ankle injuries in ballet. *Clinics in Podiatric Medicine and Surgery* 14(3): 525-532.

Frusztajer, N.T., S. Dhuper, M.P. Warren, J. Brooks-Gunn, and R. Fox. 1990. Nutrition and the incidence of stress fractures in ballet dancers. *American Journal of Clinical Nutrition* 51(5): 779-783.

Gerbino, P.G. 1999. Lower extremity overuse injuries. *Journal of Dance Medicine & Science* 3(1): 35-37.

Kadel, N., C.C. Teitz, and R.A. Kronmal. 1992. Stress fractures in ballet dancers. *American Journal of Sports Medicine* 20(4): 445-449.

Khan, K., J. Brown, S. Way, N. Vass, K. Chrichton, R. Alexander, A. Baxter, M. Butler, and J. Wark. 1995. Overuse injuries in classical ballet. *Sports Medicine* 19(5): 341-357.

Lundon, K., L. Melcher, and K. Bray. 1999. Stress fractures in ballet: A twenty-five year review. *Journal of Dance Medicine & Science* 3(3): 101-107.

Marx, R.G., D. Saint-Phard, L.R. Callahan, J. Chu, and J.A. Hannafin. 2001. Stress fracture sites related to underlying bone health in athletic females. *Clinical Journal of Sport Medicine* 11(2): 73-76.

Outerbridge, A.R., and L.J. Micheli. 1995. Overuse injuries in the young athlete. *Clinics in Sports Medicine* 14(3): 503-516.

Part III

Preventing Dance Injuries Through Biomechanically Efficient Training

Because of its medical nature, part II essentially presents the physician's perspective on injury prevention. The unifying factor in part III is the application of biomechanical (and in one case neuroanatomical) concepts to dance techniques and practices. Hence, it opens the subject of prevention to contributions from a broad range of other disciplines. It is interesting to note that this sharing of information among disciplines is the cornerstone on which the still fairly new International Association for Dance Medicine & Science (founded in 1990) rests. Especially through its journal and annual conferences, this first-of-its-kind organization is providing concrete evidence that the diverse constituencies of which the field is composed, once thought to be in many respects incapable of communicating with one another, can indeed interact to the benefit of all.

Chapter 9

An Efficient Warm-Up Based on Anatomical Principles

Ruth Solomon, Professor Emerita

The field of dance medicine and science, through its concern for preventing injuries, might be conceptualized as addressing teachers, choreographers, and heads of dance programs and companies more directly than any other segment of the dance community. As these are the people who deal most intimately with dancers, it is of the utmost importance that they be alerted to the latest developments in injury prevention research. Conversely, as a result in large part of the entrenchment of dance in university curricula, a reverse flow of information from the "front lines" to the research community has been established. This chapter demonstrates the symbiosis of medicine and dance by illustrating how anatomical principles (such as those discussed in chapters 4-8) can inform the biomechanical principles underlying the teaching of dance technique.

There is an anecdote in Eugene Herrigel's classic *Zen in the Art of Archery* (1953) that comes to mind each time I confront a new group of students in technique class. Herrigel recounts how, after several years of frustrating failure to learn the all-important Way to release the string of his Japanese bow, he happened upon a trick that simulated the desired technique and produced adequate results. He could hardly wait to shoot for his Zen master. When that day arrived, however, and the master had witnessed just one shot utilizing the bogus technique, he turned away in total disgust and refused even to speak to Herrigel for weeks.

The parallel may not be exact—I don't suppose many of our dance students knowingly deceive us—but surely most dance teachers share with me the impression that many of their students come to them with work habits that are "inappropriate" (I prefer to say "inefficient") in some respects. Even students who have had no previous instruction may, like Herrigel, seek and find ways of shortcutting what we try to achieve with them and thereby fall into faulty movement patterns or bad habits. It has always been my belief that the main business of dance technique classes is to eliminate ineffective and potentially harmful movement patterns, and get the students working in a more efficient manner (Solomon 1987). Like Herrigel's archery instructor, we must help them get out of their own way.

Indications of Inefficient Movement Tendencies

Fortunately, many of the "tendencies" that lead to movement that is aesthetically unpleasing and, from a medical point of view, potentially harmful are readily apparent because they visibly influence the contour of the body. In fact, it is one of the tenets on which my own approach to teaching technique rests and which I would like to explore here, that movement is inefficient specifically when it is initiated by the peripheral muscles that lie near the surface of the body (and are therefore highly visible) rather than by those deep in the body, most notably the psoas system, which connects the front of the spine to the thigh. I present several examples of this type of movement, discuss them especially in terms of their medical ramifications, and then describe with the aid of illustrations some exercises I use to try to overcome these tendencies.

Contracted Tibialis Anterior in Plié

Let us look first at the plié, a movement that recommends itself for my purposes because (1) it is a component of virtually every dance technique; (2) it is so central to the achievement of results that are both aesthetically and medically sound; and (3) the key to observing when it is being performed inefficiently, though small, is also very clear. The "key" I have in mind here involves the tibialis anterior, that band of tendon that runs down the lower leg and can be seen quite prominently at the front of the ankle when the muscles of the foot and leg are used in contraction (figure 9.1). When plié is performed efficiently, the weight of the body is held, as we say, "out of the legs" by the psoas system, minimizing tension in the leg muscles and allowing the feet to relax on the floor. The knee and ankle act as simple hinges, there is a strong stretch on the Achilles tendon, and *the tibialis anterior is not prominently protruding* (figure 9.2). When you see a student's tibialis anterior contract during a plié you are keyed into the fact that he or she is engaging muscle groups that ought to be released, and this in turn means that the student is relying on the legs and feet to do the work rather than using the psoas system to maintain control in the pelvis.

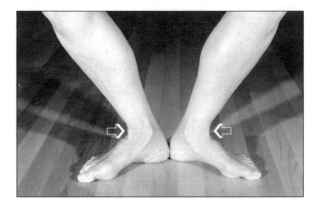

Figure 9.1 Tibialis anterior tendon incorrectly contracted as demi-plié is performed in turned-out (first) position.
Reprinted from Micheli and Solomon 1987.

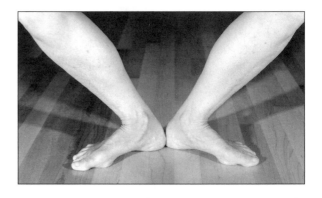

Figure 9.2 Demi-plié turned-out (first) position with tibialis anterior tendon released. Note increased flexion and stretch of Achilles tendon.
Reprinted from Micheli and Solomon 1987.

The primary use of plié is, of course, to initiate and cushion the landing from jumps. Indeed, the height of a jump or leap, and therefore to some extent its aesthetic appeal, is the direct result of power generated by the preparatory plié. Similarly, a soft, weightless landing results from a controlled, well-balanced plié. If, conversely, the feet are, as I like to say, "gripping the floor" in order to push off and regain control, the leap will be truncated, and the landing will lack resilience. The reverberation from the impact of such a landing travels up the unnecessarily tense leg and, especially given the number of times a dancer jumps over the course of weeks and months, can contribute to shinsplints and even stress fractures. So, again, keep an eye out for that protruding tibialis anterior. It is only one small factor in the plié, but it is significant.

Contracted Quadriceps Muscles in Extension[*]

Let us consider now the case of the student who is having trouble achieving full extension: The leg comes up to 90° easily enough, but beyond that whatever extension can be managed is accompanied by obvious tension. Further, if this problem has persisted long enough there may be popping sounds at the site of the hip socket and grinding sensations that may become painful enough in themselves to inhibit the student's ability (or willingness) to raise the leg.

This we readily perceive to be a positioning problem: The extended or "gesturing" leg is not moving in the proper vertical plane relative to the position of the pelvis. Normally we address this problem by simply taking hold of the leg and gently searching out the place where it can be raised without constriction (figure 9.3). This is fine as far as it goes: A high, graceful, stress-free extension requires proper positioning, and in this respect all the teacher can do is try to help the student experience where that is. I would only add the caveat that as the bony construction of the hip socket and the angle of femoral insertion in the acetabulum differ for every individual, so the "proper " position for extension will vary, however minutely, from one dancer to another. Ultimately the dancer must *feel* right when performing the extension rather than satisfying some externally imposed image of what *is* right.

However, there is another whole aspect of this problem that tends to get short shrift, if it is considered at all. If we look closely at the gesturing leg of the student who is experiencing inhibited extension, we will often see that as the leg passes 90° the quadriceps muscles along the top of the thigh are strongly contracted. In effect, what the student is trying to do is lift the leg by using the muscles of the leg itself. Unfortunately, this effort contracts not only the quadriceps but also the tendons that surround the hip socket. Far from promoting the desired elevation of the leg, this tightening of the tendons actually seems to pull the leg *down*. It is a classic example of how the body can work against itself when inappropri-

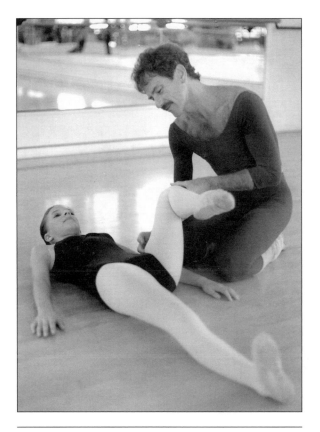

Figure 9.3 Teacher testing for release at the head of the rectus femoris and iliacus.

Reprinted from Micheli and Solomon 1987.

ate anatomical means are utilized to accomplish a task.

The quadriceps are, of course, engaged in extension, but their role is secondary to that of the "hip flexor," a lay term for the psoas. Through its attachment to the lesser trochanter at the back of the femur, the psoas provides the primary impetus for raising the leg (Ranney 1979). The muscles of the leg itself simply respond to this impulse from deeper in the body—as we tend to say, "from the pelvis." Therefore, another correction that should help the student who is having problems with inhibited extension achieve better results (in addition to placing the leg in the proper position) is to emphasize *release* of the tendons of the hip socket and the quadriceps muscles, especially at initiation of the movement (figure 9.4).

---

[*]Throughout this chapter the term "extension" is used as in the common parlance of dance. In physical therapy the movement to which it refers is generally described as "flexion."

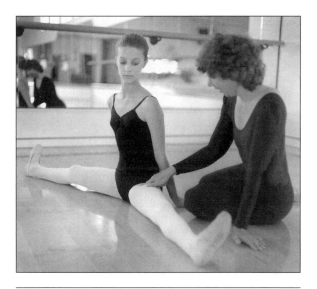

Figure 9.4 Teacher helping student to experience release of the hip socket and quadriceps in second position.
Reprinted from Micheli and Solomon 1987.

Nor should those popping sounds at the hip socket be taken lightly. They are produced when the contracted iliopsoas tendon (on the medial aspect of the hip socket) slides across the head of the femur, or the tensor fascia lata (on the lateral side) snaps across the greater trochanter, or both. The frequent repetition of this action as the femur is rotated for such movements as rond de jambe and développé can progressively irritate the tendons, causing the symptoms associated with tendinitis (see chapter 6). Once the tendons are irritated the dancer becomes reticent to lift the leg because of the pain involved; he or she tends to try to protect the hip socket by holding on even more tightly, and the tendinitis syndrome can become chronic (figure 9.5).

"Lifted" Rib Cage

A final example of movement that is inefficient and ultimately harmful can often be seen in the student who perpetually suffers from back pain, in the lumbar and thoracic areas. As I watch these students work, one movement trait frequently catches my eye. Probably responding dutifully to an injunction they have received somewhere in their training to "pull up," these students are literally trying to hold themselves up by the rib cage. That entire anatomical structure is thrust forward and up in an attempt similarly to elevate everything below it. Raising the leg in extension,

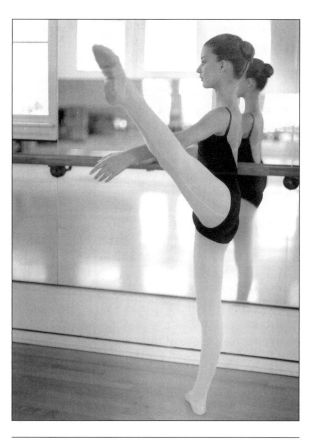

Figure 9.5 Incorrect extension in second position. The gluteus maximus is engaged, causing internal rotation of the extended leg.
Reprinted from Micheli and Solomon 1987.

for example, or going into the air, are incorrectly thought of as movements to be initiated by this lift of the rib cage.

This is another self-defeating strategy; the student is working very hard, but in the wrong area. Holding the rib cage forward and up creates a conflict of movement in that it contracts the relatively weak peripheral muscles of the back to do work that properly belongs to the large muscles on the front of the spine. What we really want our students to learn to do is *release* the rib cage, thereby enabling them to *decontract* the back muscles and in turn bring the psoas fully into play. This placement of the rib cage will be quite apparent to any experienced dance teacher. Effecting the desired realignment in this area will decrease stress in the back and reduce the likelihood of muscle spasms.

This is one manifestation of "tight back." There are others, most notably those associated with lordosis. A lordodic spine may result from a number of different causes; in dance we tend to think it is influenced by the forward tilt of the pelvis that in some dancers accompanies the attempt to increase turnout. My own feeling is that lordosis signifies a weak or underutilized psoas. At any rate, a "tight back"—whether it is related to lordosis, a malaligned rib cage, or whatever—is by definition one in which the peripheral muscles are overly contracted, causing a lack of flexibility in the spine. The antidote is exercises that encourage the student to release those muscles that impede movement in the spine and to engage those muscles that enhance it.

General Principles of the Warm-Up

As I place so much emphasis on the role of the psoas system in initiating movement, it should come as no surprise that the approach to training dancers that I have developed focuses primarily on strengthening that system and sensitizing the student to its workings. What follows is a description of the sequence of exercises with which the warm-up phase of my technique class normally begins (Solomon 1988). This is essentially floor work, that is, work done while sitting or lying on the floor. We begin with floor exercises because the support we derive from the floor helps to "unload" the bones and joints we want to articulate and to reduce tension in the muscles that support them. Further, work of this sort tends to minimize most students' concern with balance—and perhaps with the external shape of the movement generally—thus freeing them to concentrate on what is happening anatomically.

Although these exercises do not entail movement through space (locomotion) they are performed in a vigorous fashion, thus fulfilling the need to raise the heart rate, increase blood flow throughout the muscles, and lubricate the joints. An efficient warm-up should raise the body temperature about 1.5° or 2° above normal. This has the effect of increasing elasticity in the muscles and decreasing friction in the joints. Further, it facilitates the transmission of nerve impulses into the muscle fibers, and the reflexes also improve.

Throughout the warm-up, vocalization is used as an integral part of virtually every exercise; that is, the students are asked to make sounds—not

just breathing sounds, but actual words or vocalized syllables—on the strong-effort aspect of each movement. Thus, an audible breath or sound pattern is created: Allow the breath in on the release aspect of the movement, breathe (sound) out on the strong effort. This is done because, as the breathing process originates in the same area of the pelvis as does movement (what I call the "center"), the quality of the sound a student makes will emulate the quality of the movement: A clear, strong sound demonstrates that the center is being used in an uninhibited manner; a weak, constricted sound indicates that tension is limiting the movement flow. Students quickly learn to hear and interpret their own sounds, and to adjust without the instructor's having to make corrections. This holistic approach to breathing-movement has the additional advantage of making the breathing process a conditioned reflex—out on effort, in on release—so that when the dancer comes to perform, he or she will (1) not hold the breath, and (2) be free to express the movement fully, from the center.

The intention here is to present enough of this material not only to indicate how I deal with the kinds of problems discussed in the preceding sections, but also to allow those who want to work through it to experience what feels right to them and what is problematic. The next step would be to utilize these discoveries within the context of already familiar techniques. This is, of course, only one in an infinite number of approaches to training, but it is broad based enough to be applicable to virtually any other approach.

Warm-Up Exercises

Standing relaxed, with the feet in parallel position, arms above the head (figure 9.6a), we curve the lumbar spine into flexion, keeping the shoulders over the hip sockets and bending the knees as needed to deepen the curve (figure 9.6b). This articulation in the lumbar area allows the spine, from lumbar through sacrum and coccyx, to form one continuous curve—the lower end of which, if extended forward in imagination between the legs, would strike the floor at a point well in front of the feet. We are aided in this imaging by the curve of the coccyx, which, when viewed in profile, already tilts forward. The lumbar articulation simply deepens and extends that curve. By keeping the shoulders over the hip sockets

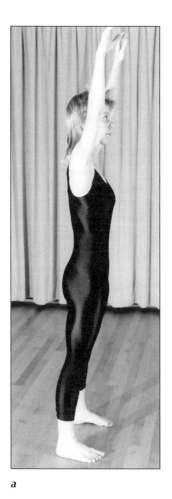 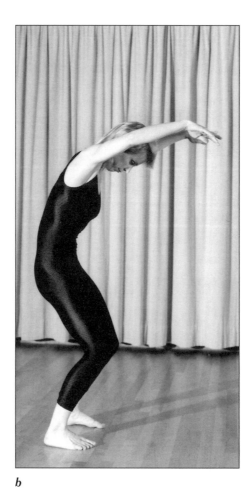 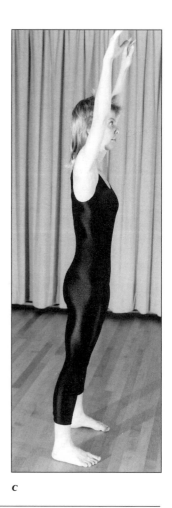

a   b   c

Figure 9.6 Exercise 1.
Photos courtesy of Bruce Berryhill.

we cause the dorsal spine to reflect the curve below it; hence, the entire spine, up through the cervical curve, is drawn into one continuous arc. Enhancing the dorsal curve has the additional advantage of releasing the rib cage—indeed, the dorsal spine can't curve if the rib cage is held forward or lifted—in turn relieving tension in the psoas, which is being pulled in the opposite direction to create the lumbar curve.

This effort cycle of the exercise is given three counts and sounded with one continuous word-exhalation, for example, "ouut." We then release for three counts, allowing the breath in and returning to the standing position, again making sure that the shoulders remain over the hip sockets (figure 9.6c). This simple exercise allows us to focus our attention on the center-of-movement area, to articulate virtually the whole spine in relation to that center, thus beginning to warm it up and align it, and to engage the psoas directly in this process.

Once we have done enough repetitions of this exercise to sense the area in which we are working, we move on to exercise 2. This begins with the same standing lumbar curve (figure 9.7a), which is maintained and lowered by bending the knees until the coccyx almost touches the floor (figure 9.7b). We hang in this position for three counts and then roll backward on the curve, keeping the knees close into the chest to deepen it; touch the floor behind the head with our toes (three counts; figure 9.7c); and roll forward on the curve until we are back on our feet (three counts; figure 9.7d). It is important that the feet, knees, and thighs remain in parallel, and the knees should be over the second toe. We again hang in this low parallel position for three counts and then rise to standing (three counts), as always making sure that the shoulders are over the hip sockets (figure 9.7e). This exercise continues using the same movement sequence with a more rapid flow of motion through six counts: three counts for rolling down

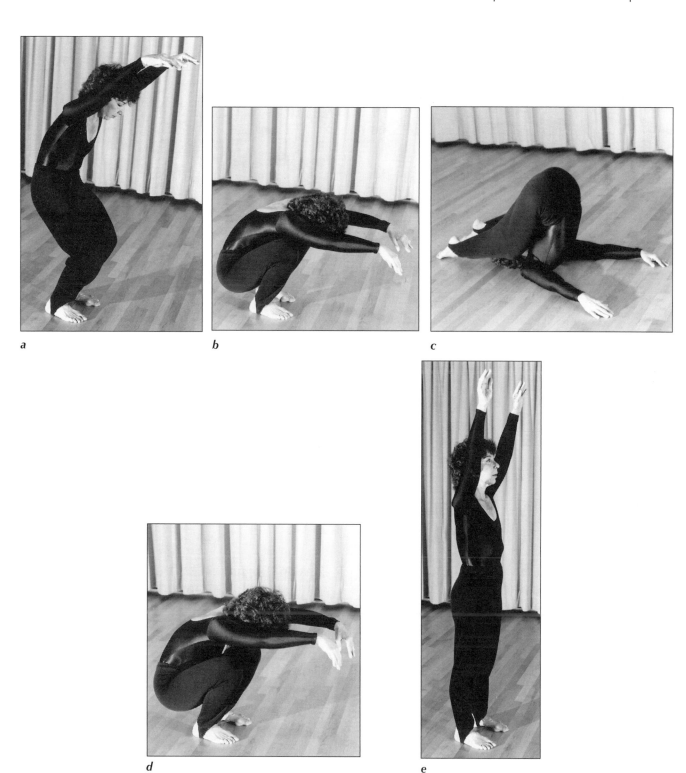

a *b* *c*

d *e*

Figure 9.7 Exercise 2.
Photos courtesy of Bruce Berryhill.

until the toes touch the floor behind the head, and three counts for rolling forward to stand. The use of the lumbar curve in this exercise—first establishing it, then controlling with it as the body's weight is lowered to the floor, then rolling on it (which we could *not* do smoothly if the spine were not consistently curved)—provides ample opportunity to experience and thereby image the spine. Throughout this first part of the warm-up we want to "think bones."

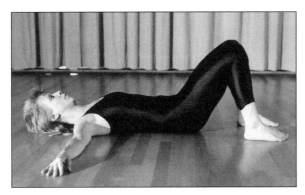

a

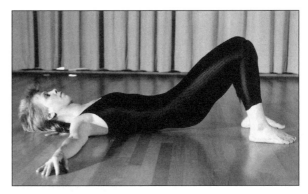

b

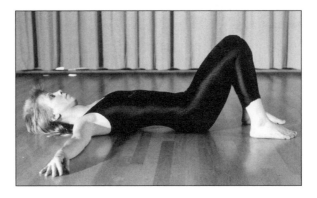

c

Figure 9.8   Exercise 3.
Photos courtesy of Bruce Berryhill.

We end exercise 2 by releasing the spine flat onto the floor (instead of completing the forward roll in the last repetition) and, with bent knees, allowing the feet to land flat in parallel (figure 9.8*a*). This places us in position to begin exercise 3, which involves what I call "pelvic rocks." First we roll the lower spine off the floor, starting with the coccyx and continuing as far as the 12th dorsal vertebra (figure 9.8*b*). This I call an "undercurve"—the equivalent of the "pelvic tilt" in many other techniques (and much physical therapy). The "rock" is completed by reversing this process into an "overcurve" (figure 9.8*c*), which requires a release in the hip socket (rectus femoris and iliacus). This exercise is performed first on two slow counts; then double-time, and then double-time again.

Exercise 4 develops on exercise 3 in much the same way exercise 2 did on exercise 1. Starting in the same position and having established the same undercurve from coccyx through sacrum to 12th dorsal (figure 9.9*a*), we extend the undercurve up the spine until we are resting on the shoulder blades, thus fully involving the dorsal spine in the articulation (figure 9.9*b*). Then we start down from the top, cascading the entire spine onto the floor (figure 9.9*c*) and ending in an overcurve (figure 9.9*d*). The breathing is especially important in this exercise and the one that follows as students tend to hold their breath through the strong-effort cycles. The movement is designed to combat this tendency; we breathe or sound out for four counts as the pelvis rises, release and allow air in for two counts at the top, breathe or sound out for four counts coming down, and release for air in on two counts in the overcurve. Exercise 5 maintains this same breathing pattern and begins in the same way, but having released for two counts at the top (figure 9.10*a*), we reverse the downward flow of the vertebrae by lowering the coccyx to the floor (figure 9.10*b*), then the sacrum and lumbar spine (figure 9.10*c*).

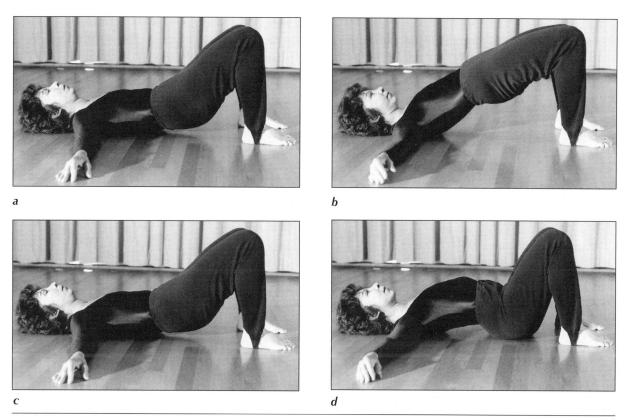

a

b

c

d

Figure 9.9 Exercise 4.

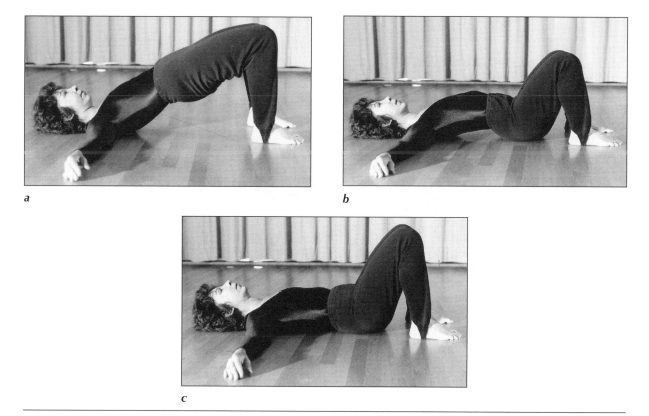

a

b

c

Figure 9.10 Exercise 5.

Photos courtesy of Bruce Berryhill.

As a relief from our focus on the spine, and in order to get some blood flowing through the limbs and joints, in exercise 6 we turn our attention to the legs and arms. Exercise 5 has left us with spine and feet flat on the floor, knees bent. We now lift the legs above us and shake them loosely for eight counts, letting air in (figure 9.11*a*). Then we flex the feet, bend the knees slightly, and, holding that basic shape, vibrate the legs vigorously, sounding the breath out for eight counts (figure 9.11*b*). We then drop the feet heavily onto the floor in parallel position and repeat essentially the same process with the arms, first shaking them loosely above us (figure 9.11*c*), then shaping them at the elbows and wrists and vibrating for eight counts (figure 9.11*d*).

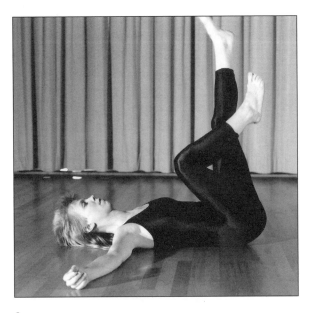

a

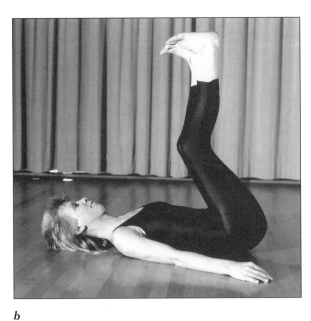

b

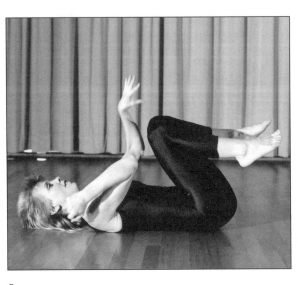

c

d

Figure 9.11   Exercise 6.

Photos courtesy of Bruce Berryhill.

Exercises 7 and 8 begin as we lift our bent legs above us, knees softly folded, and take hold of the tibia with our hands (figure 9.12*a*). Then, by pressing through the knees into the hands, we drag the head off the floor (figure 9.12*b*) and, breathing or sounding out, let it curve sequentially forward (figure 9.12*c*). This simple movement articulates the dorsal and cervical vertebrae, the ones that

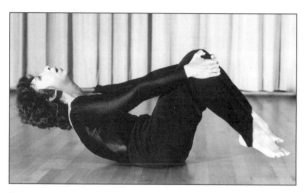

a

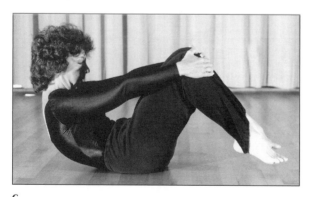

b

have been only marginally worked earlier. Then we release the spine back onto the floor, allowing the air in, and repeat. Gradually we begin to rock on the lumbar curve (figure 9.13*a*), rounding it down to a base of support in the sacrum and (exercise 8) "lever" down through this base of support to bring ourselves onto a balance point slightly behind the coccyx (figure 9.13*b*) (Sweigard 1974). The exact placement differs from one individual to another. Even when we are up on the balance point the lumbar and dorsal spine remain in an easy curve. It is important not to try to straighten the spine entirely, as to do so causes undue strain in the low back, which must then support the weight of the legs. Naturally we breathe or sound out on the levering (effort) action, and release for air in as we curve back down to the starting position.

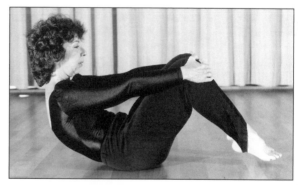

a

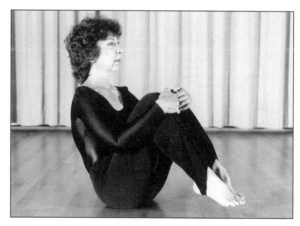

b

c

Figure 9.12 Exercise 7.
Photos courtesy of Bruce Berryhill.

Figure 9.13 Exercise 8.
Photos courtesy of Bruce Berryhill.

All of the final exercises in this sequence begin on the balance point. In exercise 9 we circle the head, first to the side (figure 9.14*a*), then forward (figure 9.14*b*), then side (figure 9.14*c*), and back (figure 9.14*d*), sounding out on the extension back, which is the long arc of the cervical vertebrae. We reverse direction each time, to make sure we are articulating the vertebrae equally on all sides. It is important throughout this exercise to maintain an open throat for easy passage of breath and voice.

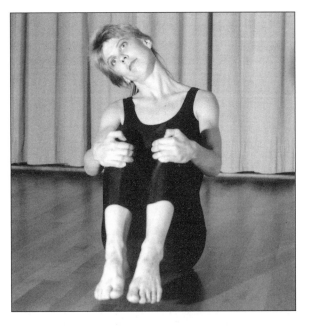

a

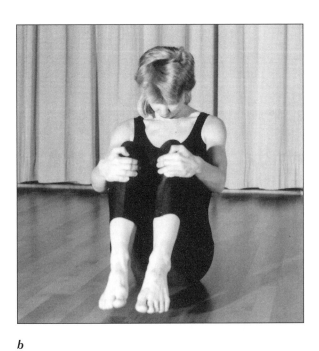

b

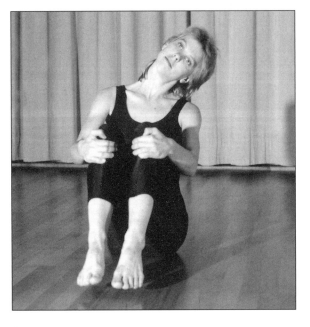

c

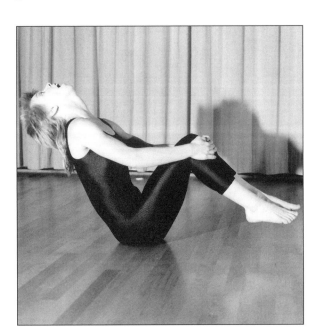

d

Figure 9.14 Exercise 9.

Photos courtesy of Bruce Berryhill.

In exercise 10 we circle the arms from the shoulders, first one at a time (figure 9.15a and b), then together, back to front, then reversing the circle (figures 9.15, c-e). This not only lubricates the shoulder joints, but has the added advantage of causing the psoas, which is already engaged in sustaining the body on the balance point, to work even harder to offset the free flow of the arms. The same effect is heightened in exercise 11, where we add the extension of the legs to the work the psoas is doing, extending them in a V shape with the torso, femurs as close to

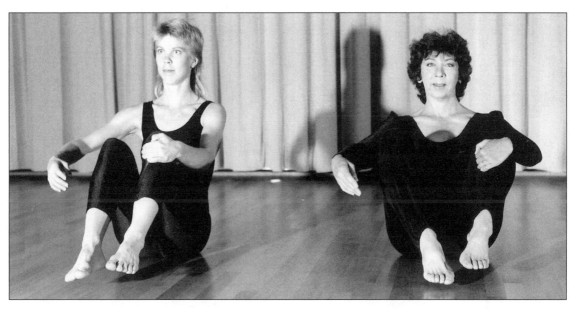

a

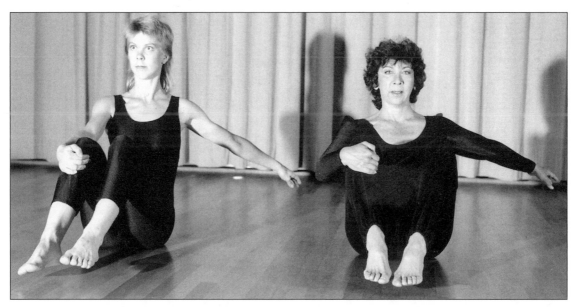

b

(continued)

Figure 9.15 Exercise 10.
Photos courtesy of Bruce Berryhill.

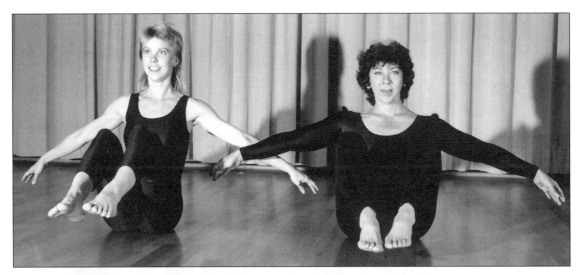

c

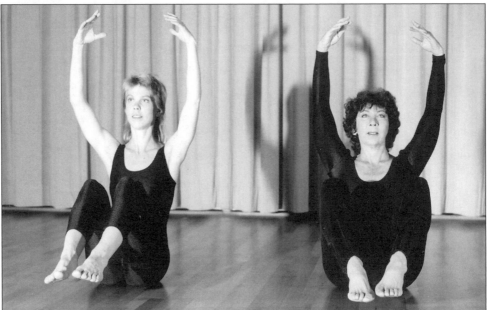

d

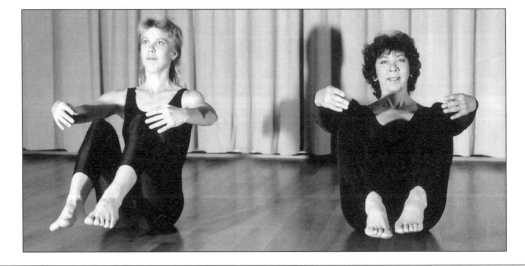

e

Figure 9.15 *(continued)*.
Photos courtesy of Bruce Berryhill.

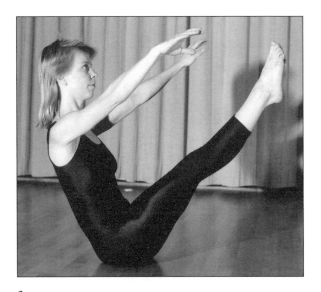

a

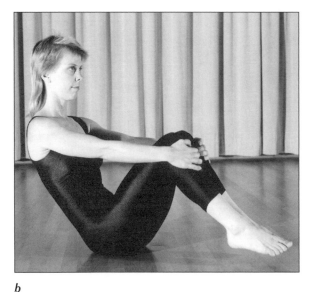

b

Figure 9.16 Exercise 11.

Photos courtesy of Bruce Berryhill.

the chest as possible and tibias articulated to line up with the femurs (figure 9.16*a*). Then we alternately fold at the knees (figure 9.16*b*) and straighten the legs, breathing or sounding out as the tibias extend and releasing for breath in as they fold. This exercise also starts to lubricate the knee joints.

Exercise 12 works primarily on lubricating and warming up the hip joints (and strengthening the psoas). From the starting position on the balance point, knees together in parallel and arms extended outside the legs (figure 9.17*a*), we open the knees to the side, bringing

the arms inside the legs (figure 9.17*b*). Then we reverse the process—knees in, arms out (figure 9.17*c*). After each set of four repetitions we catch the ankles and allow the weight of the legs to rest in the palms of the hands, releasing the hip sockets. Having performed this exercise several times with bent knees, we straighten the legs and continue, thus increasing the need for control in the pelvis (figures 9.17, *d-f*). It should be clear that the strength and facility throughout these balance-point exercises are exactly what we will use when, in standing position, we work on extension.

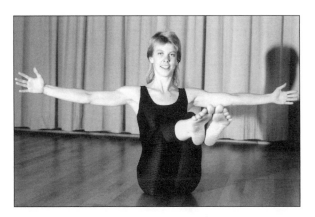

a

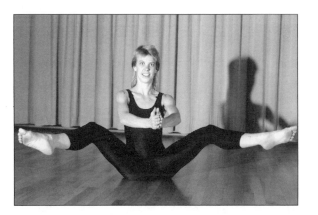

b

(continued)

Figure 9.17 Exercise 12.

Photos courtesy of Bruce Berryhill.

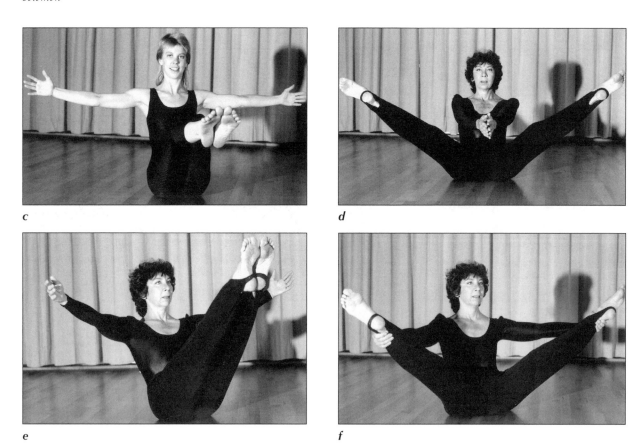

c   d

e   f

Figure 9.17 *(continued)*.
Photos courtesy of Bruce Berryhill.

The final exercises in this sequence complete the first phase in our preparation for standing work. In exercise 13, still on our balance point with the legs out straight in a raised second position, we take hold of the ankles and fold the knees in (figure 9.18*a*), then return to extended legs in second (figure 9.18*b*). As always, we breathe or sound out on the extension, in on the release. In exercise 14, with the legs together and extended in parallel, we alternately flex and point the feet (figure 9.19*a* and *b*).

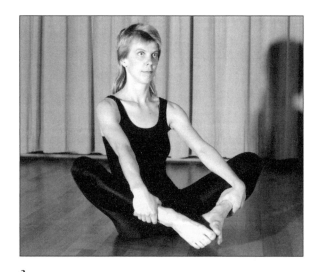
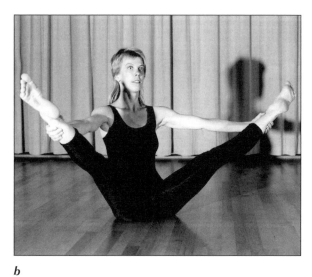

a   b

Figure 9.18 Exercise 13.
Photos courtesy of Bruce Berryhill.

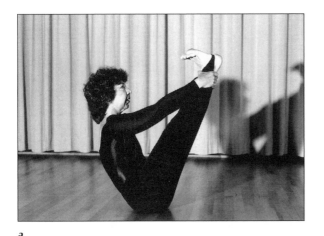

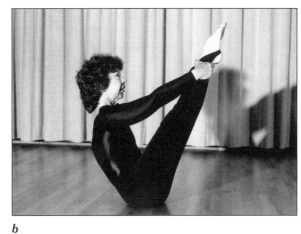

a

b

Figure 9.19 Exercise 14.

Photos courtesy of Bruce Berryhill.

This begins to warm up the ankles and feet. Last (exercise 15), we let go with the hands and, while continuing to flex and point the feet and maintaining the lumbar-dorsal curve, lower the legs until the heels are 6 to 8 in. (15-20 cm) off the floor (figure 9.20*a* and *b*). Then, with the feet flexed, we rotate the legs out from the hip sockets and cross or "beat" the legs as in entrechat for at least four sets of eight (figure 9.20*c*). Finally, lowering the legs flat onto the floor, we lever down through the sacrum, bringing the torso up to sitting position, and then, releasing in the hip sockets, allow the torso to fold over the legs (figure 9.20*d*). It is important in this final phase

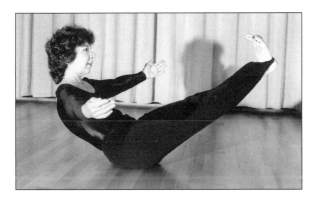

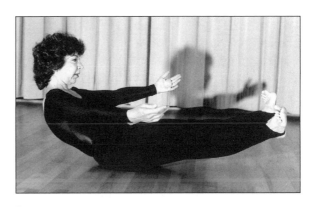

a

b

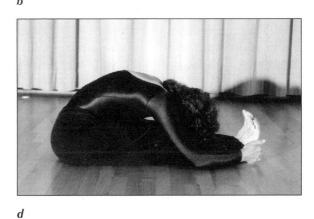

c

d

Figure 9.20 Exercise 15.

Photos courtesy of Bruce Berryhill.

to make sure that all the muscles around the hip socket—the tensor fascia lata, rectus femoris, and iliacus—are released. The principle throughout exercises 11 to 15 is to articulate the leg while maintaining a soft hip socket and *not* engaging the quadriceps as the primary motivator of the movements.

The entire sequence described here takes approximately 10 minutes when each exercise is repeated four to six times.

Conclusion

When we see movement performed in a way that evokes our admiration, one of the things we frequently say about it is that it was "effortless." More accurately, what we mean is that it *appeared* effortless because the dancer was able to find the means within his or her body to generate it efficiently. It is the search for the source of this efficiency that has shaped my approach to teaching.

"Talent" is part of the answer; genetic endowment is another part. Some bodies are by nature better equipped to dance than others. Well-formed bones, strong muscles, and pliable connective tissue are not in themselves enough, however; indeed, they can sometimes get in the way of, or be used as a substitute for, the body mechanics that actually do produce "effortless" movement. I am thinking now particularly of the use of peripheral muscles to do the work that really needs to be initiated much deeper in the body—for example, using the quadriceps as the primary motivation to lift the leg in extension, rather than as conveyors of the impulse that has originated in the psoas. Many of our students, even those (or perhaps *especially* those) who seem furthest along technically, have slipped into such habits earlier in their dance training. Fortunately, the results of movement produced in this way are sufficiently different from the effortless results of anatomically efficient movement to be instantly apparent to the trained eye.

I believe it is our primary responsibility as technique teachers to help our students find the most efficient way possible to use their bodies. I emphasize the roles of the psoas, the pelvis, and the spine because the study of anatomy has led me to believe that they are the prime motivators of movement. If the dancer is able to initiate action

by the use of these components, all else should follow and the movement produced will be relatively stress free, efficient, and safe.

References

Herrigel, E. 1953. *Zen in the art of archery.* London: Routledge.

Micheli, L.J., and R. Solomon. 1987. Training the young dancer. In *Dance medicine: A comprehensive guide,* edited by A.J. Ryan and R.E. Stephens. Chicago and Minneapolis: Pluribus Press/*The Physician and Sportsmedicine* 60, 63-64, 70-71.

Ranney, D.A. 1979. The functional integration of trunk muscles and the psoas. *Kinesiology for Dance* 9: 10-12.

Solomon, R. 1987. Training dancers: Anatomy as a master image. *Journal of Physical Education, Recreation and Dance* 58(5): 51-56.

Solomon, R. 1988. *Anatomy as a master image in training dancers* (videorecording). Santa Cruz, CA: 1 videocassette; 59 minutes; color; 1/2 inch, VHS or Beta; 3/4 inch, U-matic. (Available from Princeton Books, Pennington, NJ.)

Sweigard, L.E. 1974. *Human movement potential.* New York: Dodd, Mead.

Recommended Readings (Editors)

Buckroyd, J. 2000. *The student dancer: Emotional aspects of teaching and learning dance.* London: Dance Books.

Chatfield, S.J., W. Byrnes, and V. Foster. 1992. Effects of intermediate modern-dance training on select physiologic performance parameters. *Kinesiology and Medicine for Dance* 14(2): 13-26.

Cherveny, S.R. 1995. Practical applications of floor barre in ballet training. *Medical Problems of Performing Artists* 10(2): 70-72.

Darby, L.A. 2000. Physiology of dance. In *Exercise and sport science,* edited by W.E. Garrett Jr. and D.T. Kirkendall. Philadelphia: Lippincott, Williams & Wilkins, 771-784.

Huwyler, J. 1999. *The dancer's body: A medical perspective on dance and dance training.* McLean, VA: International Medical.

Krasnow, D., and M. Kabbani. 1999. Dance science research and the modern dancer. *Medical Problems of Performing Artists* 14(1): 16-20.

Livanelioglu, A., S. Otman, Y. Yakut, and F. Uygur. 1998. The effects of classical ballet training on the lumbar region. *Journal of Dance Medicine & Science* 2(2): 52-55.

Chapter 10

A Biomechanical Approach to Aerobic Dance Injuries

Stephen P. Baitch, PT

Although aerobics is a form of exercise rather than a performance-oriented activity, it sheds potentially useful light on the prevention of dance injuries because it involves large numbers of people in doing repetitive dance-like movement. As this chapter demonstrates, it is capable of producing the same types of injuries to which performing dancers are prone. Thus, it both reinforces our understanding of the risk factors that precipitate injuries and enlarges the population to be served by what we learn about prevention. Chapters 13 and 14 provide additional discussion of the biomechanics of the lower extremities, especially as related to pronation.

Since its inception sports medicine has focused on treating the athlete's injuries so that he or she may return to athletic participation as quickly as possible. The emphasis of treatment has been centered on alleviation of symptoms of injury, followed by an aggressive rehabilitation program. Now, due to the emergence of high technology and in-depth experimentation in biomechanics, the focus is shifting from the treatment of injury to dealing with causes. This shift is being applied to injuries in all sports, including aerobic dance. This chapter discusses the mechanisms of aerobic dance injuries and the biomechanical makeup of the lower extremities as it affects movement.

Terms Describing Anatomical Location in Chapter 10

bilateral	occurring or appearing on two sides
bisection	division into two equal lengths or parts
neutral	turned neither toward nor away from the body's midline
varus	bent or turned inward toward the midline

Injury Rates

The increasing popularity of aerobic dance has brought with it an alarming incidence of injury. According to a study performed on aerobic dancers in February 1985, 75.9% of aerobic dance instructors and 43.3% of students reported injuries (Richie, Kelso, and Bellucci 1985) with specific characteristics as to location and frequency. In a study conducted with 61 aerobic dancers at the Union Memorial Hospital Sports Medicine Center in Baltimore, 82% of the injuries reported involved the lower extremities (Vetter et al. 1985). The most common site of injury was the heel (spur syndrome or plantar fasciitis). The second most common site was the inner portion of the shin (shinsplints). The present author's experience supports these findings.

Risk Factors

Several predisposing factors of injury were observed. Of primary concern was the number of classes taken per week: The difference between the average for students (3.3) and for instructors (4.7) produced a significantly increased incidence of injury. A concrete floor covered with carpet also yielded a high injury rate (50%). (It is interesting to note, however, that a soft resilient floor did not always reduce the risk of injury; in fact, a wood-over-air-space floor covered with padded carpet had the second highest injury rate.) Shoewear was another component that was analyzed. Barefoot dancers had a 65% injury rate as compared with 49% for dancers wearing shoes. Although this speaks well for using some form of footwear, it also suggests that more work needs to be done on the construction of aerobic dance shoes. Several studies showed that excessive cushioning in shoes allows extraneous motion to occur in the foot and leg, thereby increasing the incidence

of injury (Cavanagh 1982; Nigg 1986). Training techniques were considered to be another contributing factor in aerobic dance injuries. Many aerobic dancers who were injured did not stretch adequately before and after exercise. Some injuries could also be attributed to a too rapid increase in the number of classes taken over a given period of time. This has been found to be equally true of runners who increase their weekly mileage too rapidly.

In several studies it was noted that repetitive movement combined with a hard surface definitely yielded a higher rate of injury (Francis, Francis, and Welshons-Smith 1985; Richie, Kelso, and Bellucci 1985; Vetter et al. 1985). It was hypothesized that an inability to dissipate shock might be the underlying cause for most aerobic dance injuries. However, shock reduction as a form of treatment was not always effective; nor had it proven efficacious in runners with complaints similar to those found in aerobic dancers. More recently the emphasis of treatment has been geared toward increasing control and stability of the foot while running. There is much literature to support the concept that realignment of the foot is extremely successful in treating various problems in runners (Bates et al. 1979; Botte 1981; Brody 1980; Subotnick 1976). We are now beginning to apply the same theories of realignment to aerobic dancers.

Biomechanical Analysis and Treatment

An examination of the biomechanics of the aerobic dancer's lower extremities has become crucial in our treatment approach. Characteristics such as excessive rotation of the femur and malalignment of the patella have been proven to be highly correlative with knee pain (this finding was noted previously in runners). Also observed was a correlation of tibial varum (bowed legs) and excessive foot pronation (rolling in) with symptoms of heel and shin pain as well as metatarsalgia (pain in the ball of the foot). Abnormal alignment of the foot has been known to cause problems as proximal as the hip and low back.

Many movements in aerobic dance demand the support of the entire body weight on one foot for a short period of time. The muscles of the foot, ankle, and leg contract both concentrically (shortening) and eccentrically (lengthening) in order to control the ascent and descent of the movement. At the same time, the joints of the foot and ankle must lock and unlock at precise moments to provide stability and mobility. A structural malalignment of the foot can cause excessive strain on the muscles, as well as abnormal rotation of the lower extremity. Aerobic dancers (or runners) with excessive pronation, for example, must overuse the posterior medial muscle groups of the shin in order to control the rate of ascent and descent during exercise (Viitasalo and Kvist 1983). Static evaluation reveals that when a dancer with this condition is viewed from the rear, the heel is in an everted position relative to the floor, the arch is dropped, and the tibia demonstrates bowing and rotation.

With recent advances in high technology we may enhance the static evaluation with a dynamic analysis utilizing a high-speed video camera system. The slow motion and frame-by-frame capability of this system records abnormal movement of the foot and lower extremity. The results are given in the form of a computer printout that provides angular measurements of the foot and lower leg. Once the static and dynamic results are obtained, a treatment plan is implemented. If the dancer's symptoms are occurring due to abnormal foot mechanics, a balanced orthotic (shoe insert) might be used to re-align the foot. Placing the foot in a neutral position with the orthotic can eliminate problems of the heel, shin, and knee.

It might be argued that the orthotic simply acts in this case as a shock absorber. Interestingly, however, as indicated earlier, aerobic dancers and runners have used a significant amount of cushioning in their shoes to self-treat injuries without success. In contrast, we have used a semirigid polypropylene orthosis with minimal shock absorption capability to correct alignment of the foot.

Case Study: Plantar Fasciitis

A specific case study involving plantar fasciitis will illustrate the efficacy of this treatment.

For additional information regarding the diagnosis, treatment, and rehabilitation of plantar fasciitis, see chapter 4, pages 49 and 50.

History

A 41-year-old female aerobic dancer presented with a complaint of chronic right heel pain that had developed over the past six months, apparently as a result of her participation in high-impact aerobic classes. She said that the heel pain began after she increased the frequency of her dance classes from two to three per week. The onset of the pain was gradual, and initially was noticed only after dancing. By the time the patient came to our clinic the pain was present during and after dance classes, but was most intense when she got up in the morning. Other relevant facts were that the patient had tried different types of aerobic shoes in an attempt to alleviate the heel pain, but without success; she had been dancing on wood floors covered with carpet at the time of the injury; she wore high heels frequently during the day, due to her job requirements; and prior treatment for her heel problem with anti-inflammatories and a cortisone injection had given minimal relief.

The patient's history is extremely valuable in these cases because it helps to formulate a course of treatment based on the underlying mechanism of injury. This particular history allowed the clinician to determine that the right heel pain was secondary to a gradual onset resulting from small repeated stresses after the dancer increased her activity from two to three classes a week.

Examination

Once a history is taken, a thorough static biomechanical examination is performed. The evaluation searches for limitation or excessive joint motion in the foot or lower extremity that may be the cause of a malalignment problem. The results in the case reported here showed that in the non-weight-bearing position, subtalar joint inversion and eversion range of motion

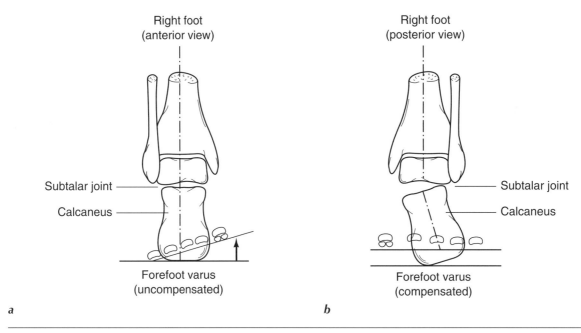

Figure 10.1 *(a)* The medial side of the forefoot is elevated in relation to the ground with the subtalar joint in neutral, indicating a forefoot varus. *(b)* The calcaneus everts past perpendicular in order to bring the medial side of the forefoot to the ground, causing excessive pronation.

Illustration courtesy of David Petrie.

measurements were within normal limits. The subtalar joint neutral position was 2° varus bilaterally. The forefoot to rearfoot relationship indicated a 4° varus on the right (symptomatic) foot and a perpendicular relationship on the left foot. Ankle dorsiflexion was measured to be 5° with the knee extended and 15° with the knee flexed, bilaterally. In the standing position, tibial varum (bowing) was noted to be 5° bilaterally. The relaxed (passive) calcaneal stance measurement indicated a 4° everted position on the right and a 2° everted position on the left foot.

To confirm these findings, a high-speed video analysis was performed during a simulated aerobic dance routine. The patient was instructed to do a series of aerobic dance movements similar to those used in her normal aerobic dance workout. Points of reference placed on the bisection of the lower legs and heel counters of both shoes (the counter is the built-up or rear part of a shoe, supporting the heel) were digitized and then analyzed frame by frame with the use of a computer. It was found that in the standing position the medial side of the forefoot was actually being raised in relationship to the ground when the subtalar joint was in the neutral position (figure 10.1*a*). However, in order to bring the forefoot to the ground, the subtalar joint had to

pronate as a compensatory mechanism, causing an everted position of the calcaneus (figure 10.1*b*). The high-speed video analysis not only verified that the abnormal pronation occurred, but demonstrated that the dynamic pronation angle (when in motion) on the symptomatic right foot (9°) exceeded the static pronation angle (when at rest) of 4°.

From a biomechanical standpoint it was determined that the excessive pronation had caused unlocking of the subtalar and mid-tarsal joint of the foot and subsequent eversion of the heel, producing hypermobility of the foot. In turn, this unlocking effect was creating an excessive strain on a band of tissue that has its attachment on the posterior medial surface of the heel (plantar fascia), thus causing heel pain. It was noted that this dancer had limited ankle dorsiflexion bilaterally. This condition, also known as equinus deformity, prevents the ankle from moving adequately in the upward direction in a non-weight-bearing situation (figure 10.2*a* and *b*). During weight-bearing activity it prevents the tibia from moving forward on the foot. In order to compensate for this problem the mid-tarsal joint of the foot must unlock and pronate so that adequate dorsiflexion can occur at the ankle joint, thus allowing the tibia to move forward over the foot.

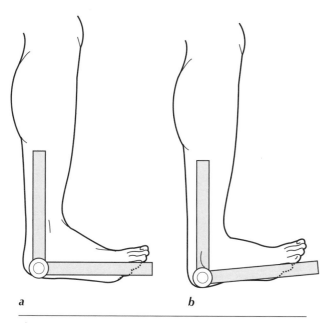

Figure 10.2 *(a)* Abnormal amount of ankle dorsiflexion indicating an equinus deformity of the ankle. *(b)* Normal amount of ankle dorsiflexion needed for adequate ambulation is 10° to 15°.

Illustration courtesy of David Petrie.

It is not unusual for dancers to have limited ankle dorsiflexion (5° or less). These same dancers often report that they frequently wear high-heeled shoes during working hours. In theory, wearing a high heel may place the gastroc-soleus muscle, located in the posterior calf, in a shortened position for a prolonged period of time (figure 10.3*a*). Conversely, wearing an aerobic dance shoe, which has minimal elevation in the heel, can be a drastic transition from wearing a 2-in. (5-cm)-high heel (figure 10.3*b*). The aerobic dance shoe, with its relatively lower inclination angle, places an undue strain on the already compromised length of the gastroc-soleus muscle during exercise. As the heel makes contact with the ground, increased mid-tarsal joint pronation may occur, allowing the tibia to move forward over its base of support (the foot), due to the inadequate amount of ankle dorsiflexion available.

Treatment

Initially, the treatment prescribed for the patient with plantar fasciitis consisted of ice massage to the right heel and stretching exercises for the gastroc-soleus muscles bilaterally. This regimen was performed before and after her aerobic dance routine. She was instructed to reduce her classes

from three to two a week. The patient was then casted for semirigid orthotic devices, which were made of high-density subortholin material. These orthotics were designed to control the abnormal subtalar and mid-tarsal joint pronation in an attempt to minimize the strain placed on the plantar fascia.

The patient gradually broke in the orthotics until she was able to wear them for her entire dance routine. After wearing them for six weeks she reported that her right heel pain had disappeared, and she had returned to her preinjury level of three classes per week. A posttreatment evaluation was performed using the high-speed video analysis system. The results indicated that initial maximum pronation angles were reduced from 9° to 5° on the symptomatic right foot. The asymptomatic left foot showed a reduction in the maximum pronation angle from 4° to 2°. It is important to note that the dancer was wearing her orthotics for the posttreatment evaluation.

Theoretically, the decrease in the maximum pronation angle with use of orthotic devices stabilizes the rearfoot and causes a locking effect of the mid-tarsal joint during gait. Limiting

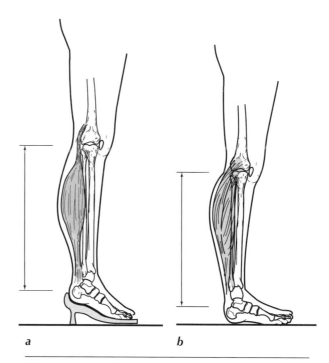

Figure 10.3 *(a)* Shortened position of the gastroc-soleus muscle when foot is in high-heeled shoe. *(b)* Length of gastroc-soleus muscle when foot is in aerobic dance shoe.

Illustration courtesy of David Petrie.

the amount of pronation at the subtalar and mid-tarsal joints prevents abnormal stretching of the plantar fascial tissue. However, the literature remains inconclusive as to whether decreasing the maximum pronation angle is the most significant contribution of orthotic devices. It must be kept in mind that the use of orthotics is only one parameter now being studied in the cause–effect relationship between pronation and injuries of the lower extremity.

Conclusion

This chapter demonstrates the systematic approach being implemented in order to evaluate and effectively treat lower extremity problems. The study of biomechanics has already had a tremendous impact on training regimens, as well as floor, shoe, and equipment design. There are still many questions to be answered regarding the role that abnormal biomechanics plays in the cause of injury. However, by shifting the focus of treatment toward the biomechanical causes of injury we anticipate being able to return many injured dancers (and athletes) to a relatively high level of activity.

References

Bates, B.T., L.R. Ostemig, B. Mason, and L.S. James. 1979. Foot orthotic devices to modify selected aspects of lower extremity mechanics. *American Journal of Sports Medicine* 7(6): 338-342.

Botte, R.R. 1981. An interpretation of the pronation syndrome and foot types of patients with low back pains. *Journal of American Podiatric Medical Association* 71(5): 243-253.

Brody, D.M. 1980. *Running injuries.* CIBA Clinical Symposia Annual 32(4). New Jersey: CIBA-Geigy.

Cavanagh, P. 1982. The shoe-ground interface in running. In *Compilation of the American Academy of Orthopaedic Surgeons symposium on the foot and leg in running sport,* edited by R.P. Mack. St. Louis: Mosby, 30-44.

Francis, L.L., P.P. Francis, and K. Welshons-Smith. 1985. Aerobic dance injuries: A survey of instructors. *Physician and Sportsmedicine* 13(2): 105-111.

Nigg, B.M. 1986. *Biomechanics of running shoes.* Champaign, IL: Human Kinetics.

Richie, D.H., S.F. Kelso, and P.A. Bellucci. 1985. Aerobic dance injuries: A retrospective study of instructors and participants. *Physician and Sportsmedicine* 13(2): 130-140.

Subotnick, S.I. 1976. The shin splints syndrome of the lower extremity. *Journal of American Podiatric Medical Association* 66(1): 43-45.

Vetter, W.L., D.L. Helfet, K. Spear, and L. Matthews. 1985. Aerobic dance injuries. *Physician and Sportsmedicine* 13(2): 114-120.

Viitasalo, J.T., and M. Kvist. 1983. Some biomechanical aspects of the foot and ankle in athletes with and without shin splints. *American Journal of Sports Medicine* 11(3): 125-130.

Recommended Readings (Editors)

du Toit, V., and R. Smith. 2001. Survey of the effects of aerobic dance on the lower extremity in aerobic instructors. *Journal of the American Podiatric Medical Association* 91(10): 528-532.

Grossman, G., and V. Wilmerding. 2000. Dance physical therapy for the leg and foot: Plantar fasciitis and Achilles tendinopathy. *Journal of Dance Medicine & Science* 4(20): 66-72.

Potter, H. 1996. Lower limb injuries in aerobic participants in Western Australia: An incidence study. *Australian Physiotherapy* 42(2): 111-119.

Potts, J.C., and J.J. Irrgang. 2001. Principles of rehabilitation of lower extremity injuries in dancers. *Journal of Dance Medicine & Science* 5(2): 51-61.

Schon, L.C., W.H.B. Edwards, F.X. McGuigan, and J. Hoffman. 2002. Pedobarographic and musculoskeletal examination of collegiate dancers in relevé. *Foot and Ankle International* 23(7): 641-646.

Sommer, H.M., and S.W. Vallentyne. 1995. Effect of foot posture on the incidence of medial tibial stress syndrome. *Medicine and Science in Sports and Exercise* 27(6): 800-804.

Chapter 11

Biomechanical Considerations in Turnout

Karen S. Clippinger, MSPE

External rotation at the hip (turnout) is a unique requirement of many dance techniques, and one of the most important. No other athletic activity emphasizes it to the same extent, and it is seldom an issue in our everyday lives. Unfortunately, as this chapter explains, (1) the biomechanics of turnout are quite complex; (2) very few dancers are endowed by nature with the ability to achieve "perfect" turnout; and (3) the practice of "forcing" turnout can cause a variety of injuries.

Turnout presents a unique challenge in many dance forms. One of the most important aspects of turnout is optimal external rotation of the femur at the hip such that the knees and feet face as close to directly side as possible. Correct turnout requires appropriate strength, flexibility, and neural activation patterns at the hip. Although anatomical constraints are an important underlying limiting factor, dancers can improve their turnout with a better understanding of proper biomechanics and with supplemental exercises. Correct turnout is essential not only for skill development but also for injury prevention. Many of the overuse injuries that occur in dance may be related to improper turnout and the resultant excessive stresses at the back, hip, knee, and foot.

Turnout is also discussed in chapters 2, 4, 5, 6, and 9.

Anatomical Constraints

"Perfect" or "ideal" turnout is classically described as a position with the feet and knees facing directly sideways (180°), such that a straight line could be drawn between the first and second toe of the right foot, right heel, left heel, and between the first and second toe of the left foot (figure 11.1). Theoretically, a large portion of this rotation should be accomplished at the hip joint rather than by excessively rotating the lower leg (tibia) outward relative to the upper leg, or by excessive twisting at the ankle-foot. Although the topic is still under investigation, one study of elite

ballet dancers (Hamilton et al. 1992) and another of ballet students (Khan et al. 1997) showed that approximately 60% of turnout came from the hip. A study of elite female ballet dancers by this author showed an average of 59° of hip external rotation, suggesting that for the average dancer approximately 66% of the ideal 90° of turnout was coming from the hip (Clippinger 1991). However, given that in reality even many elite ballet dancers do not stand with their feet facing directly side, the hip external rotation measured in two of these studies (Clippinger 1991; Hamilton et al. 1992) could represent a higher percentage of the turnout actually used in dance. Although few dancers possess perfect turnout, most strive to get as close to the ideal as their bodies will allow. Range of motion at the hip, and hence a substantial portion of optimal turnout, is determined by anatomical constraints including bony, ligamentous, and musculotendinous factors.

Bony, Musculotendinous, and Ligamentous Constraints

The orientation and shape of the acetabulum, the socket of the pelvis in which the head of the femur sits, is important in determining potential turnout (figure 11.2a). Furthermore, the angle of the neck of the femur relative to the long shaft of the femur (angle of femoral neck anteversion or retroversion) is crucial in determining the amount of external rotation at the hip (Hoppenfeld 1976). Excessive femoral neck anteversion (figure 11.2b) is commonly associated with the tendency to toe in, and is considered undesirable for dance. Femoral neck retroversion (figure 11.2c) is commonly associated with the tendency to toe out, and will allow much greater external rotation at the hip; hence, it is considered desirable for dance forms emphasizing turnout. It is commonly held that most children are born with femoral neck anteversion, and that this angle decreases with maturation (Sammarco 1983). In normal adult skeletons the range is approximately 38° anteversion to 20° retroversion, with an average of 8° anteversion (Thomasen 1982). It used to be believed that the starting angle and degree of change were in large part structurally determined; however, there is some support for the argument that function can play a powerful role. Dancers who begin train-

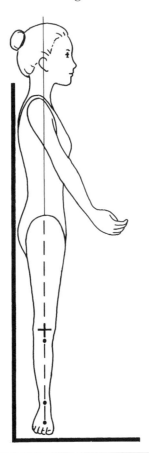

Figure 11.1 With correct turnout the midpoint of the kneecap is aligned over the long axis of the foot, while the torso remains vertical and the longitudinal arches of the foot are maintained. With perfect turnout the knees would be facing directly to the side so that a straight line is formed by the feet.

Illustration by Mary Cosenza.

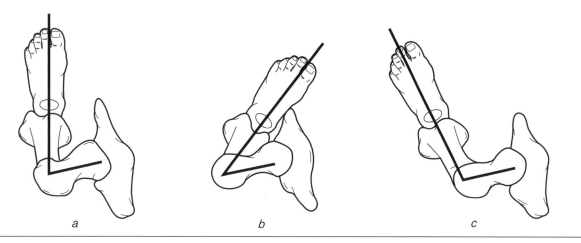

Figure 11.2   Femoral neck anteversion and retroversion with associated rotation: *(a)* normal hip, *(b)* femoral neck anteversion with associated femoral internal rotation, and *(c)* femoral neck retroversion with associated femoral external rotation.
Illustration courtesy of Karen Clippinger.

ing before 11 years of age may be able to alter the actual angle of the femoral neck to enhance turnout (Hamilton et al. 1992; Sammarco 1983). Although the issue is still under debate, careful stretching in the commonly used "frog position" (prone, double passé position), and dynamic technique training, may affect structural changes in young dancers.

Muscles and their adjoining tendons also limit motion at the hip. Increases in flexibility of the musculotendinous complex can be produced through dance movements that require a large range of motion at the hips, strengthening exercises that use a full range of motion, or stretching exercises.

After about 11 years of age it seems unlikely that the femoral neck can be molded; changes are restricted to the joint capsule, ligaments, and musculotendinous structures. The strong hip ligaments form thickened bands of the hip joint capsule, and both structures play important roles in limiting joint mobility. One particularly important ligament for the dancer is the iliofemoral ligament. This is the strongest ligament in the body, and it limits how far the femur can rotate externally and how far the leg can be brought behind the body (hip extension and hyperextension) (Gray, Pickering, and Howden 1974). Early stretching of this ligament and the closely associated capsule may be important for achieving maximal turnout. Dancers who genetically have extreme ligamental laxity may have excellent turnout even with a less than optimal angle of femoral neck retroversion.

> Figures 11.5 and 11.6 feature two effective stretches for the iliofemoral ligament.

This early plasticity of key anatomical structures provides rationale for early dance training, especially for the aspiring classical ballet dancer. Potential improvements in turnout in the older dancer are probably limited to gains allowed by the musculotendinous complex, and perhaps to some extent the joint capsule and ligaments. It is likely that the femoral neck can no longer be molded; also, the degree to which capsule and ligaments can be stretched, and whether rigorous stretching of these structures can have long-term negative effects, are controversial issues requiring further scientific investigation.

Methods of Stretching

Recommended methods of stretching include static and proprioceptive neuromuscular facilitation (PNF) techniques utilized when the muscles are already warm (i.e., after barre, center floor warm-up, or at the end of class). With static techniques, a position that places the desired muscle and related connective tissue in a position of elongation is maintained for 30 seconds. The magnitude of the stretch should be moderate, so that a sensation of stretch but not pain is experienced. An effort should be made to "relax" the muscle that is undergoing the stretch. Flexibility gains can be enhanced by repeating the same stretch about three times (Garrett 1990).

Flexibility and stretching are also discussed in chapters 9, 12, and 13.

Proprioceptive neuromuscular facilitation techniques attempt to alter neural input influencing muscle extensibility to improve flexibility. One common version, contract/relax, utilizes a 10-second contraction of the muscle followed by 10 seconds of "relaxation," during which the same muscle is passively stretched. This procedure is generally repeated three times, and a static stretch of 30 seconds or more is added at the end. For example, using the hamstring stretch shown in figure 11.3, the dancer first contracts the hamstring for 10 seconds by attempting to bring the right leg down toward the ground (hip extension) while the arms resist that motion. This contraction is followed by a conscious relaxation of the hamstrings as the arms are used to pull the leg closer to the chest, effecting a passive hamstring stretch. This procedure is repeated three times, each time with an attempt to bring the leg slightly closer to the chest. The third passive stretch should be maintained for 30 seconds to a minute. Proprioceptive neuromuscular facilitation techniques can be particularly useful for dancers having difficulty improving their flexibility.

Ballistic stretching involves bouncy movements with momentum used dynamically to stretch a muscle. An example is "flat-back bounces," which in the past were commonly

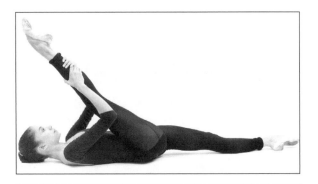

Figure 11.3 Proprioceptive neuromuscular facilitation hamstring stretch. The hamstrings are actively contracted as the dancer attempts to bring the leg away from the chest while resisting the motion with the arms. This 10-second contraction is followed by relaxation of the hamstrings as the arms are used to pull the leg closer to the chest. This sequence is repeated three times, and the final stretch is sustained for 30 seconds or longer.

Photo courtesy of Karen Clippinger.

used in jazz classes. Although ballistic stretches appear to be effective, the risk for muscle injury and muscle soreness is greater than with other stretching methods. Therefore, it is advisable (at least until further research clarifies this issue) to substitute static or PNF stretch variations that are as effective and less dangerous.

For improving turnout it is particularly important to stretch the hip internal rotators, hamstrings, hip adductors, and hip flexors. Although the latter three muscle groups may not directly limit external rotation of the hip, proper execution of many high movements to the front (e.g., grand battements or développés) requires tremendous hamstring flexibility. The hamstring stretch shown in figure 11.3 should be performed in a turned-out position as well as the parallel position shown. This variation is particularly relevant to the needs of dance and will help stretch the hip internal rotators.

Figures 11.3 and 11.4, as well as figures 12.8 and 12.9, page 161, show excellent stretches for the hip internal rotators, hamstrings, hip adductors, and hip flexors.

Correct performance of many high movements to the side requires great hamstring flexibility and marked hip adductor flexibility. One can include the adductors in the stretch shown in figure 11.3 by turning the leg out and carrying it to the side (second position). This stretch can also be performed in a side-lying position, as shown in figure 11.4. This latter variation offers an opportunity to use PNF techniques; the arms can be used to resist knee flexion, hip internal rotation, or forward movement of the leg (hip horizontal adduction). Another exercise for stretching the hip adductors is the straddle stretch (sitting with the legs in second position). To add resistance, this stretch can be carefully performed with the feet widely separated against a wall in either a sitting or supine position. Again, one can add PNF techniques by pulling the legs together as the wall resists and prevents this motion. Then, on the relaxation phase, a greater stretch can be applied by carefully bringing the pelvis closer to the wall.

Most dance movements to the back will be limited by the extensibility of the hip flexors, the hip capsule, and the iliofemoral ligament.

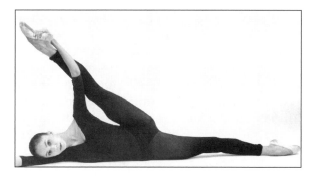

Figure 11.4 Hamstring and adductor stretch. The leg is pulled toward the head in a full externally rotated position. To add proprioceptive neuromuscular facilitation techniques, the arm can be used to resist knee flexion, internal hip rotation, or adduction.

Photo courtesy of Karen Clippinger.

Two stretches to improve hip flexor flexibility are shown in figures 11.5 and 11.6. To achieve effective gains with these stretches, particular emphasis on correct form is essential.

The most powerful hip flexor, the iliopsoas muscle, attaches onto the sides of the spine and the inside of the pelvis (ilium). Several of the other primary hip flexors, the sartorius and rectus femoris, attach onto the front of the pelvis. Due to this anatomical arrangement, either letting the low back arch or the top of the pelvis tilt forward (anterior pelvic tilt) will slacken the muscles that the dancer is attempting to stretch. To be effective, the dancer must learn to use the abdominal muscles to prevent these undesired movements. In the first stretch (figure 11.5) the dancer should concentrate on using the abdominal muscles to pull the pubic bone forward and closer to the ribs until a stretch is felt across the front of the hip (of the extended leg). As flexibility improves, the back leg can be moved farther backward and the front knee can be further bent such that the stretch is intensified. The dancer should continue to concentrate on keeping the torso vertical (rather than leaning forward) and bringing the bottom of the pelvis forward (posterior pelvic tilt). To enhance its effectiveness for dancers, this stretch should also be performed with both legs turned out.

As correct form is mastered, the more rigorous stretch shown in figure 11.6 can be added. Again, the abdominal muscles should be used to prevent an anterior pelvic tilt and emphasis should be on bringing the bottom of the pelvis forward to create the stretch. This stretch can be done with the back knee either straight or bent

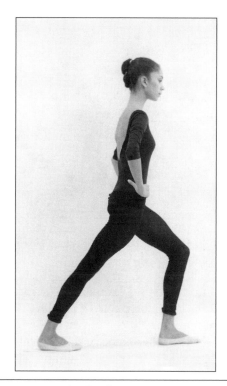

Figure 11.5 Standing hip flexor stretch. As the abdominal muscles are used to stabilize the pelvis, the dancer brings the bottom of the pelvis forward until a stretch is felt across the front of the hip.

Photo courtesy of Karen Clippinger.

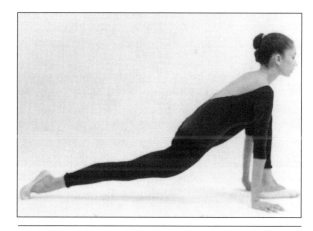

Figure 11.6 Lunge hip flexor stretch.

Photo courtesy of Karen Clippinger.

and should be performed in both parallel and turned-out positions.

Stretching of the hip internal rotators will have the most direct effect on improving turnout. This can be fostered by inclusion of an externally rotated position in each of the stretches just described (figures 11.5 and 11.6). Internal rotator flexibility can also be improved with the external

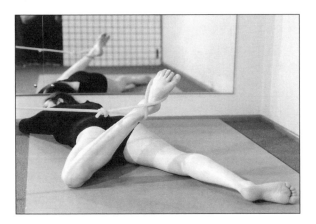

Figure 11.7   Deep outward rotator strengthening.

Photo courtesy of Karen Clippinger.

rotator strengthening exercise shown in figure 11.7. While lying prone with the knee bent to 90°, rotate outward at the hip, bringing the heel toward the opposite knee. Use surgical tubing for resistance with a "figure 8" wrapped around the ankle and the opposite end tied to something stable. Perform 10 repetitions, holding a three count with the thigh at 30°, 60°, and 90°. Allow a rest of 30 seconds to 2 minutes between sets. Be careful to keep the angle of the knee constant and rotate from the hip, rather than twisting the knee by leading with the heel. Maintain a posterior pelvic tilt and try to relax the outer gluteal muscles while emphasizing the use of the deep outward rotators.

The end position of full external rotation used in this exercise will dynamically stretch the internal rotators as well as strengthen the external rotators. However, the long-lasting effect of this dynamic stretch is unclear, and so this exercise should be used in conjunction with other static or PNF variations. For example, the PNF technique can be easily added to a standing or supine passé stretch. The standing variation can best be performed in a doorway, with the knee of the bent leg against the wall. The dancer contracts the passé leg by attempting to bring the knee forward and down (hip horizontal adduction and internal rotation) as the wall resists the motion. After relaxation of the muscles, the torso and support leg are rotated slightly farther away from the passé leg as the gesture leg is further externally rotated (i.e., greater trochanter brought closer to ischial tuberosity). The abdominal muscles should be used to maintain a neutral pelvis and prevent the low back from arching.

To perform the supine variation, the dancer uses an arm for resistance rather than the wall. It is easier to keep the hips square when performing this exercise if a double passé position is used, or if the support leg is bent with the foot pressing against the ground to lend stability. The abdominal muscles should again be firmly contracted to prevent the low back from arching. If the dancer has difficulty maintaining a neutral pelvis, a rolled towel can be placed under the bottom of the pelvis to create a slight posterior pelvic tilt. As form is perfected, the exercise can be adjusted to a neutral pelvis without the towel, focusing on using the abdominal muscles for stabilization.

For another example of a supine stretch for the internal rotators see figure 12.8, page 161.

When these positions are used to stretch the hip internal rotators or hip flexors, it should be understood that the hip capsule and ligaments often are restricting further movements, rather than the musculotendinous complex. To avoid injury it is therefore important that these stretches be performed slowly and gently, and that no hip joint pain be experienced.

Because the focus of this chapter is on improving turnout, stretches for hip extensors, hip adductors, hip flexors, and hip internal rotators have been described. However, for a rounded flexibility program for the hip, and from a perspective of injury prevention, stretches for the hip abductors and hip external rotators should also be included in the dancer's routine.

Measurement of Hip External Rotation

An estimate of the potential turnout of a dancer can be obtained by passively measuring external rotation of the hip. Three methods for doing this are shown in figure 11.8, *a* through *c*. These measures will be primarily determined by the bony, ligamentous, and musculotendinous constraints previously described. For accurate results it is vital for the pelvis to be in a neutral position, not tilted anteriorly. An anterior pelvic tilt will slacken the hip capsule and iliofemoral ligament and give a falsely high measure of external rotation. It is also important that both sides of the pelvis remain evenly in contact with the table. When the end range of external rotation of the hip is obtained, further movement of the leg will tend to produce movement of the pelvis. This is not reflective of hip external rotation, and the measurement should be taken at the point just prior to loss of a neutral pelvis. When one is performing screenings, having an assistant help maintain the pelvis in a neutral position can aid with more accurate measurement of hip external rotation.

The first measure (figure 11.8a) is performed in supine position with the knees straight and the hip extended (straight down vs. flexed). This measure will best reflect the potential turnout of the dancer when standing (with the hip in extension), and is considered the most meaningful reflection of the usual definition of turnout. When performing this measurement it is important to know that many dancers have marked ligamental laxity, which allows significant external rotation of the lower leg (tibia) relative to the upper leg (femur), and of the foot relative to the tibia. To avoid an inaccurate measurement, rotate the hip by movement of the femur rather than the foot. Also, the measure is more reflective if the examiner fully dorsiflexes the ankle with one hand to help lock the foot while placing the other hand on the inner thigh above the knee to help fully rotate the femur externally at the hip. Some examiners prefer to do this test prone with the knee flexed to about 90° (Thomasen 1982). This second technique is shown in figure 11.8b. It offers the examiner better leverage for externally rotating the hip, and is very useful for screening large numbers of dancers. However, even more care must then be taken that movement of the tibia relative to the femur is minimized and not included in the measure of rotation at the hip.

The third technique, shown in figure 11.8c, is performed with the hip flexed to 90°. Flexing the hip slackens the hip capsule and iliofemoral ligament. This measure is more reflective of turnout available in movements such as a front attitude (i.e., rotation possible with the hip in flexion). It can be performed with the dancer sitting at the edge of a table with knees flexed (as shown), or lying supine with the passive limb extended. To achieve an accurate measurement, try to isolate the rotation to the hip and limit accessory movements of the tibia relative to the femur. The examiner can help improve measurement accuracy by placing one hand above the knee to control the external rotation of the hip.

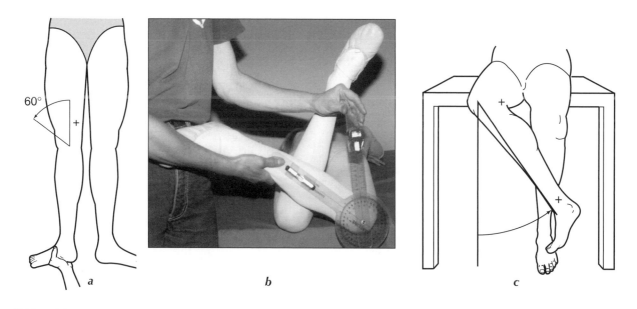

Figure 11.8 Measurement of hip external rotation (+ indicates site for placement of examiner's hands to produce external hip rotation). *(a)* Hip external rotation with the hip extended in a supine position. *(b)* Hip external rotation with the hip extended in a prone position. *(c)* Hip external rotation with the hip in flexion in a sitting position.
Photo courtesy of Karen Clippinger.

It is helpful to measure hip external rotation with the hip in both extension and flexion because the results are often quite different, and the information from both is useful in teaching students how best to maximize potential turnout. For example, many students may be lower than desired in the first measures (figure 11.8*a* or *b*), yet good with the last measure (figure 11.8*c*). In such cases, the aesthetics of the dancers' work can be significantly improved by teaching them to fully utilize their turnout in the gesture leg in the many movements performed with the hip flexed or abducted (i.e., front attitudes, extensions, kicks, ronds de jambe).

Biomechanical Constraints

Many dancers exhibit greater external rotation at the hip with the passive tests just described than they use functionally. In other words, many dancers have greater turnout than they have learned to use during dancing. This potential difference can be checked by observing a dancer (1) perform a demi-plié and rise from first position, or (2) rotate from parallel first to turned-out first position while standing with each foot on a rotator disk. The common finding of a substantial difference between these last two functional observations of turnout and the passive measurements of hip external rotation shows that factors other than bony, ligamentous, and musculotendinous constraints are involved in determining functional turnout. Two other important factors are adequate strength of key muscles and appropriate activation patterns of these muscles for optimizing correct mechanics.

Strength

The deep outward rotators and gluteus maximus are prime movers for hip external rotation, while the sartorius, biceps femoris, and gluteus medius (posterior fibers) can assist with external rotation in some positions. While some anatomists hold that the iliopsoas and hip adductors may aid slightly with external rotation, recent studies suggest this is probably not the case (Basmajian 1978; Rasch 1989; Smith, Weiss, and Lehmkuhl 1996).

When the focus is on turnout in dance, special attention should be given to the six deep outward rotators (figure 11.9). These muscles are capable

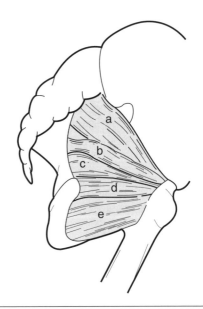

Figure 11.9 Deep outward rotators of the hip. The six deep outward rotators of the hip span the pelvis and the femur and comprise the following muscles: *(a)* piriformis, *(b)* gemellus superior, *(c)* obturator internus, *(d)* gemellus inferior, *(e)* quadratus femoris, and obturator externus (the latter is located behind quadratus femoris and not visible in this view).

Illustration courtesy of Karen Clippinger.

of producing the desired external rotation with minimal secondary actions. This capability is important both for optimizing range of motion and for achieving the desired dance aesthetic. For example, since the gluteus maximus causes hip extension as well as external rotation, when the muscle contracts it will tend to produce both of these actions. In movements such as a front attitude, where the desired action is hip flexion and external rotation, the undesired opposite action of hip extension of the gluteus maximus can limit range of motion (i.e., how high the leg can be lifted). Similarly, the sartorius and gluteus medius produce hip abduction as well as external rotation, so their unbalanced use can often produce a slight unintended hip abduction instead of the desired isolated external rotation. In dance terminology, this abduction can contribute to "lifting the hip," or "hip-hiking," and is considered an undesirable aesthetic by most schools of dance.

As specific use of the deep outward rotators enhances turnout, they should be strengthened with the exercise shown in figure 11.7. In this exercise it is important that the movement occur at the hip, that there be no twisting of the lower leg relative to the upper leg. Abdominal muscles are used throughout the exercise to prevent the pelvis from tilting forward and the spine from arching. The dancer should focus on relaxing the outer gluteus maximus and using the deep outward rotators. One can sometimes aid this muscle emphasis by having the dancer place his or her hand at the base of the buttocks while concentrating on tightening the lower muscles under the gluteus maximus.

If discomfort is felt at the knee, an exercise with the knee extended should be substituted. The dancer lies on his or her side and lifts the upper leg (hip abduction) with the knee facing toward the ceiling (i.e., in full external rotation at the hip). The heel of the top leg should be kept 1 or 2 in. (2.5 or 5 cm) behind the bottom heel (i.e., the femur of the top hip should be in about 5° of hyperextension) throughout the exercise. To achieve the desired use of the deep outward rotators the following sequence is often helpful. (1) The dancer raises the rotated leg about 10° and holds this position for three counts. (2) The dancer attempts to add hip outward rotation without letting the leg come forward (i.e., focus on rotating along the long axis of the femur to bring the heel further around). Maintaining this additional rotation, the leg is raised another 20° and held three counts. (3) The dancer adds further rotation, raises the leg 20° more, and holds a final three counts. The initial emphasis in this exercise is on maximizing the degree of rotation while limiting how high the leg is raised. Throughout the exercise, correct pelvic and torso alignment should be maintained. As strength and isolation improve, ankle weights, elastic bands, or surgical tubing can be used to provide additional resistance, and the height to which the leg is lifted can be gradually increased.

As with flexibility exercises, muscle groups in addition to the deep rotators become important for optimizing turnout in common dance movements. Movements to the front also require adequate hip flexor strength. Movements to the side require adequate strength of the hip abductors as well as the hip flexors. Movements to the back require adequate hip extensor strength. Examples of strengthening exercises for a few of these key muscles follow.

Specific Muscle Activation Patterns

When one is performing dance movements that use turnout, selection of appropriate muscles, the timing of their activation, and the relative magnitude of their activation are important for maximizing turnout.

Second Position Grand Plié

Pliés are one of the most fundamental movements in the dance vocabulary, and therefore are a good place to begin improving turnout. In performance of pliés, one can often enhance turnout by emphasizing use of the deep outward rotator muscles and hip adductors while maintaining a vertical torso and pelvis. This technique modification is usually easiest to achieve using a second position (figure 11.10a). A helpful exercise is to perform second position grand pliés with the back against a wall and the heels 1 or 2 in. (2.5 or 5 cm) away from the wall. The mid-thoracic spine and mid-sacrum should remain in contact with the wall throughout the exercise. Use of the deep outward rotators can be encouraged by (1) putting the fingertips at the base of the buttocks and feeling the muscles contract; (2) attempting to pull the outside of the thigh (greater trochanter) closer to the bottom of the back of the pelvis (ischial tuberosity); or (3) keeping the knees as close to the wall as possible throughout both the down- and up-phase of the plié.

Since proper turnout motion occurs as close to a frontal plane as the dancer's structure will allow, the hip adductors are in an appropriate location to provide assistance (figure 11.10b). Adductors potentially work eccentrically on the down-phase of the plié and concentrically on the up-phase. Most dancers are able to cue into the concentric or shortening phase of a muscle more easily. Therefore, another hint is to encourage dancers to wrap the back of the leg to the inside and pull the inner thighs together and up when rising from the plié. Once they have cued into the use of these muscles on the up-phase, they can usually transfer the muscle use to the down-phase. On the down-phase, cues such as "rotate and reach the knees directly side rather than allowing them to fall forward and inside the feet," or "stretch the inner thighs away from each other," can sometimes help emphasize the desired

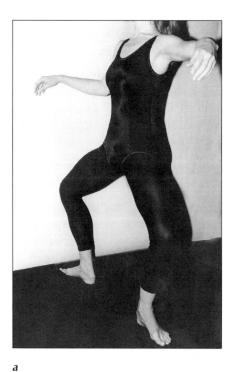

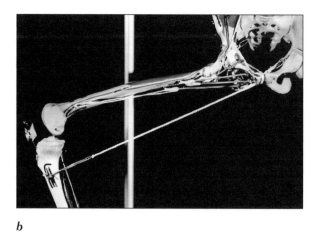

a   b

Figure 11.10 *(a)* Use of the hip adductors in second position grand-plié. The adductors are in an appropriate position to work eccentrically on the down-phase, and concentrically on the up-phase, of the plié. *(b)* Line of pull of the adductors, showing how the use of turnout puts these muscles in an appropriate position to assist with pliés.

Photos courtesy of Karen Clippinger.

adductor use. Performing these second position pliés immediately following adductor strengthening exercises, while awareness is heightened, can also encourage use of the adductors.

Lifting the lower leg while in a side-lying position can strengthen adductors. The top leg is in a passé position, with the toes just touching the ground behind the bottom knee to aid in balance. A weight can be added at the ankle or above the knee of the lower leg to increase resistance. The hip adductors can also be strengthened with the use of surgical tubing to resist bringing the leg toward the midline while in a turned-out supine position. For less isolated but more functional strengthening, second position turned-out pliés can be performed in a shuttle, on a Pilates reformer, or using a leg press.

Maintaining a vertical torso can also enhance turnout. During this exercise (second position wall plié), one ensures the vertical position by sliding the back against the wall, keeping the mid-thoracic spine and mid-sacrum in contact as the knees bend and straighten. This procedure can help counter the common tendency that many dancers have to lean forward (slight hip flexion)

during pliés. Leaning forward is often accompanied by an anterior tilt of the pelvis, decreased turnout, and use of the quadriceps femoris muscles. Although further investigation is necessary, preliminary findings suggest that a balanced co-contraction of the hip adductors, hamstrings, and quadriceps (vs. quadriceps dominance) is desirable for optimizing turnout (Clippinger-Robertson et al. 1986). When dancers are cued to bring their knees more to the side versus forward (in an effort to increase femoral external rotation at the hip), greater use of the hip adductors and hamstrings is often noted, accompanied by a decrease in quadriceps activation.

Développé à la Seconde

As with pliés, proper activation patterns are essential for optimizing turnout during movements involving lifting the leg to the side. For example, in performance of a développé à la seconde (see figure 11.11, *a-d*), specific use of the deep outward rotators is necessary to enhance elevation and minimize undesired lifting of the hip (Clippinger-Robertson 1988). Dance teachers describe this as "dropping the hip under before

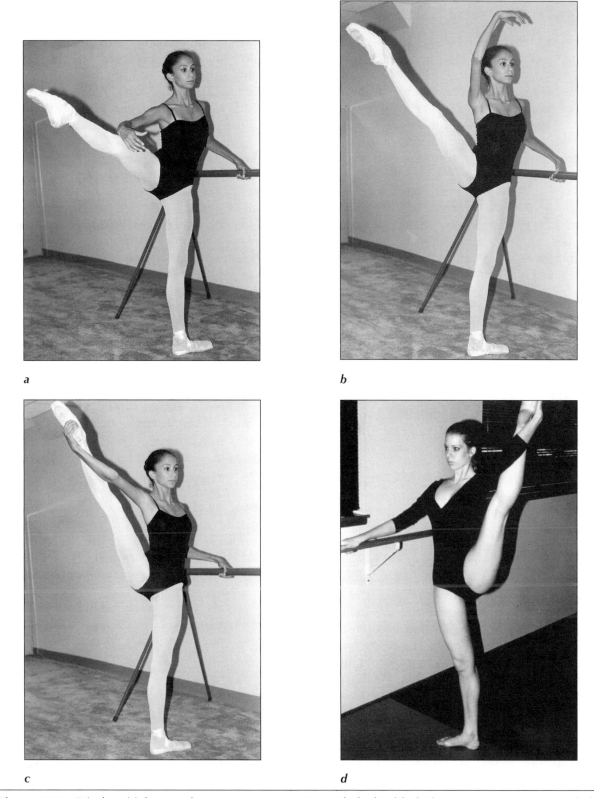

Figure 11.11 Développé à la seconde. *(a)* Incorrect execution with the hip lifted; *(b)* more correct position, with the greater trochanter of the femur coming closer to the ischial tuberosity (note that height of the leg is limited by current strength levels); *(c)* more correct position and greater height with assistance from the hand, showing potential turnout as strength develops; *(d)* ideal position.

Photos courtesy of Karen Clippinger.

145

lifting the leg up" in a développé. The anatomical correlate to this directive is to bring the projection on the outer part of the upper femur (greater trochanter) "down"—closer to the bottom of the pelvis (ischial tuberosity)—through use of the lower deep outward rotators and appropriate use of other hip muscles. With proper activation and timing, these muscles rotate the femur externally and pull the greater trochanter down, so that the process clears and maximum elevation of the leg to the side can be achieved. To help dancers accomplish these proper mechanics it is helpful to focus on the lower rotators, working to rotate the leg fully and bring the trochanter down at the very beginning of the développé. This can help counter the upward pull of the gluteal muscles. The focus can then be shifted to thinking of bringing the knee slightly behind the shoulder and reaching the foot toward the ceiling as the knee is extended. As the correctness of execution of the développé improves (figure 11.11, *a-d*), the knee faces further backward (i.e., there is greater femoral external rotation), there is less lifting of the hip (i.e., lateral pelvic tilt), and more of the desired elevation of the leg is achieved.

Activating and Strengthening the Iliopsoas

Often when dancers attempt to change their mechanics as described thus far in the chapter, they find they can bring the leg higher, but have inadequate strength to hold it in the fully extended position. This is because they are using different muscles than those that have been developed with years of training. To aid in this transition it is important to strengthen the deep outward rotators and the iliopsoas. Exercises for strengthening the deep outward rotators have already been described (figure 11.7). The iliopsoas is a powerful hip flexor that is also important in the upper ranges of hip abduction. Many of the other hip muscles are not able to produce much force above 90°, so the iliopsoas is particularly important when lifting the leg high to the side or front. Furthermore, using an externally rotated position shifts the line of pull of the muscles so the hip flexors in general become more important in producing movement that in parallel position would be carried out primarily by the hip abductors.

An exercise for strengthening the iliopsoas is shown in figure 11.12. When first performing this exercise the dancer should sit in a tucked position (posterior pelvic tilt). This increases the ability of the iliopsoas to produce force (length-tension principle) and helps isolate the muscle. The surgical tubing used for resistance should be anchored directly below the body, with the other end looped above the knee. One hand can be placed on the loop on the thigh to keep it from sliding. Relax the quadriceps and use the deeper, higher muscle (iliopsoas). Perform two sets in the upper 30° of hip flexion, and one set in the full arc from the chair. Use a three-count hold at the top of the arc. As strength and muscle isolation improve, one set with a neutral pelvis (sitting straight up vs. tucked) and one set using a turned-out position can be added. After six weeks of performing the exercise, increase the number of sets to the side and the front. This will strengthen the needed combination of hip flexors and abductors. Although the variation to the side can be done as before while sitting in a chair, it is often easier for dancers to begin by performing this exercise while lying on the side. These alterations will develop the specific strength needed when working to the side with développés, grand battements, and so on, while the initial exercise (figure 11.12) will best transfer to frontal movements. Since these exercises use a restricted range of motion, they should be followed by a stretch for the hip flexors (for example, figures 11.5 and 11.6).

To facilitate transfer of the strength aspect of these exercises to dance technique, a position can be used with the knee extended and a weight on the ankle for resistance while sitting, standing, or side-lying. To work in higher ranges use the hands to raise the leg slightly higher than it can go unaided; then let go of the leg and either hold the position for three to five counts or control the lowering back down to the barre (standing) or floor (sitting) (Clippinger-Robertson 1988). In this latter exercise the weight of the leg provides adequate resistance, so no additional weight is needed.

General Principles of Muscle Activation

Each dance movement involves a different combination of muscles with optimal timing and activation to maximize turnout and correct technique. However, some common principles apply. (1) Emphasize use of a neutral pelvis with

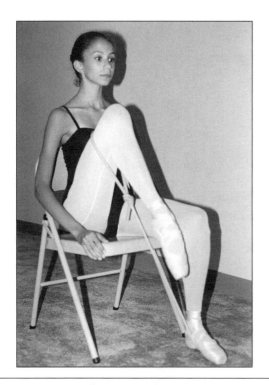

Figure 11.12 Hip flexor strengthening.

Photo courtesy of Karen Clippinger.

the body's center of gravity appropriately placed over the feet. Avoid the common errors of linking an excessive anterior pelvic tilt, posterior pelvic tilt, lateral pelvic tilt, or rotation of the pelvis with movements of the legs. (2) When performing any type of plié, emphasize using the deep outward rotators and hip adductors and keeping the knees reaching as far side as the dancer's turnout allows. (3) Begin movements involving lifting the leg by emphasizing use of the deep outward rotators first to fully rotate the femur externally in the socket (without linked pelvic compensations), and then lift the leg in the desired direction. (4) For movements to the front or side, emphasize use of the iliopsoas with the outside of the thigh "wrapping under" rather than lifting or rotating forward. (5) In work with a dancer who is having difficulty making these technique modifications, perform strengthening exercises for improving both strength and awareness of the muscle and its use (the exercises in chapter 9 are useful for this purpose). In all directions, strengthening of the deep outward rotators should be included. For movements to the front add exercises for the hip flexors (especially iliopsoas). For movements to the side (where the leg is raised in the

air) include hip abductors. For movements to the back include exercises for the hip extensors (especially hamstrings).

> Some effective exercises for hip flexors, hip abductors, and hip extensors include prone leg curls and leg presses, as well as straight-leg raises done prone, both parallel and turned out.

Implications of Improper Turnout

Although additional turnout does come from below the hip—the "normal" relative contribution of external rotation of the knee, tibial torsion, and ankle-foot motion is still under investigation (Garrick and Requa 1994; Hamilton et al. 1992; Khan et al. 1997; Worthen, Patten, and Hamill 1998)—excessive rotation from the knee downward is likely detrimental. This improper technique is sometimes termed "screwing the knee," or "forced turnout," and it can produce extreme torsion (figure 11.13). The tendency to twist the lower leg out relative to the femur can be even more pronounced if the knees are bent. Because the knee is a modified rather than true hinge joint, with 90° of knee flexion as much as 40° to 50° of external rotation of the tibia is possible (Frankel and Nordin 1980). Hence, it is easy to bring the heels forward when the knees are bent (e.g., at the base of a grand plié), which results in greater turnout of the feet, but also an extreme torsional stress to the knees when they are straightened. This torsion is conducive to injury of the knee and kneecap (Winslow and Yoder 1995). It also alters the mechanics above and below the knee and can contribute to certain injuries of the spine, hip, shin, ankle, and foot. In my clinical experience with dancers, a large percentage of the overuse injuries in the lower body are related to improper turnout.

> Overuse injuries are also discussed in chapters 1, 5, 7, 8, and 14.

Besides increasing the risk for injury, improper turnout can interfere with skill development. The

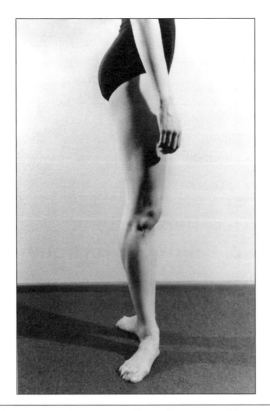

Figure 11.13 Incorrect or "forced" turnout, with greater turnout of the feet than the hips and marked twisting of the tibia relative to the femur.

Photo courtesy of Karen Clippinger.

dance student using improper turnout often develops unintentional compensations in order to maintain balance. For example, a common pattern accompanying forced turnout includes pronated feet (arches rolling in), hyperextended knees with relative internal rotation of the femur, an anterior pelvic tilt, and the ribs sticking forward (arched spine with torso in front of the desired plumb line). Such compensations distort proper alignment and the desired aesthetic, while making it hard to develop the difficult technical skills required of the advanced and professional dancer. In addition, such poor habits do not adequately develop strength, flexibility, or activation patterns of the muscles needed to improve turnout or achieve proper biomechanics.

Ankle and foot rotation is also discussed in chapters 4, 13, and 14.

In the teaching of dance, the cue is often used to guide the kneecap over the long axis of the foot (line between the first and second toes). Figure 11.14 shows correct turnout. Since the tibia tends to be slightly rotated externally at the knee, and natural toe-out of the foot relative to the tibia is generally about 15°,* the average dancer can probably turn the feet out about 15° to 20° more than the knee without creating excessive torsion stresses at the knee. Nonetheless, when working with dancers at the barre or center floor it can be helpful to cue to guide the "kneecap over the foot" as the knee bends, so that maximal development of hip external rotation is encouraged

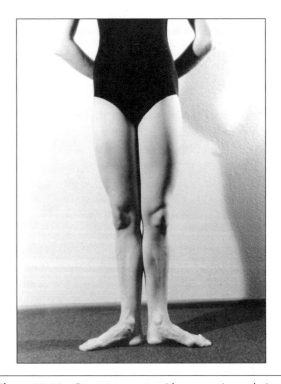

Figure 11.14 Correct turnout, with appropriate relationship between hip external rotation and knee and foot alignment.

Photo courtesy of Karen Clippinger.

*This measure refers to the degree of tibial torsion or malleolar torsion present. There is a marked individual variation with this measure and researchers differ in average values given to it, due to different measurement methods, age of subjects, and the populations studied. Thomasen (1982) uses 15° of tibial torsion as an average measure, and Gray (1984) uses 13° to 18° as average adult values. For the purpose of this chapter, 15° was chosen as average. It is interesting to note that when the femoral condyles are held in a neutral plane, Gray considers values as high as 30° of external rotation (measured relative to the hip malleolar axis) as normal (Gray 1988).

and compensations such as foot pronation are discouraged.

Using the criteria just described, the external rotation possible at the hip will determine the placement of the feet. For many dance forms, including modern and jazz, this approach is acceptable. However, for many professional training schools in classical ballet, a position of the feet close to 180° is an aesthetic prerequisite. Thomasen (1982) holds that since the lower leg is generally rotated out about 5° at the knee, and the normal ankle joint has an axis with external rotation of 15°, external rotation of 70° at the hip is needed to achieve classical turnout (Frankel and Nordin 1980). He recommends that dancers with less than 60° of hip external rotation (measured prone with the hip extended and knee bent) after age 15 be advised to stop classical ballet training. Although many experts might argue against using such a specific figure due to the difference in turnout measurement techniques and results, the lack of clarity regarding how much turnout can change with training, and the complexity of injury etiology, this perhaps harsh approach points to the difficulty of achieving the desired classical dance aesthetic and avoiding injuries if inadequate hip turnout is present (Hamilton et al. 1992, 1997; Meniel and Atwater 1988). In my experience there are dancers whose artistry and other technical expertise allow them to be successful professional ballet dancers with less turnout than this. It is probably wise, nonetheless, to counsel "ballet hopefuls" with very limited turnout to explore other options for dance or dance-related careers. Those with moderate turnout should be carefully evaluated and recommendations for training based on a composite of artistry, talent, functional considerations, and structural characteristics. It is important to remember that dance is an art form, and there is more to the form than turnout.

Conclusion

Turnout is influenced by the orientation of the acetabulum, the angle of femoral neck anteversion or retroversion, capsular constraints, ligamental constraints, and musculotendinous constraints. These anatomical factors can be improved by early training that emphasizes proper turnout from the hip and careful stretching. However, additional areas whose importance is frequently underestimated include strength and appropri-

ate muscle activation patterns to optimize biomechanics. In my clinical experience most dancers improve their use of turnout by 15° to 30° through specific strengthening of the deep outward rotators and refined muscle use. Successful optimization of turnout often requires correct mechanics, specific flexibility and strengthening exercises, and appropriate use of the muscles involved.

References

Basmajian, J.V. 1978. *Muscles alive.* 4th ed. Baltimore: Williams & Wilkins.

Clippinger, K.S. 1991. Flexibility among different levels of ballet dancers. Presented at the first annual symposium of the International Association for Dance Medicine & Science, Baltimore, MD.

Clippinger-Robertson, K. 1988. Principles of dance training. In *Science of dance training,* edited by P.M. Clarkson and M. Skrinar. Champaign, IL: Human Kinetics.

Clippinger-Robertson, K.S., R.S. Hutton, D.I. Miller, and T.R. Nichols. 1986. Mechanical and anatomical factors relating to the incidence and etiology of patellofemoral pain in dancers. In *The dancer as athlete,* edited by C.G. Shell. Champaign, IL: Human Kinetics.

Frankel, V., and M. Nordin. 1980. *Basic biomechanics of the skeletal system.* Philadelphia: Lea & Febiger.

Garrett, W. 1990. Muscle strain injuries: Clinical and basic aspects. *Medicine and Science in Sports and Exercise* 22(4): 436-443.

Garrick, J., and R. Requa. 1994. Turnout and training in dance. *Medical Problems of Performing Artists* 9(2): 43-49.

Gray, G. 1984. *When the feet hit the ground everything changes.* Toledo: American Physical Rehabilitation Network, 98.

Gray, G. 1988. Personal communication, Gary Gray Associates, Adna, MI.

Gray, H., P. Pickering, and R. Howden. 1974. *Gray's anatomy.* Philadelphia: Running Press.

Hamilton, W., L. Hamilton, P. Marshall, and M. Molnar. 1992. A profile of the musculoskeletal characteristics of elite professional ballet dancers. *American Journal of Sports Medicine* 20(3): 267-273.

Hamilton, L., W.G. Hamilton, M.P. Warren, K. Keller, and M. Molnar. 1997. Factors contributing to the attrition rate in elite ballet students. *Journal of Dance Medicine & Science* 1(4): 131-137.

Hoppenfeld, S. 1976. *Physical examination of the spine and extremities.* New York: Appleton-Century-Crofts.

Khan, K., P. Roberts, C. Nattrass, K. Bennell, W. Mayes, S. Way, J. Brown, J. McMeeken, and J. Wark. 1997. Hip and ankle range of motion in elite classical ballet dancers and controls. *Clinical Journal of Sports Medicine* 7(3): 174-179.

Meniel, K., and A. Atwater. 1988. An analysis of components of the "turnout" in beginning and advanced ballet dancers. *Medicine and Science in Sports and Exercise* 20(Suppl. 2): 2-6.

Rasch, P.J. 1989. *Kinesiology and applied anatomy.* 7th ed. Philadelphia: Lea & Febiger.

Sammarco, G.J. 1983. The dancer's hip. *Clinics in Sports Medicine* 2(3): 485-498.

Smith, L., E. Weiss, and D. Lehmkuhl. 1996. *Brunnstrom's clinical kinesiology.* Philadelphia: Davis.

Thomasen, E. 1982. *Diseases and injuries of ballet dancers.* Denmark: Universitetsforlaget I. Arhus.

Winslow, J., and E. Yoder. 1995. Patellofemoral pain in female ballet dancers: Correlation with iliotibial band tightness and tibial external rotation. *Journal of Orthopaedic and Sports Physical Therapy* 22(1): 18-21.

Worthen, L., C. Patten, and J. Hamill. 1998. A kinematic analysis of internal/external rotation at the knee joint during two ballet movements (abstract). *Journal of Dance Medicine & Science* 2(4): 153.

Recommended Readings (Editors)

Brown, T., and L.J. Micheli. 1998. Dance: Where artistry meets injury. *Biomechanics* V(9): 12-24.

Coplan, J.A. 2002. Ballet dancer's turnout and its relationship to self-reported injury. *Journal of Orthopaedic and Sports Physical Therapy* 32(11): 579-584.

Garrick, J.G., and R.K. Requa. 1994. Turnout and training in ballet. *Medical Problems of Performing Artists* 9(2): 43-49.

Gilbert, G.B., M.T. Gross, and K.B. Klug. 1998. Relationship between hip external rotation and turnout angle for the five classical ballet positions. *Journal of Orthopaedic and Sports Physical Therapy* 27(5): 339-347.

Khan, K., K. Bennell, S. Ng, B. Matthews, P. Roberts, C. Nattrass, S. Way, and J. Brown. 2000. Can 16-18 year-old elite ballet dancers improve their hip and ankle range of motion over a 12-month period? *Clinical Journal of Sport Medicine* 10(2): 98-10.

LiGreci-Mangini, L.A. 1993-1994. A comparison of hip range of motion between professional ballerinas and age-/sex-matched nondancers. *Kinesiology and Medicine for Dance* 16(1): 19-30.

Solomon, R. 1988. *Anatomy as a master image in training dancers* (videorecording). Santa Cruz, CA: 1 videocassette; 59 minutes; color; 1/2 inch, VHS or Beta. (Available from Princeton Books, Pennington, NJ.)

Stone, D. 2001. Hip problems in dancers. *Journal of Dance Medicine & Science* 5(1): 7-10.

Chapter 12

The Neuroanatomical and Biomechanical Basis of Flexibility Exercises in Dance

Robert E. Stephens, PhD

From a scientific point of view this is the most technically challenging chapter in the book. It is uniquely valuable, however, in that it offers what is, to the best of our knowledge, the most comprehensive explanation in the literature of dance medicine of the role played by the central and peripheral nervous systems in providing the impulses that allow muscles to stretch in a safe and effective manner.

Having outlined the neuroanatomical factors that contribute to flexibility, it concludes with some very practical guidelines, and a series of specific exercises (based on proprioceptive neuromuscular facilitation), for stretching those muscle groups that are most vulnerable to dance injuries. There is an interesting contrast between the stretching techniques advocated here and in the next chapter.

Flexibility is a critical factor in the overall fitness of a dancer. Although dancers are generally limber, many have limited range of motion due to tight muscles in specific areas. It is important that dancers and dance teachers understand the basics of safe and effective stretching techniques. This chapter discusses the importance of flexibility exercises, central and peripheral factors in flexibility, eight guidelines for safe and effective stretching, and four of the best flexibility exercises for dancers.

The Purpose of Flexibility Exercises

Proper performance of any dance technique requires maximum range of motion of the joints of the spine and extremities and extremely supple, flexible muscles. Understandably, professional dancers frequently develop specific muscle imbalances as a result of their dance training. The most common areas are the rotator muscles of the hips and the triceps surae (gastrocnemius and soleus muscles). This tendency to muscle imbalance should be addressed through flexibility exercises, which in turn should be *training specific* for dancers; that is, they should prepare the dancer to perform the specific movements that are characteristic of better or safer dancing. Proprioception, or position-sense, exercises should be regularly incorporated into a flexibility program. The circumduction movement involved in rond de jambe à terre (en dedans and en dehors), for example, is an excellent proprioceptive training exercise for the deep musculature of the hip joint.

If a dancer has been injured it is very important that he or she maintain strength and flexibility during the rehabilitation period. This is an optimal time to re-educate the body for returning to dance and preventing further injuries. Hence, flexibility exercises serve a therapeutic function.

Having a trained dancer visualize a mental image or images of the correct sequence of a motor movement pattern will facilitate proper performance of the movement. Intense visualization of the elements of complex movement patterns during relaxation apparently results in a sequential firing of gamma motor neurons in preparation for performance of the movement. This gamma motor activity controls proprioception sensitivity and muscle tone and has a direct positive influence upon the accuracy and quality of the potential subsequent muscle contraction. By intensely visualizing the basic components of a combination of dance steps, for example, it is possible to have a "rehearsal" effect upon the efficient sequential firing of the gamma motor system. Performance can be enhanced through this mechanism. Therefore, visualization and relaxation techniques should be incorporated into the flexibility regimen.

Motor Activity and Muscle Flexibility

The motor system portion of the nervous system is a complex intermingling of subsystems that initiate, modify, control, and coordinate all motor movement patterns, from those that are simply postural to precise movements of the limbs. The motor system controls muscle tone, which is defined as the resistance a muscle provides to passive movement or stretching of its associated limb.

Muscle flexibility is definitely affected by muscle tone. Likewise, muscle tone is the foundation for muscle flexibility and movement. For example, individuals who have had a stroke in the motor region of the cerebral cortex may exhibit plasticity of postural or limb musculature. Plasticity is the increased resistance of muscles to passive movement in one direction. The person may have chronically contracted flexors of the upper extremity (e.g., biceps brachii and forearm flexors) and extensors of the lower extremity (e.g., the psoas, quadriceps femoris, and triceps surae). The increased muscle tone (hypertonia) or "tightness" of these muscle groups would demonstrate a drastic reduction in muscle flexibility. There would be increased resistance to passive extension of the upper extremity and flexion of the lower extremity.

However, the motor system is not the only factor that controls or determines muscle flexibility. There are a number of central and peripheral factors that contribute to muscle flexibility (figure 12.1). Effective stretching techniques may utilize one or more of these central and peripheral factors in order to increase muscle flexibility. The three major mechanisms of improving flexibility involve altering the descending influences from the reticular formation in the brain through the use of relaxation and visualization techniques; utilizing spinal reflexes such as the autogenic inhibition, reciprocal inhibition, and gamma reflex pathways; and emphasizing biomechanical factors that elongate the plastic (permanent) elements of the connective tissue surrounding the muscle fibers. Each of these mechanisms is based upon the proper utilization of the central and peripheral factors that control muscle flexibility.

The Limbic System and Cerebral Cortex

Muscle tone and, to a certain degree, flexibility are controlled primarily by intricate complex neuroanatomical and neurophysiological mechanisms. Probably the most sophisticated of these—and certainly the least appreciated by dancers in terms of their contribution—are the extensive influences of the cerebral cortex and the limbic system. The prefrontal lobe of the cerebrum has a potentially powerful effect upon the initiation and modification of emotional behavior, while the limbic system tends to set the basic or primal emotional "tone" of a particular behavioral response.

Both of these areas of the brain can have an obvious effect on muscle tone, relaxation, and, ultimately, flexibility, because of their strong input into the reticular formation, which controls

FLEXIBILITY FACTORS

Central factors

Limbic system and cerebral cortex

> Emotional and behavioral input from the limbic system and the prefrontal lobes of the cerebral cortex affects muscle tone via the reticular formation.

Motor systems

> Descending pathways from the reticular formation, vestibular, extrapyramidal and pyramidal systems influence muscle tone and movement.

Sensory pathways

> ### *Proprioception*
>
> Information from receptors in the muscles as well as specialized input from the visual and vestibular systems provide essential cues as to the position of the body and limbs in space.
>
> ### *Tactile*
>
> Various types of receptors in the skin for general and discriminative touch supply information about weight distribution over the supporting body part and physical contact between body parts and with other dancers.

Spinal cord reflex pathways

> Myotatic reflex
>
> Autogenic inhibition reflex
>
> Reciprocal inhibition reflex
>
> Gamma efferent pathway

Peripheral Factors

Sensory Receptors

> ### *Neuromuscular spindles in the muscles*
>
> These receptors detect tonic (static) and phasic (changing) stretching of the muscle. The sensitivity of the NMS is controlled by the gamma efferent system.
>
> ### *Golgi tendon organs*
>
> GTO's are specialized receptors in tendons that detect tension. They are part of a protective circuit to prevent injury to the musculotendinous unit due to excessive amounts of tension.

Biomechanical

> ### *Mechanical limits to range of motion*
>
> Osseous, muscular, articular (joints), scar tissue
>
> ### *Connective tissue mechanics*
>
> Elastic (non-permanent) stretch
>
> Plastic (permanent) stretch

Figure 12.1 Flexibility factors: central factors and peripheral factors.

muscle tone. For example, when you are feeling very anxious about a particular situation, your muscle tone often increases. Remember the anxiety and nervousness of your first performances or auditions. Your muscles felt tense or tight, especially in the areas of the neck, shoulders, or lower back. Your movements were stiff, awkward, or robotic. Your timing was off. The slightest noise could cause you to nearly jump through the ceiling. This is a good example of how a psychological state (fear or anxiety) can directly influence muscle tone and physical performance. On the other hand, relaxation techniques can produce a reduction in muscle tone and a corresponding increase in flexibility. These techniques link deep breathing, positive visualization, and gentle stretching with the process of learning to "turn off" extraneous, tension-producing messages from the prefrontal and limbic cortices.

Effective stretching exercises require the use of relaxation and breathing techniques. When stretching, you should close your eyes, isolate the particular target muscle group, remove any anxiety associated with the exercise, relax and breathe slowly and deeply, and try to visualize the correct performance of the exercise. Appropriate relaxing or soothing music can help create a meditative ambience and aid in the slow progressive pacing of the exercises during a session.

The Motor System

Since muscle tone and, to some extent, muscle flexibility are controlled by the motor system, it is important for us to have a rudimentary conceptualization of how the motor system generates the complex motor movement patterns that form the basis of dance technique. The motor system may be conceptualized into six functionally interrelated parts: ideation, initiation, modification, modulation, transmission, and refinement of motor movement patterns (table 12.1).

All areas of the cerebral cortex contribute to the initial formation of the impulse or "idea" to move. How a simple idea or intent to move (e.g., "I want to do an assemblé") is transformed from a memory into a complex firing of neuronal impulses is a fascinating and little understood phenomenon. Once the idea is created, it is the job of the basal ganglia in the core of the brain to initiate a motor movement pattern that will eventually activate those muscles involved in the assemblé. The cerebellum will then modify the motor movement pattern by coordinating and synchronizing the action of each of the muscles involved in the assemblé. The cerebellum relays this information back to the motor cortex for final modulation prior to sending impulses down the spinal cord. When these descending impulses reach a specific level of the spinal cord, they are "refined" by incoming information from the spinal nerves before leaving the spinal cord to innervate the appropriate muscle groups necessary for performing an assemblé.

Motor movement patterns receive contributions and influences from five levels of the brain, and these specific patterns are subsequently superimposed upon a preexisting framework of muscle tone, which is largely under the control of spinal cord reflexes. Each system is located at successively higher levels of the brainstem and cerebrum. Generally, the higher the level, the more sophisticated or specialized the particular system. The five systems that contribute to the motor system are located at three general levels of the brain (figure 12.2). The systems at each of these levels can affect muscle tone and, therefore, via descending pathways, muscle flexibility.

The descending pathways from the motor system—along with the constant flow of incom-

Table 12.1   Neurological Analogues of Motor Movement Patterns

Conceptual components	Neuroanatomical location
Ideation	Cerebral cortex
Initiation	Basal ganglia
Modification	Cerebellum
Modulation	Motor cortex
Transmission	Descending motor tracts
Refinement	Primary sensory and reflex circuits

Medulla

 Vestibular system: Equilibrium stimuli affecting the axial muscles of the torso

Midbrain

 Tectum: Reflex responses from visual and auditory stimuli

 Reticular formation: Muscle tone via the gamma efferent system

Cerebrum

 Basal ganglia: Associative movements of the axial and proximal limb musculature

 Cerebral cortex: Movements of the distal limb musculature

Figure 12.2 Components of the motor system, listed from inferior to superior.

ing somatic sensory information—cause the continuous alterations in reflex activity that are integral to all motor movement activities. The most important of the descending motor pathways relative to muscle flexibility are the *reticulospinal tracts* from the reticular formation. These tracts or pathways play a vital role in controlling muscle tone—and, therefore, flexibility—via the gamma efferent pathway. Gamma efferent neurons control the sensitivity of the neuromuscular spindles in the muscles. These receptors detect stretch and provide the nervous system with critical information as to the position of the body and limbs (proprioception). There is an intimate relationship between proprioception and performance, and muscle tone and flexibility.

Sensory Pathways

The primary source of sensory information essential for motor activity is *proprioception*. Proprioceptive information is derived from the visual and vestibular systems and receptors located in the muscle and tendons. All motor movement activity, whether crude or precise, requires accurate proprioceptive information to the brain and spinal cord.

Tactile information from the skin plays a significant role in the successful performance of many motor activities. For example, precise tactile information from the ball of the foot is a critical factor in learning to get your weight over the supporting foot during pirouettes. All of these motor and sensory neurological factors that control muscle tone, flexibility, and proprio-

ception merge at the level of the spinal cord and assert their influence upon the numerous intrinsic spinal cord reflex pathways.

Spinal Cord Reflexes

Spinal cord reflexes form the fundamental framework for all motor movement activity, in addition to controlling muscle tone. In fact, motor activity may be thought of as a modification of basic spinal reflexes by supraspinal systems. In computer terms, the spinal cord reflexes are the "hardware", and the "software" is the brain, or supraspinal systems. In this analogy the "hardwired" reflex pathways are constantly modified by new "software programs" developed from incoming somatic sensory information and descending influences from supraspinal pathways.

All effective flexibility exercises are based upon spinal cord reflexes. There are four fundamental reflex pathways—myotatic, autogenic inhibition, reciprocal inhibition, and gamma efferent—involved in muscle flexibility and stretching exercises. All are based, more or less, upon the basic reflex pathway. There are five components to the basic reflex pathway (figure 12.3).

The key element in this circuit is the *interneuron*. It is the interneuron that determines the fundamental response pattern of the reflex arc. The interneuron may be either excitatory or inhibitory in terms of its neurophysiological function. Neuroanatomically, it may disperse the response to a stimulus to other neurons in that same segment of the spinal cord, or to other levels of the spinal cord, or to the opposite side of the spinal cord. An interneuron may also have extensive connections with the *reticular formation,* which plays a critically important role in conditioned reflex patterns (i.e., patterned motor reflex responses). The reticular formation, along with several other descending motor pathways, has a fundamental role in basic movement patterns and the control of muscle tone.

Myotatic Reflex

The myotatic reflex is a two-neuron pathway involving a sensory afferent neuron (Ia) and an alpha motor efferent neuron (figure 12.4). There is no interneuron in this circuit. The sensory fiber conveys information originating from neuromuscular spindles (NMS) embedded in the muscles. These receptors detect tonic and phasic stretching of the muscle. Information from the NMS courses

in spinal nerves to the spinal cord, where the type Ia sensory fibers will synapse upon alpha motor neurons. Alpha motor neurons will, in turn, stimulate the muscle that contained the activated NMS to contract.

The myotatic reflex arc is strongly activated by rapid stretch of a muscle. Rapid stretching of the NMS in a muscle will cause that muscle to contract. For example, when your physician strikes the patellar tendon below your kneecap, the sudden stretch of the quadriceps muscle results in its contraction and the extension of the leg (knee-jerk reflex).

In a similar way, ballistic or bouncy stretching techniques may elicit contraction of the target muscle group. These exercises activate the myotatic or stretch/contract reflex arc and increase the tightness of the target muscle. Ballistic stretches may cause microscopic tears in the connective tissue surrounding the muscle cells. Slow, pro-

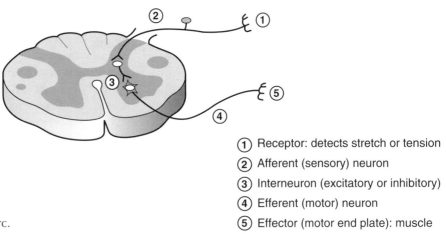

1. Receptor: detects stretch or tension
2. Afferent (sensory) neuron
3. Interneuron (excitatory or inhibitory)
4. Efferent (motor) neuron
5. Effector (motor end plate): muscle

Figure 12.3 The basic reflex arc.

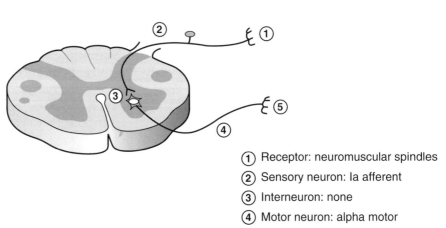

1. Receptor: neuromuscular spindles
2. Sensory neuron: Ia afferent
3. Interneuron: none
4. Motor neuron: alpha motor
5. Effector: extrafusal muscle fibers

Net effect: stretch/contract

Figure 12.4 Myotatic reflex.

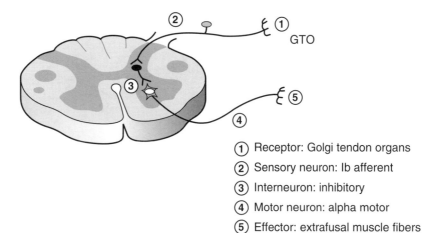

① Receptor: Golgi tendon organs
② Sensory neuron: Ib afferent
③ Interneuron: inhibitory
④ Motor neuron: alpha motor
⑤ Effector: extrafusal muscle fibers
Net effect: excessive tendon tension results in relaxation of the associated

Figure 12.5 Autogenic inhibition reflex.

gressive static stretches for 30 to 60 seconds are more effective and relaxing and should be used for most muscle groups.

Autogenic Inhibition Reflex

The autogenic inhibition reflex is more typical of a basic three-neuron pathway involving a sensory (afferent) neuron, an inhibitory interneuron, and an alpha motor efferent neuron (figure 12.5). A sensory fiber (type Ib) conveys information originating from Golgi tendon organs (GTOs) located in the tendons of muscles. These receptors detect excessive amounts of tension or physical stress in the muscle. Information from the GTOs travels in the spinal nerves to the spinal cord, where the type Ib sensory fibers will synapse upon small inhibitory interneurons. These interneurons will inhibit the function of the alpha motor neurons. The decreased influence of alpha motor neurons on the associated muscle will cause the muscle to relax. Excessive amounts of tension transmitted to the tendon by muscular contraction tend to cause neurophysiological inhibition of that same muscle. There are specific minimum thresholds for activation and central engagement of this reflex arc.

Autogenic inhibition protects the muscle from being injured by excessive amounts of tension. This tension/relax circuit can be utilized quite effectively in certain stretching techniques. In the specialized exercises at the end of this chapter, autogenic inhibition is intentionally activated in order to induce muscle relaxation. During the contraction phase of the proprioceptive neuro-muscular facilitation (PNF) stretching technique, the autogenic inhibition (tension/relax) reflex is activated in the working muscle.

Reciprocal Inhibition Reflex

Reciprocal inhibition is also representative of a basic three-neuron pathway involving a sensory (afferent) neuron, an inhibitory interneuron, and an alpha motor efferent neuron (figure 12.6). A type Ia sensory fiber conveys information originating from NMS located in the muscles. Information from the NMS in a contracting muscle (agonist) travels in the spinal nerves to the spinal cord, where the type Ia sensory fibers will synapse upon small inhibitory interneurons. These interneurons will *inhibit* the function of the alpha motor neurons to the antagonistic muscles. The decrease in alpha motor neuron activity to the antagonistic muscle will cause the muscle to relax.

Contraction of a particular muscle, such as the quadriceps on the front of the thigh, will activate the reciprocal inhibition reflex and induce relaxation of antagonist muscle, in this case the hamstring. While you are performing certain flexibility exercises you should concentrate on contracting the muscle group that is antagonistic to the stretching muscle. This technique should provide an additional amount of relaxation of that muscle. Reciprocal inhibition is used naturally in dance when, for example, during the demi-plié the anterior tibialis muscle on the front of the legs is contracted in order to stretch the gastrocnemius and soleus muscles, resulting in a deeper demi-plié.

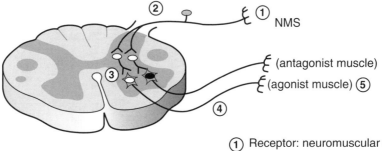

(1) Receptor: neuromuscular spindles

(2) Sensory neuron: Ia afferent

(3) Interneurons to agonist (+) and antagonist (–)

(4) Motor neuron: alpha motor

(5) Effector: extrafusal muscle fibers

Net effect: contraction of agonist muscle results in corresponding relaxation of antagonist muscle

Figure 12.6   Reciprocal inhibition reflex.

Gamma Efferent Pathway

Muscle tone and proprioception are controlled by the gamma efferent pathway. The key neuron in this circuit is the gamma motor neuron located in the spinal cord (figure 12.7). Gamma motor neurons are directly influenced by descending information from the reticular formation (reticulospinal tracts), in addition to receiving input from the basal ganglia (rubrospinal tracts) and cerebral cortex (corticospinal tracts). Output from the gamma motor neuron leaves the spinal cord, courses in a spinal nerve, and finally terminates in the specialized muscle fibers (intrafusal) that are encapsulated in the NMS.

Intrafusal muscle cells control the amount of tension and, therefore, sensitivity of the NMS. In other words, "tighter" spindles are more sensitive to being stretched. Information from the spindles is conveyed to the spinal cord via type Ia sensory fibers in the spinal nerves. Inside the spinal cord these fibers participate in a myotatic reflex, which will result in the contraction of some of the regular (extrafusal) muscle cells in the originating muscle, thus providing the muscle with tone.

The net result of the gamma efferent pathway is an alteration in muscle tone and the maintenance of accurate proprioceptive (position sense) output from the NMS. Increased gamma motor activity causes a corresponding increase in muscle tone, or hypertonia. Decreased gamma motor activity results in a reduction of muscle tone, or hypotonia. Both hypertonia and hypotonia result in a decrease in the degree and accuracy of movement performed by an affected muscle. Optimal muscle tone, a dynamic balance between the two,

is essential to the proper performance of the precise movements characteristic of dance technique.

However, while performing flexibility exercises it is possible and, indeed, preferable to induce some degree of hypotonia in order to enhance the stretching of the muscle. Since gamma motor activity is controlled by the brain—primarily through the reticular formation—it is possible to decrease muscle tone by incorporating the relaxation, visualization, and breathing techniques mentioned earlier. The gamma efferent pathway, along with the previously mentioned reflexes, forms the neuroanatomical basis of the highly effective stretching technique of PNF.

Proprioceptive neuromuscular facilitation, or contract/relax stretching techniques, involves three phases: (1) passive stretch for 20 seconds; (2) an 8-second isometric contraction; and (3) an increase in the amount of passive stretch. Contract/relax stretching exercises take advantage of the decreased muscle tension (hypotonia) that immediately follows an isometric contraction of a stretched muscle (phase 2). During this hypotonic phase the muscle can be stretched even more (phase 3). Proprioceptive neuromuscular facilitation techniques are very effective for stretching larger muscle groups, such as the hamstrings, adductor muscles, quadriceps femoris, and triceps surae (gastroc-soleus).

Proprioceptive neuromuscular facilitation utilizes four basic neuroscientific principles: resistance, reflex, irradiation, and successive induction. Voluntary isometric contraction of the passively stretched muscle, along with adjacent muscle groups, activates the GTOs and the auto-

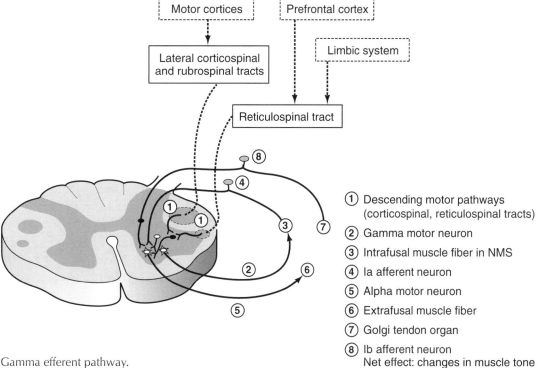

Figure 12.7 Gamma efferent pathway.

① Descending motor pathways
(corticospinal, reticulospinal tracts)
② Gamma motor neuron
③ Intrafusal muscle fiber in NMS
④ Ia afferent neuron
⑤ Alpha motor neuron
⑥ Extrafusal muscle fiber
⑦ Golgi tendon organ
⑧ Ib afferent neuron
Net effect: changes in muscle tone

genic inhibition reflex. The subsequent inhibition of the contracted muscle is overridden by the powerful descending influences from the brain, which are causing the contraction. Stretching adjacent muscle groups (irradiation), voluntary concentric activation of antagonistic muscles, and alternating agonist muscle groups against antagonist groups on both sides of the body will induce increased inhibition of the stretched muscle after the voluntary contraction is complete. During the passive stretch phase of the exercise it is important to utilize mental relaxation and deep-breathing techniques in order to decrease gamma efferent activity and its effect upon muscle tone. Proprioceptive neuromuscular facilitation techniques for the hamstrings, adductor muscles, quadriceps, and gastroc-soleus muscles are described in the exercise description section of this chapter.

Biomechanical Factors in Flexibility

There may also be mechanical limits to range of motion, such as osseous, muscular, or articular structures. Osseous (bony) or scar tissue limitation may affect flexibility by physically restricting or impeding the movement of a joint. Muscles that are excessively tight from training, or as a result of neurological factors, may also limit flexibility. Finally, the type of joint may limit range of

motion according to its function and structure.

When stretched, connective tissue surrounding the muscle cells (endomysium) exhibits permanent (plastic) and nonpermanent (elastic) elongation. Under normal conditions, when the stretch is removed the elastic elongation recovers, but the plastic elongation remains. When connective tissue is stretched, the relative proportion of elastic and plastic elongation within a particular muscle can vary widely, depending upon how, and under what conditions, the stretch is performed. The principal factors that influence the proportion of elastic/plastic elongation are the amount of applied force, duration of applied force, and the temperature of the tissue.

Elastic elongation response is affected by high-force, short-duration stretching, and normal or colder tissue temperatures. Ballistic or bouncy stretching techniques without warm-up of the muscle are representative of conditions that affect elastic elongation. These conditions also activate the myotatic (stretch/contract) reflex and may cause microscopic tears in the tissue. Furthermore, they do not result in permanent elongation of the target muscle.

Plastic deformation is enhanced by low-force, long-duration stretching at elevated temperatures (113° F), with cooling taking place before release of the tension. Sustained gentle stretching of a muscle in a whirlpool, followed immediately by icing while the muscle is still stretched, produces permanent elongation of the muscle. This method of stretching greatly reduces the risk of tissue trauma.

Guidelines for Flexibility Programs

What follows is a list of some basic practices that will enhance most stretching routines. The actual use that is made of them on any given occasion will be dictated by circumstance—essentially, when and where the routine is performed. Optimally, the dancer will regularly structure his or her days in such a way as to accommodate as many of these practices as possible.

1. Keep your program simple, painless, and soothing. Develop a fixed routine—including a set sequence of stretches—and stick with it.

2. Warm up for 5 to 10 minutes before starting your flexibility training. Ride a stationary bike, go for a brisk walk, or perhaps just take a nice hot bath or whirlpool before stretching. The resultant elevation in body temperature will make stretching more effective and comfortable and reduce the possibility of injury.

3. Use static (30-60 seconds) stretches for most muscle groups, and PNF for hamstrings, adductors, and the triceps surae. Alternate stretching agonist–antagonist muscle groups. Your program should integrate gentle progressive exercises with slow, deep breathing and a relaxed mental state.

4. Perform these exercises in a quiet, warm, and comfortable environment. Limit the possibility of interruptions. The morning is usually the optimal time for flexibility and proprioceptive training. Therapeutic exercises are best performed in the morning because generally a person concentrates better at that time and has a decreased sensitivity to physical discomfort or mild pain.

5. Concentrate on correct form and alignment of the body. The benefits of any exercise are greatly diminished when it is performed improperly, and the risks of injury are significantly increased.

6. Keep your eyes closed, breathe slowly and quietly, and concentrate on relaxation and isolation of the mind and body. Learn to "turn off" extraneous gamma efferent activity from the spinal cord by removing the elements of anxiety and forceful determination from the exercises. Let the exercises work for you; relax and enjoy the sensation of stretching your muscles.

7. The exercises that follow are for serious dancers; they are not recommended for the general public, who have no need or preparation for the extreme flexibility demanded by high-performance dance training. If one of these exercises is too difficult or uncomfortable to perform, you should check with an expert to find an alternative exercise or modification.

8. Use common sense when doing these exercises; *if it hurts, don't do it.* Ask yourself why it hurts (are you performing the exercise incorrectly, or is there a structural or functional problem?), and if necessary seek the advice of a qualified health professional.

Selected Flexibility Exercises

The flexibility of the adductor, hamstring, and calf muscles is important to all dancers. Tightness of any one of these muscle groups will hamper the development of proper dance technique and seriously predispose the dancer to injury. The following four exercises demonstrate the utilization of basic spinal cord reflexes and the fundamental principles of flexibility training that were discussed in this chapter. A more detailed and complete program of stretching and strengthening exercises for dancers may be found in *The Dancer's Complete Guide to Healthcare and a Long Career* (Ryan and Stephens 1988).

1. Partnered Diamond Stretch (Adductors)

The partnered diamond exercise is an advanced stretching exercise that uses the contract/relax technique. Your adductor muscles should be warmed up prior to performing this exercise. You and your partner should be very cautious and aware of the possibility of overstretching. The adductor muscles are very sensitive to excessive tension and stretch; be careful and go slowly.

While you are in the diamond position, a partner blocks your feet with his or her knees and *gently and carefully* presses down on your knees until your adductor muscles are mildly stretched

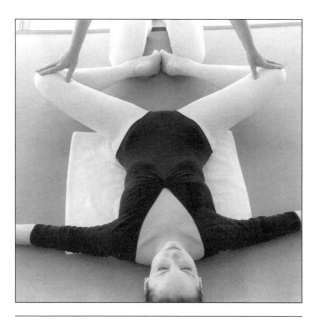

Figure 12.8 Partnered diamond stretch (adductors).
Photo courtesy of Robert Stephens.

(figure 12.8). After 20 seconds of static stretch (do not increase the stretch during this phase), very slowly start to push your knees against the resistance of your partner's hands. Gradually increase the intensity of the contraction for 6 seconds, sustain a maximal contraction for about 2 seconds, and then relax. Your partner then presses gently to increase the stretch. This initial passive stretch (phase 1), your isometric contraction (phase 2), and the relaxation and final stretch (phase 3) constitute one set of this exercise.

Your partner must be ready for the relaxation that initiates phase 3 and avoid applying excessive tension on your knees. A mild stretch is sufficient in this exercise, and your partner and you need to be very aware of excessive amounts of tension in the groin muscles. If you perform the exercise properly, you should not experience pain or discomfort. If you do, stop immediately. The abdominal muscles must maintain the proper alignment of the pelvis and of the lower spine during this exercise.

After 20 seconds of relaxation the contraction can be repeated, and a total of three sets can be performed in a continuous series. Your partner should be aware that during the third set the extremely stretched adductor muscle will be able to generate little force, and he or she should be very careful not to overstretch. It is best to do three or four sets at lesser intensities rather than one or two sets at maximal tensions. At the end

of this exercise your knees are slowly brought back together by your partner.

2. Contract/Relax Hamstring Stretches

Contract/relax techniques are safe and effective methods for stretching the hamstrings. You may use a partner or perform this exercise on your own. The partnered hamstring stretch is most effective when your hamstrings are warmed up and you have a very trustworthy, responsible partner. As with all partnered exercises you should be very cautious and aware of the possibility of overstretching during this exercise.

While you are lying on your back, a partner supports your right leg with his or her right hand or shoulder. Your partner *gently and carefully* applies pressure to your leg in order to stretch the hamstring muscles on the back of the thigh (figure 12.9). After 20 seconds of static stretch (do not increase the stretch during this phase), very slowly start to push your right leg against the resistance of your partner's hand or shoulder. Gradually increase the intensity of the contraction for 6 seconds, sustain a maximal contraction of the hamstring muscles for about 2 seconds, and then relax while your partner gently applies pressure to increase the stretch. During the contraction phase, the agonist (hamstring and gluteals) and antagonist (quadriceps) muscle groups of both extremities should be activated.

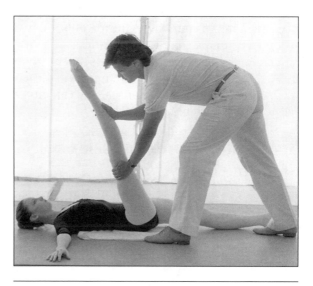

Figure 12.9 Contract/relax hamstring stretches.
Photo courtesy of Robert Stephens.

As in the previous exercise, your partner must be ready for the relaxation and avoid applying excessive tension on your hamstrings (maintaining a staggered stance is important for the partner's balance). A moderate stretch is sufficient in this exercise, and your partner and you need to be very aware of excessive amounts of tension on the hamstrings.

Your partner's initial passive stretch, followed by your isometric contraction, relaxation, and the final stretch, constitutes one set of this exercise. Three continuous sets are usually performed without release of the stretch. By the third set the hamstrings will be so stretched that they will not be able to generate very much force; therefore, your partner should be very careful not to overstretch. It is best to do more sets at a lower intensity rather than one or two sets at maximal tension. At the end of this exercise the dancer's leg is slowly returned to the floor by the partner.

As an alternative to partnered hamstring stretches you can perform the same type of stretching technique by using a modified contraction/relaxation exercise. Lying on your back, bring the right leg up to hip level and support it by holding the back of the thigh with both hands (make sure you have a good grip). If your hamstrings are too tight to reach comfortably, use a towel to sling around the thigh. Stretch the hamstrings by gently pulling the right thigh toward the chest, keeping the knee straight. The left leg should not lift off of the floor, and the left knee should be straight. Maintain a moderate stretch for about 20 seconds. Perform an isometric contraction by pushing against your hands (or towel) for 6 to 8 seconds. After the contraction, continue to gently stretch the hamstrings. Repeat the sequence two more times and change sides. If the tension is too much at any point in the exercise, you can either reduce the stretch or bend the knee.

3. Modified Contract/Relax Standing Calf Stretch

In order to stretch the superficial calf muscle (gastrocnemius) simply lean toward the barre in a lunge, keeping the heel of the straight leg on the floor (figure 12.10). Continue leaning forward until the heel begins to lift off the floor, and then press the heel down by using the tibialis anterior muscle and pushing against the barre with your hands. Hold the stretch for about 20 seconds,

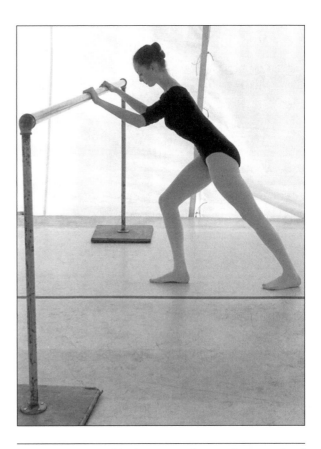

Figure 12.10 Modified contract/relax standing superficial calf stretch for the gastrocnemius.
Photo courtesy of Robert Stephens.

slowly rise to demi-pointe position against resistance, then slowly lower from the demi-pointe position while resisting this action. The *resistance* to relevé, produced by using one set of muscles to offset the action of another, is the key factor in inducing muscle stretch in this exercise. Repeat the sequence two more times.

4. Modified Contract/Relax Standing Deep Calf Stretch

Continue your calf stretches by slowly bending the knee of the back leg, while leaning forward and keeping the heel on the floor (figure 12.11). Lean forward until the heel barely begins to lift off the floor, and then press the heel down by using the tibialis anterior muscle and pushing against the barre with your hands. Hold the stretch for about 20 seconds, slowly rise to demi-pointe position against resistance, and then slowly lower from the demi-pointe position while resisting this action. Once again, the resistance to relevé

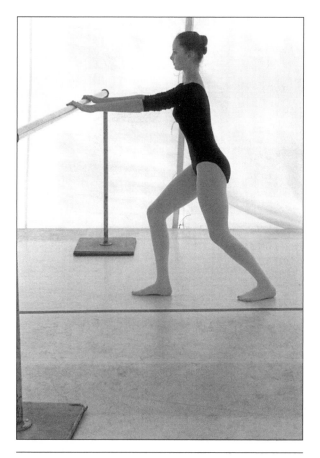

Figure 12.11 Modified contract/relax standing deep calf stretch for the soleus.
Photo courtesy of Robert Stephens.

is the key factor in inducing muscle stretch in this exercise. Repeat this sequence two more times. After working one side, repeat the calf stretches on the other side.

Conclusion

All dancers stretch, based on a generalized belief that in the short term this will prepare their bodies for class, rehearsal, or performance, and that in the long term it will increase their flexibility. One suspects, however, that it is only a very small percentage of the dance population that has had an opportunity to investigate the subject of flexibility in depth. As this chapter attempts to illustrate, the perhaps somewhat forbidding field of neuroanatomy contains much of the information one might reasonably seek not only about flexibility but also about how mind and body interact to produce movement in general, and is not as inaccessible as might be imagined.

It is hoped that, armed with an understanding of principles like those discussed here, tomorrow dancers will be more capable than their predecessors of assuming responsibility for their own advancement and safety.

Reference

Ryan, A.J., and R.E. Stephens, eds. 1988. *The dancer's complete guide to healthcare and a long career.* Chicago: Bonus Books.

Recommended Readings (Author)

Carpenter, M.B., and J. Sutin. 1983. *Human neuroanatomy.* 8th ed. Baltimore: Williams & Wilkins.

Gowitzke, B.A., and M. Milner. 1988. *Understanding the scientific bases of human movement.* 3rd ed. Baltimore: Williams & Wilkins.

Noback, C.R., and R.J. Demarest. 1981. *The human nervous system: Basic principles of neurobiology.* 3rd ed. New York: McGraw-Hill.

Pansky, B., D.J. Allen, and G.C. Budd. 1988. *Review of neuro-science.* 2nd ed. New York: Macmillan.

Ryan, A.J., and R.E. Stephens, eds. 1987. *Dance medicine: A comprehensive guide.* Chicago and Minneapolis: Pluribus Press/Physician and Sportsmedicine.

Sapega, A.A., T.C. Quedenfeld, R.A. Moyer, and R.A. Butler. 1981. Biophysical factors in range-of-motion exercise. *Physician and Sportsmedicine* 9: 57-65.

Stephens, R.E. 1989. *Clinical neuroanatomy: A case history approach.* 5th ed. Kansas City: University of Health Sciences.

Recommended Readings (Editors)

Alter, M.J. 1996. *Science of flexibility.* Champaign, IL: Human Kinetics.

Gamboa, J.M., and S.P. Gallagher. 1996. Developing a warm-up and conditioning program for performing artists. *Orthopaedic Physical Therapy Clinics of North America* 5(4): 515-545.

Huwyler, J. 1999. *The dancers body: A medical perspective on dance and dance training.* McLean, VA: International Medical.

Knudson, D. 1998. Stretching: From science to practice. *Journal of Physical Education, Recreation and Dance* 69(3): 38-42.

Volianitis, S., Y. Koutedakis, and R.J. Carson. 2001. Warm-up: A brief review. *Journal of Dance Medicine & Science* 5(3): 75-81.

Chapter 13

Strengthening and Stretching the Muscles of the Ankle and Tarsus

Sally Sevey Fitt, EdD

This chapter takes a somewhat different approach from the preceding one to stretching as an element in injury prevention, emphasizing the development of strength to at least the same extent as flexibility. It augments the medical and more classically biomechanical studies of the ankle in chapters 4 and 14.

Many surveys of dance injuries indicate that the body region with the highest rate of injury is the lower leg and foot, including traumatic injuries (i.e., fractures, sprains, and strains) and chronic conditions (i.e., tendinitis, shinsplints, recurring muscle spasms, and persistent muscle soreness) (Bachrach 1988; Fuller 1975; Miller et al. 1975; Nagrin 1988; Ryan et al. 1976; Schneider et al. 1974; Shaw 1977; Washington 1978). However, because movement occurs only at joints (the articulations of adjacent bones), the focus of this chapter is on the ankle and tarsus joints, where the movement that precipitates pain experienced in the lower leg and foot actually occurs. The terms lower leg and foot are used in this discussion until the more specific terminology related to the ankle and tarsus joints (figure 13.1) has been defined.

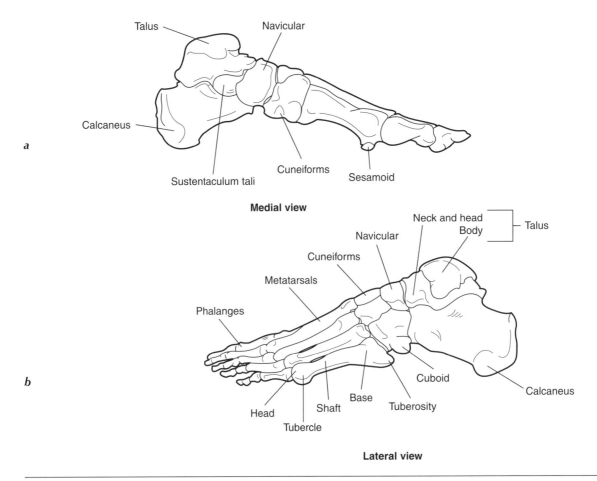

a

Talus — Navicular

Calcaneus —

Sustentaculum tali

Cuneiforms Sesamoid

Medial view

Neck and head
Navicular Body Talus

Cuneiforms

Metatarsals

Phalanges

b

Cuboid

Calcaneus

Head Shaft Base Tuberosity

Tubercle

Lateral view

Figure 13.1 Bones of the foot, dorsal and plantar views.
Reprinted from Behnke 2001.

Traumatic injuries often occur because the musculature lacks the strength to adjust readily to extreme and immediate demands. For example, when one "falls off balance" there is a need for greater strength than normal to pull back to the balanced position. If strength is insufficient, traumatic injuries can result. Likewise a misaligned landing from a jump or leap requires greater strength than a properly aligned landing. In an ideal world dancers would never fall off balance, nor would they ever land in a misaligned position, but in the real world they do. For this reason they need more strength in the muscles of the lower leg and foot than is developed in the normal dance class.

Chronic injuries occur because the baseline capabilities of the muscular system (both strength and flexibility) are insufficient to meet everyday demands. For example, tendinitis may be caused by one of two major training errors. First, asking

more from a muscle than it has to give, either in strength or in muscular endurance, can temporarily "wear out" the musculotendinous unit (muscles and tendons are not separate entities, but rather different components of the same unit), causing a reaction of the body of the muscle (muscle soreness or spasm) or the tendon of the muscle (tendinitis). Second, tendinitis can be caused by insufficient stretching of a muscle after an intensive exercise bout, leaving the muscle in a state of partial contraction. (It should be noted that the two causes of tendinitis listed here are the hypotheses of this author and have not been systematically studied by her under controlled conditions. However, William Stanish 1984 supports these hypotheses.)

Chronic injuries seem to respond positively to conditioning for strength and stretch when exercises are specifically targeted to the exact muscle involved. The problem for the technique teacher is deciding exactly which muscle needs attention. Unfortunately, these people seldom have time to study surveys of injuries or textbooks and articles on efficient and effective conditioning practices. As a result, the gap between current conditioning theory and actual practice in the dance studio widens. The purpose of this chapter is to narrow that gap between conditioning theory and common practices in dance technique classes in an attempt to reduce the rate of dance injury at the foot, ankle, and lower leg. Information is presented on the conditioning process in four sections: principles of conditioning, anatomical and kinesiological information about the possible actions of joints, evaluation of the present status of conditioning for the lower leg and foot in technique classes (including evaluation of injuries), and description of exercises to increase strength and mobility of the muscles of the ankle and tarsus.

Conditioning for Strength and Elasticity (Flexibility)

There are five fundamental types of conditioning that build the capacities of the human body: (1) muscular strength, (2) muscular elasticity or flexibility, (3) muscular endurance, (4) cardiorespiratory endurance, and (5) neuromuscular coordination (Fitt 1996). Although this chapter focuses only on increased strength and elasticity to prevent injury and to speed rehabilitation, it is helpful to define each of the types of conditioning. *Strength* is the ability to contract a muscle or muscle group against resistance. *Flexibility* is the ability of a muscle to be stretched to its maximum length. *Muscular endurance* is the ability of a muscle to continue contraction over time. *Cardiorespiratory endurance* is the ability of the cardiovascular and respiratory systems to support over time the increased demands caused by exercise. *Neuromuscular coordination* is the establishment of neuromuscular patterns necessary for performance of specific tasks.

Strength and elasticity are the focus of this chapter because they are often neglected in dance classes. Some dancers and teachers of dance may say, "Neglected? That's impossible! Look at all the time we spend on our feet!" However, this time is not necessarily spent in exercises that are effective for increasing strength and elasticity. Most

exercises conducted in dance technique classes are focused on neuromuscular coordination or muscular endurance for the foot and lower leg.

Building Strength

The fundamental rule for building strength is to contract the target muscle maximally for 5 to 10 repetitions (Fleck and Kraemer 1987). When one hears the term maximal contraction one often thinks of isometric contractions—that is, those that are produced by pressure against a nonmovable resistance. However, strength is specific to the angle of the joint in which the maximal contractions are performed, and to the velocity of the contraction—slow or quick repetitions (Fleck and Kraemer 1987). For this reason, isometric contractions (with no movement through the range of motion) are less effective than exercises that require maximal contraction throughout the entire range of motion. The most effective exercises for strength are isokinetic; that is, they involve movement against a graded resistance, which modulates the resistance depending on the strength of the musculature at the specific joint angle. The major problem with isokinetic exercises is that the highly refined equipment needed to do them is very expensive. The second best type of exercise to build strength is isotonic exercise (movement through the range of motion) against an external resistance, performed at both slow and quick tempos.

Increasing Muscular Elasticity

Every dancer knows how to stretch, but not every dancer knows how to stretch effectively. Like strength, flexibility or muscular elasticity is specific to the joint position. This is because the muscles of a given joint have highly specified roles in the production of motion. One must reverse the joint action that is normally produced by a muscle to achieve the most effective stretch position. A muscle that flexes and outwardly rotates a given joint is most effectively stretched when the joint is placed in a position of extension and inward rotation. While the muscle will also be stretched in a position of extension without rotation, the stretch is not as effective as when all of the actions of the muscle are reversed. Consequently, different muscles will be stretched if a slight shift is made in the joint position. Information about joint actions and the musculature that produces those actions is necessary to design effective, efficient stretches.

The process used to stretch muscles is as important to increasing the range of motion as the accurate identification of the joint position for the stretch. Ballistic or bouncing stretches are potentially injurious, as they utilize body momentum to force effort into a partially contracted muscle, causing microscopic tears of the muscle tissue. Therefore, they are to be discouraged. One effective method for stretching a muscle is the use of reciprocal inhibition to facilitate the stretch (Fitt 1996). Reciprocal stretches are most effective when the muscle mass of the opposing muscle groups is approximately equal. Unfortunately, the muscle mass of opposing muscle groups is not equal for the ankle and tarsus joints, and this reduces the effectiveness of reciprocal stretches for these muscles. Second in effectiveness to reciprocal stretches are the long, slow, sustained stretches described by DeVries (1966) as "static stretches."

A long, sustained stretch involves (1) identifying the joint position that produces the most efficient stretch for the targeted muscle, (2) assuming that position in such a way that gravity can assist in the stretch, (3) maintaining the position while consciously relaxing the target muscle and giving in to gravity to increase the stretch, and (4) continuing the stretch for at least 30 seconds to 1 minute. Because of the imbalance of muscle mass of opposing muscle groups in the ankle and tarsus, the long, sustained stretch is most effective for stretching in that region.

Stretching has several objectives. One already mentioned is to increase the range of motion of a joint. Other objectives of stretching include cooling down of the musculature after class, reducing the level of residual contraction in a muscle after a heavy exercise bout to reduce subsequent muscle soreness, general relaxation, and correcting muscular imbalances. The nature of stretching shifts somewhat according to the objective of the stretch. The long, sustained stretch is thought to be most effective for all objectives at the ankle and tarsus. The stretches described in this chapter are for the purposes of increasing range of motion

and stretching muscles after heavy exercise bouts. Therefore, the long, sustained stretch is recommended. (Editors' note: For another discussion of flexibility and stretching see chapter 12.)

Ankle and Tarsus Joints and Possible Actions

The foot is a miraculous architectural structure. Just imagine: You walk, run, jump, and leap off and onto some of the smallest bones of the body. The reason they last for a lifetime is that they incorporate the strongest of architectural structures, the arch. Moreover, there are many joints in the foot to disperse the force of landings.

The toes are made up of a proximal and distal phalanx for the great toe and proximal, middle, and distal phalanges for the second to fifth toes, with joints between the bones (the interphalangeal joints). The proximal phalanges articulate with the metatarsal bones at the phalangeal-metatarsal joints. The proximal ends of the metatarsal bones articulate with the distal tarsal bones, forming the metatarsal-tarsal joints.* There are seven bones in the tarsus region (cuboid, three cuneiforms, navicular, talus, and calcaneus) that articulate with each other and cumulatively provide the actions of the tarsus. The talus, of the tarsus region, articulates with the tibia and fibula (bones of the lower leg) to form the ankle joint. Motion potential is increased by the number of joints in the foot, making the foot resilient to stresses of locomotion, but also susceptible to injury.

Ligaments (inelastic, connective tissue that connects bone to bone) of the foot and ankle stabilize the joints and protect them against the hypermobility that produces injuries. However, strength in the muscles of the ankle and tarsus is also needed as support against the extreme demands that dancers place on their feet. In addition, these muscles must be elastic to meet the dancer's need for mobile feet.

The ankle and tarsus joints are crucial to all locomotion. The ankle joint has two possible actions: plantarflexion (pointing the foot) and dorsiflexion (flexing the foot). The tarsus joints also have two possible actions: pronation

---

*Proximal and distal are terms used to describe relative positions: Proximal means closer to the "center" of the body, and distal means farther from the center of the body.

(a combination of abduction and outward rotation) and supination (a combination of adduction and inward rotation). The ankle and tarsus work synergistically to produce the familiar motion of what is normally called the ankle, but what is actually the combination of ankle and tarsus.

Dancers seem to learn best when the kinesthetic sense is used to fortify the definition of terms such as dorsiflexion, plantarflexion, supination, and pronation. Hence, the intent in this section is to clarify, in motion, the definitions of the movements possible at the ankle and tarsus.

Dorsiflexion of the Ankle

Sit on the floor with the legs stretched straight in front of you (the "long-sit" position) and with no rotation at the hip (have the kneecaps pointing straight at the ceiling). Pull the heels down on the floor, causing the toes to point straight up toward the ceiling without moving the heels on the floor and without turning the feet outward or inward. Some people call this a flexed foot, but in truth it is dorsiflexion of the ankle joint. Often dorsiflexion of the ankle is accompanied by extension of the toes (pulling the toes up toward the body).

Plantarflexion of the Ankle

In the same long-sit position as you used to feel dorsiflexion, press the feet down toward the floor, attempting to touch the toes or the balls of the feet, or both, to the floor. Make sure the feet are in alignment for pure plantarflexion—that is, that there is no pronation or supination of the tarsus. Plantarflexion of the ankle is often accompanied by flexion of the metatarsophalangeal joint (gripping of the toes).

Supination of the Tarsus

Sit on a table with the thighs on the table, the knees bent, and the lower legs hanging off the table in a relaxed fashion. Turn the soles of your feet toward each other as if you were going to clap them together. There is both inward rotation and adduction (movement of each foot toward the midline between the feet) of the tarsus or foot. In dance classes the action of supination of the tarsus is often called a "sickled foot." With the legs dangling from the table and with both tarsal joints supinated, the appearance of the lower leg and foot is like closed parentheses: ().

Pronation of the Tarsus

Still sitting on the table with the legs dangling off the table from the knee down, turn the soles of the feet away from each other, out toward the sides. There is both outward rotation and abduction (movement away from the midline) of the tarsus in this action. In dance classes the action of pronation of the tarsus is often called a "beveled foot." With the legs dangling and both tarsal joints pronated, the appearance of the lower leg and foot is like an open set of parentheses:)(.

Neutral Position of the Tarsus

In addition to the actions of pronation and supination, it is important to point out that a tarsus that is neither pronated nor supinated is considered a neutral tarsus. In the neutral position of the tarsus the second toe is approximately aligned with the true center of the ankle joint. This position of the tarsus places the least stress on the lateral and medial ligaments and muscles of the ankle and tarsus, particularly in weight-bearing positions or in locomotion.

Combined Actions of the Ankle and Tarsus

In the demonstrations just described you were asked to focus your attention on the actions at either the ankle or tarsus joints. Now we will combine the actions at the two joints.

Dorsiflex both ankles and supinate both tarsal joints (soles of the feet together). Next, still maintaining dorsiflexion of the ankles, pronate both tarsal joints (turn the soles of both feet out and away from each other). You have been holding dorsiflexion of the ankle joint constant while moving at the tarsal joints in actions of supination and pronation.

Plantarflex both ankles and supinate both tarsal joints. Then try plantarflexion and pronation. For many dancers this action is quite difficult to find, which is unfortunate because it is the muscles that plantarflex and pronate that stabilize the outside of the foot in relevé or pointe position. Without strength in these muscles the likelihood of sprains of the tarsus is greatly increased.

Now that you have kinetically examined all of the possible motions of the ankle and tarsus region, do "ankle circles" and observe how the ankle and tarsus work in a close partnership to

Fitt

Actions of the tarsus	Actions of the ankle
Pronation	Plantarflexion
Supination	Dorsiflexion

Figure 13.2 Combined actions of the ankle and tarsus.

allow all of the possible actions of what is normally called the ankle. On figure 13.2, enter key words that describe the feel of the combined actions listed.

Muscle Groups That Perform the Actions of the Ankle and Tarsus

Muscles are generally grouped and identified by the actions that they perform on the joints they cross. The joint determines what actions are possible, and the muscles produce the force for the actual movement. Joint actions are opposites, such as plantarflexion and dorsiflexion, or pronation and supination. Likewise, the muscle groups have opposite actions. Agonist muscles perform a given action at a particular joint; the antagonists perform the opposite action at that joint. For example, the plantarflexor muscles are agonistic for the action of plantarflexion and antagonistic for the action of dorsiflexion. How-

ever, because the ankle and tarsus joints operate in close synergy, one must consider paired actions to determine the antagonistic muscles. Three of the muscles that cross the ankle joint have action only at the ankle joint (the gastrocnemius, the soleus, and the plantaris). All of the other muscles acting on the ankle joint also act on the tarsus. These are multijoint muscles, and the combined actions at the two joints must be considered when strength and stretching exercises are designed for these muscles. There are some muscles that cross the ankle and tarsal joints and also cross the toe joints (flexor hallucis longus, extensor hallucis longus, extensor digitorum longus, and flexor digitorum longus). For these three-joint muscles, in addition to considering the actions at the tarsus and ankle one must take into account the agonistic actions produced at the toes when designing strengthening exercises, and the antagonistic actions for the toes when designing stretching exercises.

Simply put, the principles described thus far are as follows: (1) To strengthen a muscle, do all of the joint actions performed by that muscle against resistance and through the full range of motion; (2) to stretch a muscle, reverse all of the joint actions performed by the muscle and do a long, sustained stretch in that position. Figure 13.3 gives the specific muscles that perform the isolated joint action. The muscles *indicated in italics* are those that have only that action. All the other muscles have actions at more than one joint.

Plantarflexion (ankle joint): *gastrocnemius, soleus, plantaris,* tibialis posterior, peroneus longus, peroneus brevis, flexor digitorum longus, flexor hallucis longus

Dorsiflexion (ankle joint): tibialis anterior, peroneus tertius, extensor hallucis longus, extensor digitorum longus

Pronation (tarsus joints): peroneus longus, peroneus brevis, peroneus tertius, extensor digitorum longus

Supination (tarsus joints): tibialis anterior, tibialis posterior, flexor digitorum longus (slight action of supination by the flexor hallucis longus and the extensor hallucis longus)

Note: Intrinsic muscles are those muscles that do not cross the ankle joint; they have both proximal and distal attachments on the bones of the foot. None of the intrinsic muscles of the foot are included in the list above. However, there is one exercise given for these muscles in the exercise section.

Figure 13.3 Muscles by joint action.

Pronators and plantarflexors: peroneus longus, peroneus brevis

Pronators and dorsiflexors: peroneus tertius, extensor digitorum longus

Supinators and dorsiflexors: tibialis anterior, extensor hallucis longus

Supinators and plantarflexors: tibialis posterior, flexor hallucis longus, flexor digitorum longus

Note: The gastrocnemius and soleus are not listed because they do not have an action at the tarsus; they do not cross that joint.

Figure 13.4 Ankle/tarsus muscles listed by combined actions.

While the listing of muscles and single-joint actions gives a sense of which muscles do what, the more important information for designing exercises combines the actions of the ankle and tarsus (figure 13.4).

These lists of specific muscles are included for those who wish to refer to anatomy books for illustrations and further information. Actually, all that is needed to design exercises is to understand the four combined actions of the ankle and tarsus, and to have done a systematic evaluation of strength and elasticity of the relevant muscle groups.

Common Conditioning Practices in Dance Classes

Strength conditioning of the lower leg and foot in dance technique classes is commonly minimal; no progressive resistance exercises are used to increase the strength of the musculature. Relevés on one foot approach maximal contractions for the plantarflexors, but no maximal contractions are done for dorsiflexors, pronators, or supinators in dance classes.*

Conditioning for muscular endurance receives attention in technique classes due to the repetitive nature of tendues, pliés, and relevés, but this

conditioning is insufficient when one considers that time constraints limit the number of repetitions necessary to achieve the desired results.

Conditioning for muscular elasticity of the muscles of the lower leg and foot is usually limited to stretches of the dorsiflexors of the ankle to increase the pointe of the foot, with an occasional "token" stretch of the gastrocnemius (calf muscle and Achilles tendon). Generally, stretches in class are based more on tradition than on the structure of the muscular system or the particular needs of the students in the class.

Warm-ups are fairly common in dance classes, but the focus is often on familiar exercises rather than what is needed to prepare the body to dance. Also, it is rare to find dancers spending time in cool-down exercises, or stretching out overworked muscles at the end of class.

Dance teachers have depended on tradition to determine the content and structure of their classes. In certain components of any dance class, tradition—and adherence to it—is appropriate. However, ignoring the principles of conditioning that have been shown to be effective in building strength and muscular elasticity is not useful. Recent research clearly demonstrates an unusually high incidence of injuries to the lower leg and foot; therefore, dance educators may want to reevaluate the conditioning practices that are in common use.

Principles of Conditioning Versus Actual Practices in Dance Classes

A number of gaps are immediately obvious when one compares conditioning theories and common conditioning practices in dance classes. It is clear that dance classes do not employ the *overload principle* (enhancing the strength and endurance of muscles by subjecting them to training loads that exceed the accustomed workload). Occasionally one might find a maximal contraction in a dance class when a dancer is about to fall off a balance, or when all of the body weight is on one foot, but the systematic use of overload to build

---

*I have in mind throughout this discussion the basic ballet technique class. Some modern techniques provide a wider range of conditioning for the foot and ankle—significant contractions of the dorsiflexors, for example—though few, I believe, systematically use weights or maximal contractions for strength training.

strength is notably absent. There is *lack of specificity* in conditioning the musculature of the ankle and tarsus to increase either strength or stretch. Whatever strength or muscular elasticity is built into the technique class is seldom intentionally directed at specific muscle groups. What is taught frequently encourages marked muscular imbalances of strength or elasticity, or both, of opposing muscle groups. To affect this tendency it would be expedient to integrate the principles of efficient conditioning into dance classes.

Dancers' Specific Demands on the Ankle/Tarsus Joints

In a normal standing position, gravity is a dorsiflexor of the ankle joint and a pronator of the tarsus. Maintaining a simple standing position requires counteraction of the effect of gravity by the plantarflexors of the ankle and the supinators of the tarsus. The pronators and plantarflexors are the key muscles to counteract gravity in the half-toe position; the muscle groups shift as the position (relation to gravity) changes. The examples given (normal standing and half-toe balances) are only two of the possible demands on these joints. As the dancer moves through a complex combination, different demands are placed upon the musculature of the ankle and tarsus to counteract the ever-changing effect of gravity on those joints. In all locomotion (except the most stylized of walks, runs, jumps, leaps, and hops), the plantarflexors of the ankle are the key muscles for opposing gravity. If a dancer has excessive range of motion in plantarflexion, strength in the dorsiflexors of the ankle, as antagonists, is necessary to stabilize the ankle joint in half-toe or pointe position. Functionally, the optimal position of the tarsus is neutral: neither pronated nor supinated. Neutral alignment of the tarsus allows for direct transference of weight from one segment of the foot to another, and it produces less stress on the ligaments and tendons. A balance of strength between pronators and supinators is therefore necessary to maintain a neutral position of the tarsus.

Results of Insufficient Conditioning

Lack of strength in the muscles of the ankle/tarsus region severely reduces the capacity to stabilize the joint, a critical factor in the demanding bal-ances executed by dancers. In the worst-case scenario, lack of strength in these muscles can lead to debilitating strains, sprains, or fractures. In less traumatic instances, lack of strength can be a contributing factor in the occurrence of tendinitis or shinsplints when demands exceed the capabilities of specific muscles or muscle groups.

Lack of muscular endurance has the same effect as lack of strength in that the demands placed on the musculature can no longer be met. The need for muscular endurance is most pronounced in rehearsals, where the dancer is required to perform the same combinations over and over. Without sufficient muscular endurance, injuries can be the result.

Lack of muscular elasticity (flexibility) can cause tearing of muscles when the joint is moved beyond its normal range of motion. These tears can be severe, as in the case of a ruptured Achilles tendon, or relatively mild, as in minor strains. Lack of muscular elasticity is also an important factor in the everyday aches and pains the dancer experiences. These minor strains are one cause of aches and pains, but another is the excessive demands inherent in standard dance movements. When one muscle group is inelastic, the opposing muscle group must work harder to accomplish motion than if the inelastic muscle group were stretched out. Thus, increasing muscular elasticity makes motion easier and less stressful than working with limited mobility. A prime example of this principle is stretching the hip extensors to make dance "extension" (flexion of the hip joint) more efficient.

Specific stretching of a muscle group immediately following a demanding exercise bout with that muscle group can reduce the level of muscular stress that may lead to tendinitis or other chronic conditions. A regular "cool-down" procedure after pointe class—or any class that emphasizes plantarflexion of the ankle (such as relevé, jumps, or leaps)—should include specific stretching of the gastrocnemius and the soleus muscles (see exercise section of this chapter). Stretching to increase muscular elasticity is a critical factor for all phases of a dance class, rehearsal, or performance.

Evaluation of Pain

Dancers have a keen kinesthetic awareness. Even if they don't know the names of the muscles or the joint actions, they still can begin to identify a particular pain and deal with it effectively. They need to identify *where, when,* and *how* the pain occurs. This information will be valuable whether or not it is necessary to see a physician for precise diagnosis and treatment. While the following guidelines for analyzing pain are addressed to the ankle and tarsus region, these principles can also be applied to other regions of the body.

Where Do You Hurt (Localization of the Pain)?

- Is the pain anterior or posterior (front or back)?
- Is the pain on the medial or lateral side of the lower leg (inside or outside)?
- If the pain radiates, what is its path?
- Is the pain isolated in the foot? Where in the foot?

When Do You Hurt (Functional Analysis)?

- When performing the possible combinations of actions of the ankle and tarsus, which action makes it hurt?
- Does it hurt differently when you perform different actions (see "How Do You Hurt?")?
- Which actions in technique class (or everyday activities) cause the most pain? What kind of pain (how does it hurt)? Is it different for different activities?

How Do You Hurt (The Nature of the Pain Itself)?

- What does the pain feel like? Try to find words that describe the "feel" of the pain. Some words that are often used are sharp, shooting, isolated, diffuse, prickly, burning, jabbing, crunching, grating, deep, superficial, and grabbing.
- Is the pain related to stretching the muscle (hot, prickly, pulling, or lengthening) or is it contraction pain (shortening, gripping, or cramping)?

After analyzing the pain the dancer has an information base for identifying different types of injury. The most common injuries to the ankle and tarsus are tendinitis, shinsplints, muscle spasms, sprains, strains, and fractures. A brief description of each of these common conditions is given here to assist the dancer who is evaluating an injury.

Common Injuries to the Ankle and Tarsus

Tendinitis is inflammation of the tendon (the attachment of muscle tissue to bone tissue). It often occurs when the strength of a muscle is inadequate to meet the demands being made on it, or when muscles are not stretched out following intense exercise bouts. The location of the tendinitis follows the location of the muscle and the path of the tendon. In order to determine which tendon is inflamed, the dancer can go through the combined actions of the ankle, tarsus, and toes (contracting the muscle against resistance and stretching the muscle) to identify which actions cause stretching pain and which cause contracting pain. Knowing the joint actions that cause pain helps in determining what activities to avoid in the acute stages of tendinitis. Gentle stretches should be done using the joint actions opposite to the contraction pain. Once the pain is gone, the muscle groups causing the pain should be strengthened. Home remedies for tendinitis include icing, rest, and gentle stretching of the muscle. Aspirin can be taken as an anti-inflammatory drug, with dosages of two with each meal and two before bedtime (please consult a physician before taking any drugs). If tendinitis persists, it is essential to see a physician.

The term *shinsplints* once had a very specific meaning: It referred to the microscopic pulling of muscle fibers away from the bone where the belly of the muscle attached directly to the bone. Over the years, shinsplints has become a general term that includes any pain in the area of the tibia (Gans 1985), and the original concept has been redefined as medial tibial stress syndrome (MTSS). Functionally the cause of this syndrome is similar to that of tendinitis: asking more from the muscle than it has to give. As with tendinitis, the treatment for MTSS follows the pattern of rest, icing, and gentle stretching. To determine how to stretch for MTSS one can use the same technique as is used for tendinitis: Run through the possible combinations of joint actions and identify which actions produce stretch pain and which produce contraction pain. Gentle stretches should be done using the joint actions opposite to the contraction pain. Once the pain is gone, the muscle groups causing the pain should be strengthened. If MTSS persists for more than a week or two, one should examine the possibility that the injury may be a stress fracture.

Sprains are injuries to soft tissue (muscle, nerve) and connective tissue (ligaments, joint capsules, tendons, and other connective tissue) that are caused by excessive movement of a joint. The most common sites of sprains are on the lateral side of the tarsus (excessive movement in the direction of supination usually caused by landing on an improperly aligned tarsus) and in the toes (caused by stubbing). It is prudent to always have a sprain examined by a physician to rule out the possibility of a fracture. General treatment of a sprain includes icing, compression, elevation, and rest. Sprains, which usually include injuries to the ligamentous structure, often take as long as 18 months to heal completely. Even then there may be some residual loss of range of motion from a sprain. Following recuperation, muscles around the sprain should be strengthened and stretched to prevent recurrence and to regain lost capacities.

Strains are, like sprains, injuries caused by excessive movement of a joint. However, in strains the injury is limited to the soft tissue (it does not include connective tissue). Treatments similar to those used for sprains can be used for strains. Reconditioning the muscles after recovery from a strain is essential, or the injury will likely recur. Without rehabilitative exercises the muscles are even weaker than they were when the original injury took place.

Fractures fall into several categories, including simple, compound, green stick, and stress fractures. All fractures exhibit loss of integrity of the bone structure: a break, crack, chip, or shattering of a bone. The belief that if one can move a body part it is not broken is simply not true. A physician should always direct treatment for fractures.

Any discussion of pain would be incomplete without mentioning its value. Pain is an ally because it aids in identifying and treating an injury. Pain tells us when movement activities are asking too much of the body, and when to stop.

Self-Assessment of Strength and Range of Motion

The first step in using this information to guide conditioning is the assessment of capabilities, especially strength and elasticity (or range of motion).

There are many technical tools for measuring strength, but the easiest is manual strength test-ing. This technique involves manually resisting the joint action while contracting against the resistance. For example, testing the strength of the plantarflexors and pronators involves manually pushing the foot toward dorsiflexion and supination while muscularly trying to pronate and plantarflex. Manual testing is far from the most precise measurement of muscular strength, but it is practical because no special equipment is necessary. With appropriate training the person doing the testing can identify the contraction as "strong," "average," or "weak."

In range of motion testing of the ankle and tarsus, the subject relaxes the foot and lower leg while the tester manipulates the foot into different positions. Similar to the rough but informative assessment of strength, manual testing can provide gross identification of range of motion as "marked," "average," or "limited." Figure 13.5 is an assessment sheet for recording the results of strength and range of motion testing. Once completed, this chart becomes a guide for the tested dancer's conditioning program. Weak muscles should be strengthened and inelastic muscles stretched.

Guidelines for Increasing Strength

Exercises for building strength require maximal contractions that move through the full range of motion. In the initial phases of some of the exercises described further on, the weight of the body alone, or the simple movement of a joint through an unfamiliar action, is sufficient to achieve a state of maximal contraction. That is because the muscles in the first phases of conditioning are not yet very strong. However, as strength increases it becomes necessary to find a way to add resistance to the performance of the exercise to continue building strength.

Increasing Resistance

Certain systems of increasing resistance are more effective than others for this area of the body. Free weights are difficult to use because they do not attach readily to the foot. Elastic bands, in many forms, can serve this purpose. As strength increases, one might use different color-coded

Assessment of Strength and Range of Motion

Strength	Strong	Average	Weak
Plantarflexors (neutral tarsus)			
Dorsiflexors (neutral tarsus)			
Plantarflexors/pronators			
Plantarflexors/supinators			
Dorsiflexors/pronators			
Dorsiflexors/supinators			
Range of motion	**Marked**	**Average**	**Limited**
Plantarflexors (neutral tarsus)			
Dorsiflexors (neutral tarsus)			
Plantarflexors/pronation			
Plantarflexors/supinaton			
Dorsiflexors/pronation			
Dorsiflexors/supinaton			

Figure 13.5   Sample form for recording the results of testing.

strengths of Theraband, which are available at any medical supply house.

These forms of resistance are effective for strengthening the muscles of the tarsus (pronators and supinators) and the dorsiflexors of the ankle. For the muscles that exclusively plantarflex the ankle joint (those that are already strong in most dancers), other systems that add greater resistance are appropriate. One method for building strength in the plantarflexors is to shift the weight to one foot in performing normal dance exercises such as pliés and relevés. This action doubles the load on the muscles.

Match the Weak to the Strong

The specific nature of the exercises that are needed is determined by the manual assessment of strength performed previously. If there is a major imbalance between opposing muscle groups in the ankle and tarsus, bring the strength of those muscles more closely into balance by exercising the weakest muscles. In the process one may identify a difference in strength between opposing muscle groups or between the same muscle group of the right foot and the left foot. This information is valuable, as one goal of any conditioning program is to achieve balance of muscular capacity. When an imbalance of muscular strength is discovered, the general

rule is to do a few extra repetitions with the weak muscles or muscle group to work toward more balanced strength. If the action is hard to do, do more—within reason.

Condition by Muscle Groups

Approach conditioning by muscle groups, starting with those that control the joint actions of the ankle and tarsus (plantarflexors, dorsiflexors, pronators, and supinators), and then isolating the combined actions of the ankle and tarsus (plantarflexors and pronators, plantarflexors and supinators, dorsiflexors and pronators, and dorsiflexors and supinators). The exercises described later are designed to build strength according to muscle groups. In doing any exercise to build strength, be aware of how much is enough and how much is too much. One must go beyond existing capacities to build strength, but going too far can lead to excessive muscle soreness, or even injury.

Stretch After Strengthening

Maximal contractions are beneficial and build strength with amazing speed, but always stretch out after a strength-building exercise bout. Without stretches the residual neuromuscular tension remains, and tends to increase the normal level of muscle soreness. In addition, stretching the active muscle group after an intense exercise bout seems to reduce the buildup of excessive muscle bulk (Fitt 1981-1982; Koutedakis, Cross, and Sharp 1996; McDougall et al. 1980). The principle for stretching out is to reverse the combined joint actions used in the strengthening exercises with a long, sustained stretch. Specific positions for stretching the different muscle groups are identified in the stretching section of this chapter.

Vary the Tempo of Strength Exercises

Increased strength is specific to the angle of the joint and the velocity of the contraction used in conditioning. Therefore, it is necessary to do the exercises for strength at both slow and fast tempos to achieve the maximum benefit.

Exercises to Increase Strength

The Ankle/Tarsus Series (For Strengthening All Combined Actions of Ankle and Tarsus)

This series can be done in a long-sit position or lying on one's back. Dorsiflex the ankle joint. Press the soles of the feet out to the sides (pronate), without rotating at the hip joint and without lessening the degree of dorsiflexion. Then press the soles of the feet inward (supinate), isolating the action to the tarsus. Alternate the in-and-out action and repeat to the point of fatigue. Repeat the sequence with the ankle joint in a position of plantarflexion. As strength increases, add more repetitions until about 40 or 50 are done easily. Then go on to the advanced ankle/tarsus series.

The Advanced Ankle/Tarsus Series (For Strengthening All Combined Actions of the Ankle and Tarsus)

Add resistance to the previous series by the use of surgical tubing. The tubing is placed around the balls of the feet, and the exercises are performed against the resistance. Do the exercises for the action of pronation in both plantarflexion and dorsiflexion (figure 13.6*a* and *b*, respectively) and supination (figure 13.6*c* and *d*).

The "Mouth" (For Strengthening the Dorsiflexors of the Ankle)

In the long-sit position, place the right heel on top of the left ankle joint. Place a circular, elastic resistance device behind the toes (figure 13.7). Holding the elastic in place with the left foot, pull straight up against the resistance with the toes and foot on the right side. Repeat the exercise with the left foot on top, dorsiflexing it against the resistance. If one foot (ankle) is stronger than

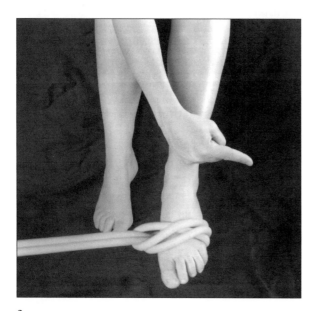

a

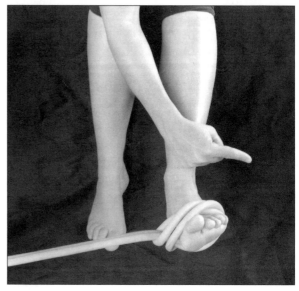

b

(continued)

Figure 13.6 Ankle/tarsus strengthening exercise: *(a)* pronation in plantarflexion; *(b)* pronation in dorsiflexion; *(c)* supination in plantarflexion; *(d)* supination in dorsiflexion.

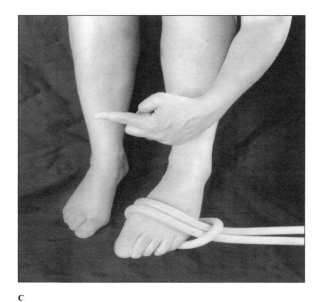

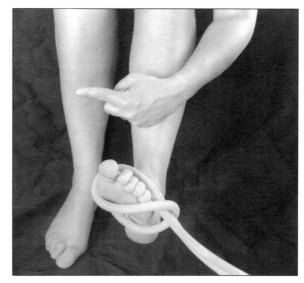

c   *d*

Figure 13.6   *(continued)*.

Photos courtesy of Rosalind Newmask.

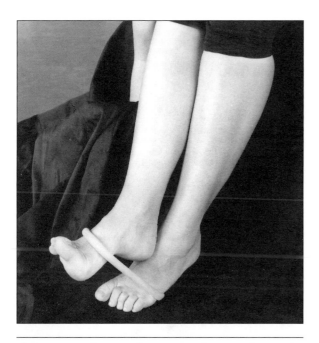

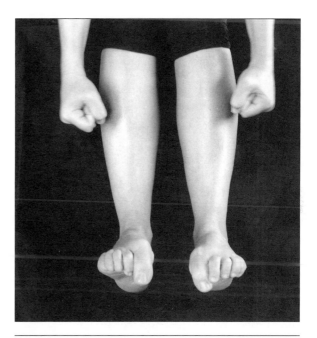

Figure 13.7   The "mouth": exercise for strengthening the dorsiflexors of the ankle.

Photo courtesy of Rosalind Newmark.

Figure 13.8   Toe gripper: exercise for strengthening the intrinsic muscles of the foot.

Photo courtesy of Rosalind Newmark.

the other, one or two extra repetitions should be done on the weak ankle to begin the process of equalizing strength.

Toe Gripper (For Strengthening the Intrinsic Muscles of the Foot)

In a long-sit position, flex the knees slightly, dorsiflex the ankle, and grip the toes as hard as

possible (figure 13.8). Simultaneously grip the hands into tight fists (this fortifies the contraction of the foot muscles by activating the flexor reflex). Hold the contraction about 15 to 20 seconds, but not to the point of cramping the muscles of the foot. Release, stretch, and wiggle the toes. Repeat the whole exercise, including the stretch.

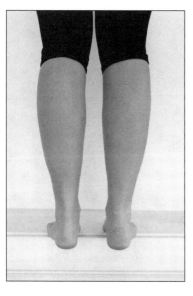
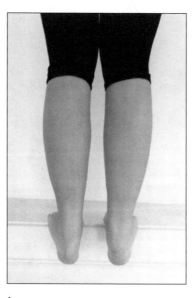
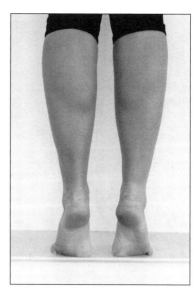

a   b   c

Figure 13.9 The stair step: exercise to strengthen the plantarflexors of the ankle.

Photos courtesy of Rosalind Newmark.

Stair-Step Full Relevés (To Strengthen Plantarflexors of the Ankle and Increase Awareness of a Properly Aligned Tarsus During Action of the Ankle)

Stand on a stair step with the balls of the feet on the edge of the step, the heels unsupported (figure 13.9*a*). Allow the heels slowly to descend as far as possible, while keeping the tarsus in a neutral position (figure 13.9*b*). Then rise through the normal standing position and, maintaining neutral alignment of the tarsus, go on to full relevé or half-toe (figure 13.9*c*). Lower the heels to the starting position. Repeat this exercise to fatigue. When your strength has developed to the point that it is easy to do 30 repetitions, try this exercise with all your weight on one foot. Reduce the number of repetitions accordingly.

Weighted Pliés/Relevés (To Strengthen the Plantarflexors of the Ankle As Well As All the Muscles Involved in Plié and Relevé)

Do a complete plié/relevé sequence in all positions with weight added to the normal body weight. A scuba diver's weight belt can be used, or free weights, or even a dance bag held in the hands with the arms hanging at the sides (figure 13.10). As strength increases, do more repetitions or add more weight. With more strength, reduce

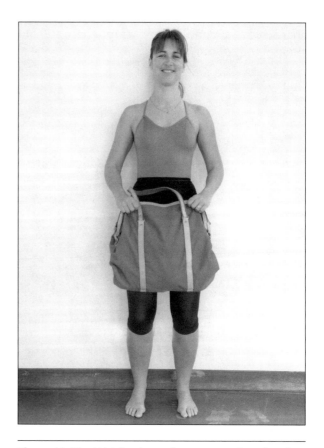

Figure 13.10 Weighted exercise: to strengthen the plantarflexors of the ankle.

Photo courtesy of Rosalind Newmark.

the amount of weight and repetitions and do the sequence on one foot at a time. Increase weight or repetitions as strength increases.

Note: Pay careful attention to alignment in the torso and legs as you would in an unweighted plié series.

How Much Strength Is Enough?

There may come a point when the dancer says "This is enough." There is no pat answer to the question of how much strength conditioning is enough. Each dancer must review the demands he or she makes on the body. These demands serve as a guide for strength conditioning, but it is important to remember that one should always have a reserve of extra strength so that the body can accommodate to unusual demands. Also, it is important to explain to the dancer that there are phases in the conditioning process—an initial phase, an improvement phase, and a maintenance phase—so that conditioning simply becomes an integral part of one's regimen.

Guidelines for Increasing Elasticity

The use of the long, sustained stretch for the muscles of the ankle and tarsus was recommended earlier in this chapter. The rationale is based on the fact that the ankle and tarsus do not have a balance of muscle mass between agonists and antagonists. The long, sustained stretch is therefore most effective in this region.

Balance the Elasticity of Opposing Muscle Groups

Imbalance in the muscular elasticity of opposing muscle groups at the ankle and tarsus has just as serious consequences as does an imbalance of strength. Having more range of motion in one direction than another (for example, more supination than pronation) means that the agonists are less elastic (in this case, the supinators) and the antagonists (the pronators) are more elastic. Given the different standard range of motion potential inherent in these two actions, the tarsus will take

a neutral muscular position between the greater possibility of supination and the lesser possibility of pronation. This is a muscular neutral, not the neutral position of the tarsus joint, which is considered the ideal. It means that the foot will fall into a position of supination whenever it is not bearing weight. Landing on a supinated tarsus greatly increases the likelihood of sprains and strains of the tarsus, commonly called ankle sprains.

Stretch by Joint Action

The most effective and efficient way to stretch any muscle is to reverse all of its joint actions. It is possible to stretch effectively by performing all of the combinations of actions possible at the relevant joints. Thus, stretching of the ankle and tarsus muscles requires stretching in the following combinations of actions: pronation and plantarflexion; pronation and dorsiflexion; supination and dorsiflexion; and supination and plantarflexion. Because there are four muscles that cross the ankle, tarsus, and the toe joints, the addition of flexion and extension of the toes as another feature of the stretch ensures that one has stretched all of the muscles of the ankle and tarsus.

Stretch Past the Comfort Zone

It is not unusual to find dancers doing what I call "token stretches"—stretches of very short duration that stay within the comfort zone, never going past the point of pain. For a stretch to be effective—that is, to increase the elasticity of the muscle—it is necessary to go beyond the existing capacities of the muscle to stretch. Hence, the stretches that are least comfortable to do tend to be the ones that are needed the most.

Use Gravity or Other External Forces to Increase the Stretch

The long, sustained stretch is most effective if the target muscles are in a passive state (i.e., not contracted at all). For this reason it is helpful to place the joint in a position where gravity will increase the stretch on the target muscles. If the plantarflexors are the target muscles, for example, a joint position should be taken that allows gravity to assist in the dorsiflexion of the ankle joint.

If it is difficult to use gravity in this way (as it is for some of the combined actions of the ankle and tarsus), other sources of external force can be used to increase the stretch, as long as the person experiencing the stretch has control over them. One easy way to provide external assistance for a stretch is by manually pushing the joint into the stretch position. Doing this for oneself is the safest technique for using manual stretches. With another person doing the pushing it is difficult to control the pressure, so extreme caution must be exercised to avoid injury.

How Long Is Long Enough?

Holding a stretch for less than 20 to 30 seconds is a "token" stretch. There is not enough time in short-duration stretches for the connective tissue of the muscle to be stretched. Hold a stretch for at least 1 minute, particularly when the muscles have been inelastic for some time. Moreover, each stretch should be repeated at least three or four times during the day to reinforce the sense of stretch in the muscles and the new position of the joint allowed for by the stretch.

Relax and Reassemble After a Stretch

A period of relaxation and reassembly is critical after a long, sustained stretch. This is particularly true of stretches that are new to the dancer, and are focused on muscles that have not been intensively stretched in the past. The body needs time to adjust to the new information given to it by a long, sustained stretch. Allow that time by relaxing and paying conscious attention to the changes that have occurred. Relaxation should be followed by imaginary movements of the joint, and then gentle movements of the joint to reawaken the muscles around it to the demands of contraction.

Stretching Exercises

Gastrocnemius and Soleus (Achilles Tendon)

Assume a parallel lunge position with the right leg forward and the hands reaching out to rest against a wall. Keeping the left knee straight and the left heel on the floor, press forward through

the hips onto the right leg, taking more weight on the hands. Hold this position for 30 seconds to 1 minute (figure 13.11a). Then slowly bend the left knee, still keeping the left heel on the floor, and hold this stretch position for 30 seconds to 1 minute (figure 13.11b). Come out of the stretch of the left

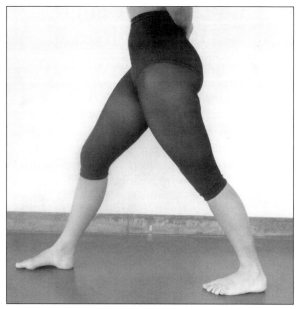

a

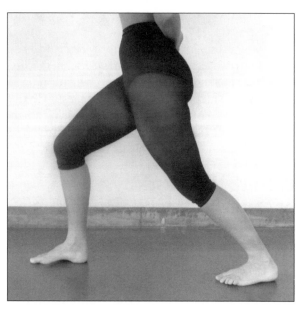

b

Figure 13.11 Stretches for the *(a)* gastrocnemius and *(b)* soleus.

Photos courtesy of Rosalind Newmark.

*Editors' note: For another opinion on partner stretching, see chapter 12.

180

ankle slowly, taking time to assess the changes and process the new information. Repeat the exercise on the other side, with the left foot forward and the right ankle the focus of the stretch.

Note: Always do this stretch in both positions of the knee, as different muscles are stretched when the knee is straight (gastrocnemius) and bent (soleus).

Stretch for Pronators and Plantarflexors

Sitting in a chair with the right lower leg resting on top of the left thigh, assume a position of dorsiflexion and supination of the right ankle and tarsus. Place the right hand on the inside of the right ankle joint and take hold of the foot with the left hand (figure 13.12). Pull with the left hand and push with the right, thereby applying an external force to increase the stretch in the direction of dorsiflexion and supination. Hold the stretch for 30 seconds to 1 minute. Relax for a moment before repeating the exercise on the other side.

Stretch for Pronators and Dorsiflexors

Sitting in a chair with the right lower leg resting on top of the left thigh, assume a position of plantarflexion and supination of the right ankle and tarsus. Place the right hand on the inside of the right ankle joint and take hold of the foot with the left hand (figure 13.13). Push with the right hand and pull with the left hand to increase the joint actions of supination and plantarflexion. Relax for a moment before repeating the exercise on the other side.

Adding the Toe Muscles

While doing the previous stretch, add powerful gripping of the toes, or manually pull the toes into flexion (figure 13.14).

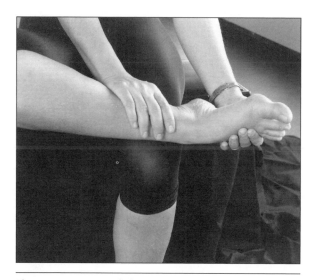

Figure 13.13 Stretch for pronators and dorsiflexors.
Photo courtesy of Rosalind Newmark.

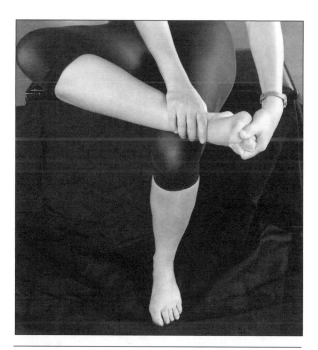

Figure 13.12 Stretch for pronators and plantarflexors.
Photo courtesy of Rosalind Newmark.

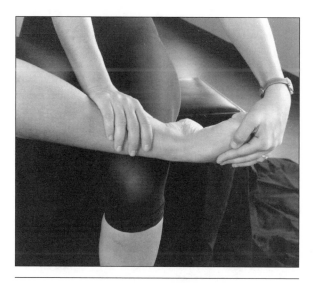

Figure 13.14 Stretch for toe muscles.
Photo courtesy of Rosalind Newmark.

Stretch for Supinators and Plantarflexors

Sitting either in a chair or on the floor, draw the right knee up to the chest and take hold of the right foot with the right hand on the little-toe side of the foot (figure 13.15). With the hand, pull the foot up (into dorsiflexion) and to the outside (into pronation). Hold the stretch for 30 seconds to 1 minute and relax for a moment before repeating the exercise on the left side.

Adding the Toe Muscles

To include the muscles of the toes in the previous stretch, maintain dorsiflexion and pronation with the right hand and pull the toes up into a position of extension with the left hand. Add stretch of the toe muscles to the left side of the stretch as well.

Stretch for Supinators and Dorsiflexors

Sitting in a chair with the right lower leg resting on top of the left thigh, assume a position of plantarflexion of the ankle and pronation of the tarsus with the right foot. Hold the right ankle with the right hand, the thumb toward your chest and the fingers on the outside of the ankle. Place the heel of the left hand on the most medial aspect (toward the middle) of the ball of the foot. Press with the left hand and pull with the right

hand while maintaining a plantarflexed position of the right ankle. Hold the stretch for 30 seconds to 1 minute and then relax for a moment before repeating the stretch on the other side.

Anterior Shinsplint Stretch

Kneel and sit back on the heels with the ankles plantarflexed. Place the hands on the floor on either side of the knees. Lift the knees off the floor, taking the weight of the body on the hands and on the tops of the feet while keeping the buttocks close to the heels (figure 13.16). Allow gravity and the weight of the body to increase the plantarflexion of the ankle joints. Keep the tarsus in a neutral position (neither supinated nor pronated) throughout this exercise. Hold the position for 30 seconds to 1 minute. Relax and do some easy ankle circles on completion of the exercise.

Stretch for Shinsplints on the Posterior and Medial Aspect of the Lower Leg

Do the soleus stretch described previously with the back foot turned out (figure 13.17). As usual, hold the stretch for at least 30 seconds to 1 minute and relax for a moment before doing the second side. Then do the soleus stretch with the back foot turned in (figure 13.18).

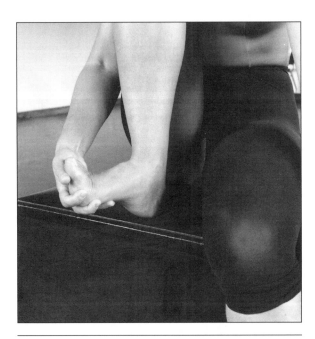

Figure 13.15   Stretch for supinators and plantarflexors.
Photo courtesy of Rosalind Newmark.

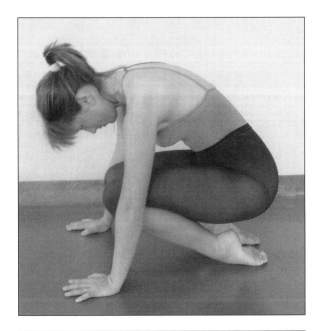

Figure 13.16   Anterior shinsplint stretch.
Photo courtesy of Rosalind Newmark.

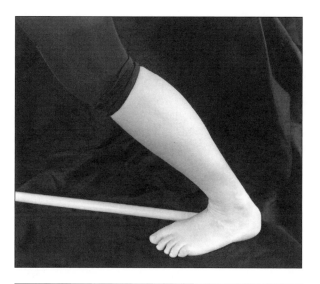

Figure 13.17 Stretch for shinsplints, turned-out position.
Photo courtesy of Rosalind Newmark.

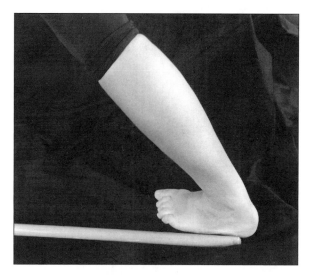

Figure 13.18 Stretch for shinsplints, turned-in position.
Photo courtesy of Rosalind Newmark.

Conclusion

The primary rationale for this chapter is that dance classes do not sufficiently focus on building strength and elasticity in the foot and lower leg to prevent injuries to that region. Efficient and effective conditioning practices are often ignored, and the injury rate in this region, for dancers, is inordinately high. A simple system for increasing strength and elasticity of the muscles of the ankle and tarsus is presented. The general steps of the system include (1) identification of areas of weakness, inelasticity, or injury; (2) identification of joint actions in those areas; (3) identification of key muscle groups; (4) analysis of present conditioning practices and special demands on those areas; (5) assessment of strength and range of motion; and (6) using the principles of conditioning to design exercises to balance strength and mobility of agonist and antagonist muscles of the right and left sides. I believe that effective strengthening and stretching exercises can be incorporated into technique classes, working toward the central goal: *to dance.*

References

Bachrach, R.M. 1988. The relationship of low back/pelvic somatic dysfunctions to dance injuries. *Orthopaedic Review* 17(10): 1037-1043.

DeVries, H.A. 1966. *Physiology of exercise for physical education and athletics.* Dubuque, IA: Brown.

Fitt, S.S. 1996. *Dance kinesiology.* 2nd ed. New York: Schirmer Books.

Fitt, S.S. 1981-1982. Conditioning for dancers: Investigating some assumptions. *Dance Research Journal* 14(1 and 2): 32-38.

Fleck, S.J., and W.J. Kraemer. 1987. *Designing resistance training programs.* Champaign, IL: Human Kinetics.

Fuller, P.E. 1975. An identification of common injuries sustained in ballet and modern dance activities. PhD diss., Texas Woman's University, Denton, TX.

Gans, A. 1985. The relationship of heel contact in ascent and descent from jumps to the incidence of shin splints in ballet dancers. *Physical Therapy* 65(8): 1192-1196.

Koutedakis, Y., V. Cross, and N.C.C. Sharp. 1996. Strength training in male ballet dancers. *Impulse* 4(3): 210-219.

McDougall, J.D., G.C.B. Elder, D.G. Sale, and J.R. Sutton. 1980. Effects of strength training and immobilization on human muscle fibers. *European Journal of Applied Physiology* 43: 25-34.

Miller, E.H., H.J. Schneider, J.L. Bronson, and D. McLain. 1975. A new consideration in athletic injuries: The classical ballet dancer. *Clinical Orthopaedics and Related Research* 111: 181-191.

Nagrin, D. 1988. *How to dance forever.* New York: Morrow.

Ryan A.J., R.S. Gilbert, R. Schuster, and S.I. Subotnick. 1976. Ballet dancers' injuries pose sportsmedicine challenge. *Physician and Sportsmedicine* 4: 44-57.

Schneider, H.J., A.Y. King, J.L. Bronson, and E.H. Miller. 1974. Stress injuries and developmental change of lower extremities in ballet dancers. *Diagnostic Radiology* 113(3): 627-632.

Shaw, J.L.H. 1977. The nature, frequency and patterns of dance injuries: A survey of college dance students. MA thesis, University of Utah, Salt Lake City.

Stanish, W. 1984. *Tendinitis: Its etiology and treatment.* Lexington, MA: Collamore Press, Heath.

Washington, E.L. 1978. Musculoskeletal injuries in theatrical dancers: Site, frequency and severity. *American Journal of Sports Medicine* 6(2): 75-98.

Recommended Readings (Editors)

Kravitz, S.R., and C.J. Murgia. 1999. The mechanics of dance and dance-related injuries. In *Sports medicine of the lower extremity edition 2*, edited by S.I. Subotnick. New York: Churchill Livingstone, 645-655.

Liederbach, M., and R. Hiebert. 1997. The relationship between eccentric and concentric measures of ankle strength and functional equinus in classical dancers. *Journal of Dance Medicine & Science* 1(2): 55-61.

Macintyre, J., and E. Joy. 2000. Foot and ankle injuries in dance. *Clinics in Sports Medicine* 19(2): 351-368.

Ménétrey, J., and D. Fritschy. 1999. Subtalar subluxation in ballet dancers. *American Journal of Sports Medicine* 27(2): 143-149.

Miller, C., J. Gooch, and M. Haben. 1992-1993. Lower extremity range of motion in advanced-level ballet dancers. *Kinesiology and Medicine for Dance* 15(1): 59-68.

Potts, J.C., and J.J. Irrgang. 2001. Principles of rehabilitation of lower extremity injuries in dancers. *Journal of Dance Medicine & Science* 5(2): 51-61.

Shrader, K.E. 1996. Biomechanical evaluation of the dancer. *Orthopaedic Physical Therapy Clinics of North America* 5(4): 455-475.

Wiesler, E.R., D.M. Hunter, D.F. Martin, W.W. Curl, and H. Hoen. 1996. Ankle flexibility and injury patterns in dancers. *American Journal of Sports Medicine* 24(6): 754-757.

Chapter 14

Pronation As a Predisposing Factor in Overuse Injuries

Steven R. Kravitz, DPM

Part III on biomechanics concludes with a concise explanation of how the forces generated at the foot and ankle by dance movement, in conjunction with anatomic malalignment, can cause some of the most common injuries in dancers. This chapter is closely related through its subject matter to chapters 4 and 13.

From early on a major theme of the dance medicine literature has been that injuries to dancers result most often from overuse. By this we mean simply that the constant repetition of prescribed movements required by the practice of dance can wear body parts to the point that they give way. Research in biomechanics has been particularly useful in explaining how this happens. Using everything from the common tools of measurement to state-of-the-art computer and laser technology, biomechanists have demonstrated how the body's natural configurations—especially its malalignments—interact with stresses applied by dance training to produce injuries.

The anatomical region where these stresses are most intense in all dance forms is the foot and ankle. Many common malalignments result in excessive pronation; hence, from an injury prevention point of view, pronation is a subject of particular concern to dancers. This chapter looks at the mechanisms by which pronation predisposes the dancer to injury, and some of the things that might be done to counteract them.

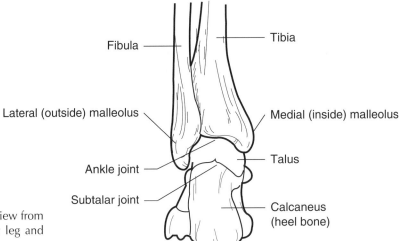

Figure 14.1 Ankle and subtalar joints: view from the back (posterior) aspect of the lower leg and foot.

Biomechanics of the Ankle Joint

Anatomically, the ankle joint consists of the articular aspects of the distal tibia and fibula surrounding the articulating joint surface of the talus (figure 14.1). This joint primarily allows dorsiflexion and plantarflexion of the foot on the leg. The joint just below the talus, the subtalar joint, allows for articulation between the talus and the calcaneus. This joint has three facets, or joint surfaces, where the two bones lie in direct contact with one another. These three areas, as with all movable joints, have a smooth surface of hyaline cartilage over bony areas at the corresponding facets, which decreases friction and allows opposing bones to move with respect to one another. The structure of the anterior, middle, and posterior facets of the subtalar joint classifies it as a "saddle joint"; that is, it allows the talus to rotate and slide as well as plantarflex or dorsiflex relative to the calcaneus.

Thus, articulations at the ankle and subtalar joints allow for motion in all three cardinal body planes—frontal for eversion/inversion, sagittal for dorsiflexion/plantarflexion, and transverse for inward rotation (adduction)/outward rotation (abduction). This range of available motion is possible because the axis around which it occurs is oblique to all three cardinal body planes, and thus not parallel to any one plane (figure 14.2).

The athlete and dancer should note that, due to the structural and dynamic factors briefly

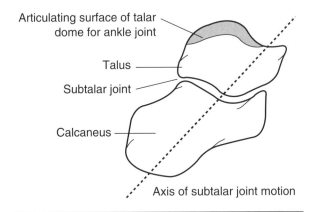

Figure 14.2 Sagittal plane view of the talus and calcaneus. The axis of the subtalar joint is near 45° to the frontal and transverse planes, producing equal motion in the two planes.

described, the various mechanical aspects of the subtalar joint complex allow the foot to pronate and supinate, thereby affecting the foot's stability. This mechanical action causes the foot to function both as a mobile shock absorber (when pronated) and as a rigid lever (when supinated). The latter function can be used to propel one forward from step to step, off the ground to perform a jump, or, in the case of a ballerina, on to her pointe stance.

Biomechanics of Pronation

Pronation describes a foot that collapses medially as one bears weight on it. Pronation at the subtalar joint allows the calcaneus to evert, leading

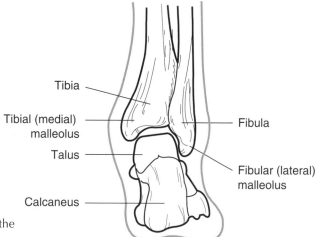

Tibia

Tibial (medial) malleolus

Talus

Calcaneus

Fibula

Fibular (lateral) malleolus

Figure 14.3 Excessive pronation as viewed from the rearfoot, with marked calcaneal eversion.

to the foot's rolling in upon itself (figure 14.3). Small amounts of calcaneal eversion during heel contact may occur normally, but the calcaneus should reduce to perpendicular during the middle of the stance phase of the walking cycle. Calcaneal eversion in this period of the walking or running cycle is often indicative of excessive pronatory motion, and should be evaluated for biomechanical instability.

As the calcaneus everts, the talus is forced to rotate internally and plantarflex. As already mentioned, motion at the subtalar joint occurs in all three body planes; thus, as the heel everts relative to the calcaneus the talus is forced to perform the other two motions described. Heel eversion cannot occur by itself; the other two movements must simultaneously develop in a weight-bearing attitude.

Potentially Injurious Effects of Pronation

The internal rotational force of the talus transfers through the ankle joint to the lower tibia and fibula, forcing the leg to rotate internally. The leg rotates at a faster rate than the thigh (when not extended and locked), leading to a significant shearing force at the knee and a tendency to pull the patellar tendon internally, directing the kneecap off its normal track. The resultant effect may produce chondromalacia, or "dancer's knee," as the undersurface and the surrounding tissues around the kneecap become inflamed.

Furthermore, plantarflexion of the talus can lead to anterior movement of the upper tibia, thus increasing strain to the foot as well as the knee. As the talus plantarflexes, the inside column of the arch unlocks, enhancing the collapsing effect on the foot. This produces the typical "rolled-in foot" appearance, and can encourage the development of many overuse injuries, such as heel pain, medial tibial stress syndrome, and stress fractures.

Heel Pain (Plantar Fasciitis)

The mechanism for heel pain is easily demonstrated. Make an arch out of your hand and picture a rubber band attached around the end of the thumb and forefinger. Opening this arch, imagine the rubber band being stretched. Similar mechanisms occur on the plantar aspect of the foot, where a traction or stretch is placed on the multiple tissues located there, especially the fascia. The plantar fascia is a thick piece of tissue that is attached as a narrow band to the calcaneus and then broadens as it runs distally toward metatarsal heads 1 through 5. Collapse of the arch structure places considerable strain on this tissue, and is a common cause of arch and heel pain.

Shinsplints

Shinsplints may also be associated with these mechanisms. This is especially true of strain involving the tibialis posterior muscle, which will often overwork to maintain the arch in an appropriate functioning position. Muscles generally serve to provide motion to bones where they interact at joints, and are not designed to support unstable structures. One function of the tibialis posterior muscle is to provide foot supination; thus the collapsing foot places excessive strain on this muscle and can initiate a posterior shinsplint.

Stress Fractures

Excessive pronation can also contribute to stress fractures. The internally rotating leg establishes torque forces relative to the internally rotating talus, and may develop a type of stress fracture that often presents as pinpoint pain over bone 1.2 to 2 in. (3 to 5 cm) proximal to the fibular malleolus. Second metatarsal stress fractures are also commonly associated with this pathology. The mechanisms here relate to the only way the foot can truly "roll in." Calcaneal eversion with excessive subtalar joint pronation causes the first metatarsal to become hypermobile, and ultimately to dorsiflex. As this occurs the first metatarsal moves toward the top surface of the foot, and the inside pillar of support to the foot is lost. The rolled-in appearance with associated calcaneal eversion is the result. As the first metatarsal dorsiflexes, it loses its ability to maintain weight-bearing function. Weight that normally would have been absorbed by the first metatarsal is transferred to the much thinner second metatarsal. During aggressive propulsive activity, too much force may be received on the second metatarsal bone, causing it to develop a small hairline fracture known commonly as "stress fracture," or "march fracture."

> Chapter 8 includes more detailed discussion of stress fractures.

Preventing Excessive Pronation

A small amount of pronation is normal and needed to absorb shock; however, excessive pronation can lead to overuse injuries of the type commonly seen in dancers. These injuries may occur at anatomic sites from the lower lumbar spine distally through the plantar aspect of the foot.

The overly pronated foot can be treated with support to decrease injury potential. The athlete, dancer, and athletic trainer should note that all means of foot support might be helpful in decreasing symptoms associated with the problems described in the previous sections. Thus, foot strapping and padding applied to stabilize the arch is often an effective means of adjunctive therapy. Shoes with strong heel counters and longitudinal arch pads can be helpful. Shoe inserts (orthotics) can be professionally made from a cast impression of the foot, and are the best device for providing needed support. Orthotics can help decrease multiple overuse injuries and the rate of deformity development—for example, bunions, hammertoes, and heel spur syndrome—to which the pronated foot is especially susceptible. This holds true for the pediatric patient as well as the individual with a more developed foot. That is not to say that all children need orthotic support; indeed, most do not. However, professional opinion must be sought when the need is in question.

> For a case study in the use of orthotics, see chapter 10, page 133.

One last point: Appropriate muscle balance with well-toned leg musculature is an excellent shock absorber and may be adjunctively helpful in decreasing shock transmission between foot and leg, thus decreasing potential injury associated with excessive pronatory mechanisms. Hence, a well-developed dance regimen should serve this preventative function. Virtually the whole of chapter 13 is devoted to describing a regimen to combat such malalignments as excessive pronation by stretching and strengthening the muscles that control the subtalar joint. Further information regarding the causes and effects of excessive pronation is to be found throughout this book, especially in chapter 4.

Conclusion

Foot pronation is an important shock-absorbing mechanism. The subtalar joint, just below the ankle, is a primary factor in transmitting forces from the foot to the leg, and defines how the foot pronates in reaction to these forces. Excessive pronation is commonly associated with "malalignment," as well as with overuse injuries and developmental foot deformity. Controlling the degree of pronatory factors may decrease the deformity rate, and is advantageous in reducing the potential for overuse injury. Supporting the foot with appropriate footwear and, when necessary, orthotics, can be very helpful.

Recommended Readings (Editors)

Brown, T., and L.J. Micheli. 1998. Dance: Where artistry meets injury. *Biomechanics* V(9): 12-24.

Grossman, G., and V. Wilmerding. 2000. Dance physical therapy for the leg and foot: Plantar fasciitis and Achilles tendinopathy. *Journal of Dance Medicine & Science* 4(20): 66-72.

Marshall, P. 1989. The rehabilitation of overuse foot injuries in athletes and dancers. *Clinics in Podiatric Medicine and Surgery* 6(3): 639-655.

Potts, J.C., and J.J. Irrgang. 2001. Principles of rehabilitation of lower extremity injuries in dancers. *Journal of Dance Medicine & Science* 5(2): 51-61.

Solomon, R., E. Trepman, and L.J. Micheli. 1989-1990. Foot morphology and injury patterns in ballet and modern dancers. *Kinesiology and Medicine for Dance* 12(1): 20-40.

Sommer, H.M., and S.W. Vallentyne. 1995. Effect of foot posture on the incidence of medial tibial stress syndrome. *Medicine and Science in Sports and Exercise* 27(6): 800-804.

Part IV

Psychological Concerns

In recent years the concept of "mind–body synthesis" has increasingly influenced our understanding in matters pertaining to the health, general well-being, and everyday lives of dancers. This is demonstrable in the volume of dance medicine and science research now being devoted to such subjects as personality, perception, memory, motor memory, pain coping strategies, stress coping strategies, performance anxiety, gender differences, career transitions (especially retirement), the special needs of adolescent dancers, diet, nutrition, body image, and the female athlete triad (eating disorders, menstrual irregularities, osteoporosis). The three chapters of part IV offer a brief introduction to this trend, with emphasis on its relevance to injury prevention.

Chapter 15

Stress, Performance, and Dance Injuries

Raymond W. Novaco, PhD

Chapter 15 can be thought of as groundbreaking in its early recognition of the role stress plays in affecting the dancer's general well-being and causing such specific problems as performance anxiety (or "stage fright"). It points to a number of factors in the dancer's lifestyle that promote stress, and suggests some strategies for minimizing their effect.

To a greater extent than is true of other artistic performers, the dancer's training and performance regimens present risk for incapacitating injury. Gelsey Kirkland, in her *Dancing on My Grave* (1986), poignantly described the toll taken on her body by the need to meet choreographers' demands. Enduring perpetual inflammation and traumatic injuries, as well as Balanchine's and Robbins's insensitivity to such matters, stretched her physical and psychological resources beyond the limit.

One suspects that nothing could have helped Kirkland—hers is clearly the extreme case—but generally speaking, stress coping skills can both help prevent injuries and facilitate recovery from them. They can also contribute to performance enhancement. These skills, based on psychological techniques corroborated by research, are widely used in sport psychology. This chapter explores potential applications of stress reduction to dance. First, however, basic ideas about the nature of stress and how we are affected by it are discussed.

Stress and Arousal

In everyday usage stress refers to forces and feelings "out there" that put pressure on us, and also to something "in here" that is akin to a nervous disorder. This dual reference point creates some ambiguity in how we envision and discuss the subject. Scientific views of stress are not without ambiguities either, but they generally represent it as a condition inherent in the organism or system, stimulated by exposure to environmental demands, resulting in impairments to health and performance. Stress remains defined as a condition of imbalance between perceived demands and our resources for coping with them (Lazarus 1966; Mostofsky and Barlow 2000; Selye 1976).

The casual incorporation of stress into common parlance, in part through the marketing of stress management techniques, has induced some people to claim that there is both "positive" and "negative" stress. Selye (1976) inadvertently promoted this distinction by introducing the term "eustress" (as opposed to "distress") to describe those external conditions—work pressures, life challenges, performance demands, and various crises—that can motivate one to exceptional achievement levels. Despite its appeal to management consultants, no one has substantially developed the concept of "eustress," and the concept of positive stress has no scientific standing (Fink 2000). The confusion arises from failing to distinguish stress from coping (i.e., skills we acquire to produce beneficial outcomes in the struggle with adversity), and mistakenly treating stress as equivalent to arousal.

Arousal is very much a part of stress, but many things that produce arousal are not stressful. The prolongation of arousal does have a great deal to do with health, for example in affecting blood pressure, eating habits, or sleep patterns. The ability to regulate arousal, especially that associated with emotional reactions, is a central part of stress management, and bears heavily on matters like the rehabilitation of injuries. Tension, frustration, and demoralization are common reactions to injury that inevitably impair the recovery process.

Heightened physiological arousal can have a detrimental effect on performance. If arousal is too high or too low, performance suffers. In stress literature this is represented as an "inverted-U function" for the relationship between arousal and performance. This concept, known as the Yerkes-Dodson law, was elaborated by Duffy (1932, 1957) and Hebb (1955), and was later adopted in research on anxiety. While Duffy focused on the relationship between muscle tension and performance, Hebb discussed the arousal function in information processing. Easterbrook (1959) explained the arousal-caused impairment of performance in terms of "cue utilization"; arousal narrows the range of cues a person can use in doing a task. The more complex the task, the more cues are involved and the more disruptive become the effects of high arousal. Therefore, the idea of maintaining an "optimum level of arousal" appears. This implies that the level of arousal needs to fit the task and its performance requirements. Sport psychology makes great use of these principles (LeUnes and Nation 1989).

When a task has many mental components, or if there are precise movements to be performed (as in dance), the importance of moderating arousal is greatest. If arousal is too low, there is little effort and no intensity. If arousal is too high, there is decreased concentration and poor execution. The way a particular level of arousal will affect performance very much depends on the requirements of the task and the skill level of the performer. High arousal should be less disruptive to gross motor movements that have become automatic in the performer's repertoire.

Another aspect of the significance of physiological arousal as a component of stress is its intrinsic role in the disruptive emotions. Arousal is closely associated with such emotions as fear, anger, and disappointment, and it is in this realm of our thinking about this association that we have come farthest in defining our beliefs about the activation and control of stress. Prior to the 18th century, emotions were understood as passions by which we are "gripped," "seized," or "torn" (Averill 1974). This view suggests that emotional reactions are strictly the result of things that happen to us. However, more recently we have come to see ourselves as architects of our experiences, and only rarely as their victims. We construct our experience, and much of that construction takes place in the head, while the rest is produced by our own behavior. This belief in human volition is a major theme of stress reduction interventions. Cognitive control techniques are widely used for stress management and in the regulation of pain. Knowing how to use the power of the mind as a coping skill is partly dependent on recognizing dysfunctional thought processes for what they are, such as conquering the potentially paralyzing effects of depression, anxiety, and shame (Greenberger and Padesky 1995).

Cognition, Performance Anxiety, and Pain Management

Among the early pioneers of sport psychology was Timothy Gallwey (1974), who recognized the importance of what goes on in our head for successful performance. His research, and that of others who followed in his footsteps, raises a number of important issues for dancers.

Performance Anxiety

In Gallwey's analysis, performance anxiety springs from self-doubt. The lack of trust in one's ability to perform to full capacity leads to anxiety and to physiological "tightening." Otherwise smooth, efficient movements become halting and self-conscious. Furthermore, this relationship between self-doubt, anxiety, and performance is what system theorists would call a "deviation-amplification" process: self-doubt produces anxiety, which leads to performance errors, which create further self-doubt. Sensations of weakness in bodily joints, light-headedness, and general loss of muscle tone can be symptoms of self-doubt. Commonly, people in this state compensate by trying too hard.

Stage fright is an amplification of normal anxiety reactions that have escalated to debilitating levels. It is normal to be nervous before performing in front of an audience, but if the performer gives undue attention to anxiety symptoms (e.g., "butterflies," dizziness, rapid breathing, excess perspiration, trembling) nervousness can escalate into panic. The dancer may fear losing control, become hypercritical, and dwell on expectations of failure.

Being on stage means, of course, being the center of attention with few places, if any, to hide. "Dancing in front of an audience involves risk—a slip, misstep, gesture offbeat, forgetting what is supposed to be done. Fear of failure is most troubling. Dreadful apprehension may also occur when the theme of the dance threatens to become real, that is, the roles the dancers enact are too close to the performers' immediate personal life experiences" (Hanna 1988, p. 125). Some accomplished dancers experience stage fright throughout their careers, but they are able to focus on the performance, preventing the anxiety from becoming debilitating. This is an application of the idea of being task oriented, which is a fundamental coping skill in controlling disruptive emotions.

Pain Management

Besides producing certain emotional episodes like stage fright, our cognitions play an important role in the experience of pain. Perception and tolerance of pain are psychologically mediated processes. As Melzack and Wall (1965) theorized, pain is a multidimensional phenomenon involving sensory, motivational, and cognitive-evaluative components. Because of intense desires to excel and the pressures of competition, dancers may ignore pain signals from their bodies that warn against continued exertion. Kirkland (1986) gives numerous examples of subjecting herself to chronic strain. In describing the compulsory regimens for turnout, she recalls, "There was no regard for the knees or hips, which in my case were distorted to the breaking point." Despite advice from an orthopedic surgeon regarding her feet, which had turned purple from inflammation, she "danced through the pain and compensated" (p. 34). As perhaps in this instance, a dancer's attitude toward physical injury may sometimes involve a touch of self-destructiveness, or be a way to cover career disappointments (Horosko and Kupersmith 1987).

The influence of mind on body has been recognized at least since the Greek and Roman Stoic philosophers. Hence, one can say that such mental processes as attention, expectation, appraisal, and reflection have a significant bearing on stress responses. Important determinants of stress and coping include the allocation of attention; our expectations of self and others; the appraisal or interpretation of events and circumstances; and our reflection, reconstruction, and rehearsal of experiences. Recurrent stress responses, such as the activation of the stress hormones cortisol and corticosterone (produced by the adrenal glands), have a detrimental effect on physical well-being, including the aging of the brain (Porter and Landfield 1998).

Stress Interventions

Considerable work in cognitive-behavior therapy spearheaded progress in the development of stress intervention techniques (Meichenbaum and Jaremko 1983), which are being used extensively in sport psychology (Williams 1986) and in the treatment of a wide range of health problems (Mostofsky and Barlow 2000). Across the now vast body of clinical research, stress reduction interventions are understood in terms of remediation procedures, regulatory techniques, and preventive strategies. *Remediation procedures* are interventions implemented to curtail and treat stress reactions. Psychological and medical procedures are available for such therapeutic action. *Regulatory techniques* are psychological coping tactics utilized to counteract precursors or elements of stress reactions, particularly with regard to tension, emotion, and cognition predisposing to stress. Behavior patterns linked with recurrent stress episodes may be modified in a self-regulatory effort. *Preventive strategies* involve proactive personal and organizational actions designed to reduce exposure to stressors, to develop skills for dealing with environmental demands, and to augment environmental and social resources that promote well-being.

The full scope of stress interventions cannot be described here, but two basic principles—arousal reduction and cognitive restructuring—and a number of associated techniques will be briefly discussed.

Arousal Reduction

Procedures designed to reduce arousal are commonly part of stress management programs. Both mental and physical relaxation are emphasized to control and regulate tension. The first structured approach in the medical and psychological literature was Jacobson's progressive relaxation method of systematically tensing and then relaxing sequential sets of skeletal muscles (Jacobson 1929).

Programs of this sort share roots in such ancient Eastern practices as yoga and tai chi, but it was not until the emergence of Transcenden-

tal Meditation (TM) in the 1960s and 1970s that Eastern ideas about relaxation gained widespread recognition. In TM technique the person sits comfortably in a quiet place with eyes closed, focuses on breathing, and repeats a mantra silently for 10 to 20 minutes, once or twice daily. Significant degrees of arousal reduction across many physiological channels have been found to be associated with TM practice.

Another relaxation induction procedure is autogenic training, developed by Schultz and Luthe (1959). Autogenic training was conceived by Schultz, a German psychiatrist, as a form of self-hypnosis that could be used to create mental resolve for behavior change, as well as to modify physiological conditions in specific organ areas. The technique emphasizes smooth, rhythmic breathing, self-instructions of calmness, and the use of suggestions of "heaviness" and "warmth" for body regions, especially limbs.

Besides these self-administered techniques of arousal reduction, more technical procedures, such as biofeedback and hypnosis, have demonstrated utility. There is indeed a wide array of relaxation induction techniques, including the use of music and massage, that have demonstrated their efficacy (Seaward 1994). The goal of each method is to teach the subject to control troublesome internal states. Having the capability to regulate arousal and tension improves the likelihood of optimum performance. Yoga, tai chi, massage, and meditation would seem to have particular value for dancers.

Cognitive Restructuring

Various procedures are used extensively in clinical work to modify cognitive dimensions of stress disorders. Changing belief systems, modifying perceptions, altering the focus of attention, eliminating intrusive thoughts, and adjusting expectation are among the tactics utilized to help clients restructure how they view the world and themselves. The treatment efficacy of such procedures has been extensively documented in clinical psychology research journals. Problems involving anxiety disorder, depression, assertiveness, pain, eating disorders, anger, alcoholism, and smoking have all been successfully treated with cognitive-behavioral therapies, often in a brief psychotherapy program (Bond and Dryden 2002).

With regard to stress, the process of coping effectively entails the ability to ascertain the nature of problems, think of alternative solutions, identify steps to solution, anticipate obstacles, and utilize feedback from coping efforts. These elements correspond to the necessities of injury rehabilitation. However, not all sources of stress are amenable to mastery. Natural disasters, aging, serious injury, disease, and the death of loved ones are examples of such conditions. Hence, the concept of coping acknowledges that there may well be constraints on possible outcomes and the availability of means. The severity of an injury (e.g., a joint sprain vs. a total rupture of a major tendon) may indeed limit the dancer's ability to regain preinjury proficiency.

Imagery and Visuo-Motor Behavioral Rehearsal

One cognitive technique that has extensive use in sport psychology is imagery and visuo-motor behavioral rehearsal (VMBR). This involves relaxation, visualization of performance, and performance in a simulated stressful situation. It is important that the person have an accurate mental image of optimum performance and be able to visualize the details of the behavioral sequence. Suinn (1972) developed this technique to remove emotional obstacles to performance and used it effectively with Olympic skiers. Other investigators then applied it to tennis and basketball players and to karate competitors in tournament situations (DeWitt 1980; Hall and Erffmeyer 1983; Noel 1980; Weinberg, Seabourne, and Jackson 1981). It is widely used to enhance performance and in injury rehabilitation (LeUnes and Nation 1989; Williams 1986).

Goal and Value Modification

Regarding stress arising from economic and occupational experiences, the most effective forms of coping involve the modification of goals and values. Goal setting is a cognitive-behavioral skill that has been incorporated into stress reduction programs and other approaches to performance enhancement. It involves an assessment of personal values, and a clear specification of short-term goals. Journal writing and establishment of a timetable with realistic expectations are useful tools.

The dancer experiencing stress from competitive pressures, along with the intense desire to perform to perfection, can be helped by a goal-setting strategy. The success of this hinges on an accurate knowledge of the performance requirements and a realistic assessment of the dancer's capabilities. Training procedures can be designed to improve diet, strength, flexibility, and conditioning. The visualization of goals to be achieved through practice can also be useful.

Time Management

Work stress is often generated by unrealistically high expectations of personal capacity. Trying to accomplish too much in a short time creates overload, which is highly stressful; therefore, time management is an important stress coping skill. Intense, unpredictable, and uncontrollable stressors disturb concentration, so the first step is overload avoidance. Learning to avoid excessive obligations can be difficult for high achievers, but peak performance is more likely to occur through relaxed concentration than through frenzied strain. Concentration on the here and now requires quietude of mind, undistracted by preoccupations. A lapse in concentration because of worries or fatigue detracts from proper technique, which raises the probability of injury.

Dance Injuries, Commitment, and Coping

Just as conditions of stress present risk for injury, being injured becomes a major stressor in itself. As Kirkland states, at the moment of injury the question "Will I ever dance again?" shoots through the brain of every dancer (Kirkland 1986). This is in large part a product of the sense of commitment that is deeply ingrained in most dancers, and that commitment has both positive and negative aspects. On the one hand it enforces the pursuit of goals in the face of obstacles and thereby blunts the pain experience, making the injured person more apt to sustain the requisite coping efforts (Lazarus and Folkman 1984). However, it also renders the person vulnerable to threat. The dancer who is deeply committed to a distinguished career is more threatened by an injury than one who has less lofty ambitions. The difference is between conditions of motivation or determination and those of anxiety or insecurity. It is one thing to endure discomfort, but it is quite another to cause greater tissue or structural damage by ignoring bodily signals.

Although injury denial is a normal way of coping among intense persons dedicated to achievement, the persistence of pain dictates taking the longer view of injury, sacrificing ego for recuperation and rehabilitation. Stress coping skills are useful in dealing with the frustration and demoralization that can ensue. We are affected emotionally by what we pay attention to and how it is appraised or interpreted. Cognitive restructuring combined with a sensible goal-setting strategy, including the visualization of renewed performance strength, can be an effective combination. Having an image of a long-term goal (as, for example, Roger Bannister had an image of breaking the 4-minute mile) is one way to start, but the goal should be realistic. Imagery can then be used to envision step-by-step the achievement of that goal, including the overcoming of anticipated obstacles. Because the recovery from injury is often complicated by setbacks of a physical or psychological nature, visualization can facilitate coping. In visualizing dance performance itself, kinetic, tactile, auditory, and scenic images can be utilized.

Among the most important stress-mitigating factors is the availability and utilization of supportive social relationships. While social relations can have negative as well as positive effects on psychological well-being (Rook 1984), it has been found that social support has a "buffering" effect on stressful life experiences. Supportive relationships can enhance coping with stressful events and perhaps reduce exposure to such events; they may even directly benefit physical and psychological health. Although the psychological mechanisms remain to be understood, social support protects us from otherwise debilitating forces associated with life crises and daily hassles. When one is faced with a serious injury, friends and colleagues can provide the best antidote to demoralization and prolonged distress. Using those valued relationships will help to maintain self-esteem and provide encouragement during rehabilitation.

Conclusion

Stress has been neglected as a subject relevant to dance performance and dance injuries. This chapter has pointed to several areas of stress involvement, including arousal functions, dis-

ruptive emotions, cognitive interference, and coping with injury itself. There are many stress regulatory interventions, shown to be efficacious by clinical research, that hold promise for enhancing dance performance and promoting well-being among dancers. It is to be hoped that the field of dance medicine will incorporate research on stress and coping.

References

Averill, J.R. 1974. An analysis of psychophysiological symbolism and its influence on theories of emotion. *Journal for the Theory of Social Behavior* 4: 147-190.

Bond, F.W., and W. Dryden, eds. 2002. *Handbook of brief cognitive behaviour therapy.* Chichester, England: Wiley.

DeWitt, D.J. 1980. Cognitive and biofeedback training for stress reduction with university athletes. *Journal of Sport Psychology* 2: 288-294.

Duffy, E. 1932. The relation between muscular tension and quality of performance. *American Journal of Psychology* 44: 535-546.

Duffy, E. 1957. The psychological significance of the concept of "arousal" or "activation." *Psychological Review* 64(5): 265-275.

Easterbrook, J.A. 1959. The effect of emotion on cue utilization and the organization of behavior. *Psychological Review* 66(3): 183-201.

Fink, G., ed. 2000. *Encyclopedia of stress.* San Diego: Academic Press.

Gallwey, W.T. 1974. *The inner game of tennis.* New York: Bantam Books.

Greenberger, D., and C.A. Padesky. 1995. *Mind over mood.* New York: Guilford.

Hall, E.G., and E.S. Erffmeyer. 1983. The effect of visuo-motor behavior rehearsal with videotaped modeling on free throw accuracy of intercollegiate female basketball players. *Journal of Sport Psychology* 5: 343-346.

Hanna, J.L. 1988. *Dance and stress: Resistance, reduction and euphoria.* New York: AMS Press.

Hebb, D.O. 1955. Drives and the c.n.s. (conceptual nervous system). *Psychological Review* 62(4): 243-254.

Horosko, M., and J.R.F. Kupersmith. 1987. *The dancer's survival manual.* New York: Harper & Row.

Jacobson, E. 1929. *Progressive relaxation.* Chicago: University of Chicago.

Kirkland, G. 1986. *Dancing on my grave.* New York: Doubleday.

Lazarus, R.S. 1966. *Psychological stress and the coping process.* New York: McGraw-Hill.

Lazarus, R.S., and S. Folkman. 1984. *Stress, appraisal and coping.* New York: Springer.

LeUnes, A.D., and J.R. Nation. 1989. *Sports psychology.* Chicago: Nelson-Hall.

Meichenbaum, D., and M.E. Jaremko, eds. 1983. *Stress reduction and prevention.* New York: Plenum Press.

Melzack, R., and P. Wall. 1965. Pain mechanisms: A new theory. *Science* 150(699): 971-979.

Mostofsky, D.I., and D.H. Barlow, eds. 2000. *The management of stress and anxiety in medical disorders.* Boston: Allyn and Bacon.

Noel, R.C. 1980. The effect of visuo-motor behavior rehearsal on tennis performance. *Journal of Sport Psychology* 2: 221-226.

Porter, N.M., and P.W. Landfield. 1998. Stress hormones and brain aging: Adding injury to insult? *Nature Neuroscience* 1(1): 3-4.

Rook, K.S. 1984. The negative side of social interaction: Impact on psychological well-being. *Journal of Personality and Social Psychology* 46(5): 1097-1108.

Schultz, J.H., and W. Luthe. 1959. *Autogenic training: A psychophysiologic approach in psychotherapy.* New York: Grune & Stratton.

Seaward, B.L. 1994. *Managing stress: Principles and strategies for health and well-being.* Boston: Jones and Bartlett.

Selye, H. 1976. *The stress of life.* New York: McGraw-Hill.

Suinn, R. 1972. Removing emotional obstacles to learning and performance by visuo-motor behavior rehearsal. *Behavior Therapy* 3: 308-310.

Weinberg, R.S., T.G. Seabourne, and A. Jackson. 1981. Effects of visuomotor behavior rehearsal, relaxation and imagery on karate performance. *Journal of Sport Psychology* 3: 228-238.

Williams, J.M., ed. 1986. *Applied sports psychology.* Mountain View, CA: Mayfield.

Recommended Reading (Author)

Auerbach, S.M., and S.E. Gramling. 1998. *Stress management: Psychological foundations.* Upper Saddle River, NJ: Prentice Hall.

Benson, H. 1975. *The relaxation response.* New York: Morrow.

Garfield, C.A. 1984. *Peak performance: Mental training techniques of the world's greatest athletes.* Los Angeles: Tarcher.

Recommended Reading (Editors)

Bouten, K., and A. Koops. 2001. Prevention of physical and mental overload. In *Not just any body.* Owen Sound, Ontario, Canada: Ginger Press, 81-83.

Gratto, S.D. 1998. The effectiveness of an audition anxiety workshop in reducing stress. *Medical Problems of Performing Artists* 13(1): 29-34.

Greben, S.E. 1992. Dealing with the stresses of aging in dancers. *Medical Problems of Performing Artists* 7(4): 127-131.

Hamilton, L. 1997. The emotional costs of performing: Interventions for the young artist. *Medical Problems of Performing Artists* 12(3): 67-71.

Hamilton, L., and W.G. Hamilton. 1994. Occupational stress in classical ballet: The impact in different cultures. *Medical Problems of Performing Artists* 9(2): 35-38.

Hamilton, L., J.J. Kella, and W.G. Hamilton. 1995. Personality and occupational stress in elite performers. *Medical Problems of Performing Artists* 10(3): 86-89.

Krasnow, D., L. Mainwaring, and G. Kerr. 1999. Injury, stress, and perfectionism in young dancers and gymnasts. *Journal of Dance Medicine & Science* 3(2): 51-58.

Liederbach, M., G.W. Gleim, and J.A. Nicholas. 1994. Physiologic and psychologic measurements of performance stress and onset of injuries in professional ballet dancers. *Medical Problems of Performing Artists* 9(1): 10-14.

Mainwaring, L., G. Kerr, and D. Krasnow. 1993. Psychological correlates of dance injuries. *Medical Problems of Performing Artists* 8(1): 3-6.

Marchant-Haycox, S.E., and G.D. Wilson. 1992. Personality and stress in performing artists. *Personality and Individual Differences* 13(10): 1061-1068.

Patterson, E., R.E. Smith, J.J. Everett, and J.T. Ptacek. 1998. Psychosocial factors as predictors of ballet injuries: Interactive effects of life stress and social support. *Journal of Sport Behavior* 21(1): 101-112.

Ramel, E.M., and U. Moritz. 1998. Psychosocial factors at work and their association with professional ballet dancers' musculoskeletal disorders. *Medical Problems of Performing Artists* 13(2): 66-74.

Sataloff, R.T., D.C. Rosen, and S. Levy. 1999. Medical treatment of performance anxiety: A comprehensive approach. *Medical Problems of Performing Artists* 14(3): 122-126.

Smith, R.E., J.T. Ptacek, and E. Patterson. 2000. Moderator effects of cognitive and somatic trait anxiety on the relation between life stress and physical injuries. *Anxiety, Stress, and Coping* 13: 269-288.

Taylor, J., and C. Taylor. 1995. *Psychology of dance.* Champaign, IL: Human Kinetics.

Weinberg, R., and D. Gould. 2003. *Foundations of sport and exercise psychology.* 3rd ed. Champaign, IL: Human Kinetics.

Chapter 16

The Role of Dance Teachers in the Prevention of Eating Disorders

Niva Piran, PhD

The rise to prominence of dance psychology owes far more to the growing concern with eating disorders and recognition that these conditions rest on a psychological base than to any other subject. This chapter is a product of its author's involvement in a program at an elite ballet school in Canada designed to help students avoid eating disorders. As a result of her experience she concludes that dance teachers everywhere play a key role in promoting this cause.

Almost all North American women are dissatisfied with their weight in what has been described as a "normative discontent" (Rodin, Silberstein, and Striegel-Moore 1984). Preoccupation with body weight and shape occurs on a continuum, from mild body dissatisfaction to severe clinical eating disorders (Shisslak, Crago, and Estes 1995). Approximately 70% of high school girls in North America, from different ethnic and racial groups and diverse socioeconomic backgrounds, report dieting to lose weight despite being within the normal weight range (Pike and Striegel-Moore 1997). It has been estimated that 15% of schoolgirls engage in extreme weight control efforts, including self-induced vomiting and laxative abuse (Phelps et al. 1993). Within this "normative" context of women at large, some studies have singled out dance schools as "high-risk" environments for the development of body weight and shape preoccupation, disordered eating patterns, and eating disorders. This may be particularly the case in "elite" training schools (Smolak, Murnen, and Ruble 2000).

All of these problems have been associated with significant morbidity, with a host of medical complications, and, in severe cases, with an elevated potential for death (Pomeroy and Mitchell 2002). Specific risks related to an early age of onset of eating disorders include growth retardation, pubertal delay and interruption, and osteopenia (Katzman 1999). Eating disorders have also been found to predict the development of psychological difficulties such as depression (Stice 2001) and social withdrawal, affecting both peer and intimate relationships (Sullivan 2002). The combination of physical, psychological, and social complications may further lead to disrupted scholastic or vocational performance (Sullivan 2002). The prevention of eating disorders among dancers in training is therefore clearly indicated.

To date little has been published about the prevention of eating disorders in schools of dance or about the outcome of such efforts. This author has implemented and evaluated a prevention program in a world-class co-ed residential ballet school for students ages 10 to 18 (Piran 1999, 2000). The program emphasizes the need to work with everyone involved in the school community, and to introduce school-wide changes in order to prevent eating disorders among students. It also highlights the particular role of a mental health consultant (normally a psychologist or psychiatrist) in such an endeavor. Interestingly, in the general literature on prevention of eating disorders and in the literature pertaining to dance, the role of teachers in promoting prevention has tended to be overlooked (Piran in press). This is a significant omission, since teachers and coaches spend a lot of time with their students and, especially in dance and athletics, are highly influential in relation to their trainees (Powers and Johnson 1999). Regarding teachers' concern with prevention, three surveys conducted with teachers in general schools found that they were mainly interested in learning how to prevent eating disorders by interacting more constructively with their students on a daily basis, and in information that would guide them in the early identification of eating disorders (Piran in press).

This chapter aims to describe the role of dance teachers in primary and secondary prevention of eating disorders. *Primary prevention* refers to the elimination of risk factors and the enhancing of protective practices to reduce the number of students who begin to display severe preoccupation with body weight and disordered eating patterns (Mrazek and Haggerty 1994). *Secondary prevention* aims at the early identification of disordered eating patterns and severe body dissatisfaction (Mrazek and Haggerty 1994). In discussing these issues the chapter draws on general risk and protective factors research (for a review, see Piran 2001a, 2002), on the findings of a qualitative study conducted in a ballet school (Piran 2001b), and on intensive dialogues with students, teachers, and teachers-in-training conducted by the author over the past 15 years. Throughout, the teacher's role in prevention as an aspect of the larger social world of dancers in training (including such influences as family members and peers) is emphasized.

The Teacher in Context

As multiple sources of pressure on students' body esteem have been identified in and outside of the domain of dance, the task of the dance teacher is to create an environment that both protects against adverse influences and allows for the acquisition of critical skills to withstand injurious pressures. Teachers' familiarity with the different levels of social influence that shape their students' experience can help clarify their role in caring for the well-being of their students. Four levels of social context are briefly outlined here: the larger culture, the dance culture, the school culture, and the professional and social contexts that have shaped the teacher's own approach to dance and training.

The Body in the Context of the Larger Western Culture

Pressures for thinness have been widely recognized as a risk factor for the development of negative body esteem, which in turn may lead to disordered eating patterns. These pressures are transmitted not only through the mass media, but also through close social interactions, such as weight-related peer teasing or critical comments by parents or other adults. Women, in particular, have experienced the pressures of objectification (the learned tendency to hold an observer's perspective toward one's own body), of devaluation of a fully feminine body (likely an aspect of social inequity for women), of constricting images of the idealized woman (constraining not only their appetites and body size, but also their ability to express needs and emotions, such as anger), and a higher rate of sexual harassment and violence. Both men and women have been influenced by consumerism and mass marketing that presents bodies as "projects" in need of shaping and repair. Perfecting the body is a greater task for women, as their social worth is more highly connected to appearance. These factors, among others, have been found to lead to disruption in the experience of positive connection with the body, or disembodiment (for a more comprehensive review, see Piran 2001a). Disembodiment interferes with one's ability to practice self-care, silences internal dialogue, and disrupts relationships, while enhancing one's tendency to manage or control the body from the "outside." Within this context it is hard to arrest the development of eating disorders and other potentially harmful behaviors (Piran et al. 2002).

The Body in the Context of Dance

Social pressures leading to disembodiment, or disrupted positive connection with the body, may become accentuated in the dance world. Pressures for thinness are greater, especially for female ballet dancers. The ongoing monitoring of dancers' bodies as they practice and perform intensifies the objectified experience of the body, and the continual verbal and physical corrections of movements by teachers and choreographers further challenge the experience of body boundaries. Girls and women generally feel a greater need to perfect all aspects of their appearance and performance because they are subjected to stiffer competition. The ballet world tends to reinforce traditional roles for women and men, with the idealized social image of the female ballerina even more restrictive than that of women in general (Vincent 1979). While strength, muscularity, power, and athleticism are admired in the male partner, the female ballerina is expected to be ethereal, thin, and controlled. Puberty in early adolescence, naturally associated with weight gain and breast development, in itself yields deviations from the idealized image of the ballerina. Under these circumstances even monthly cyclical hormonal changes, leading to temporary water retention, can be experienced as major disruptions to the idealized image. Being fully feminine in ballet can therefore be

challenging. Some girls in ballet who used to enjoy their athletic abilities and strength prior to adolescence find that these qualities are now a liability. Boys and young men, in contrast, may experience pressure related to lack of upper body strength, an experience that may compel some to try performance-enhancing substances. Overall, in the dance world an uncommonly large number of factors intersect to intensify pressures in the body domain.

The Body in the Context of the Dance Training Site

Dance schools and companies may differ greatly from one another with regard to factors relevant to the development of eating disorders among trainees, including the role of teachers in prevention. First, schools that aim at training world-class dancers tend to apply greater pressures not only in the domain of dance performance, but also in the domain of appearance. There are, however, exceptions to this rule; some local community schools, with no stated agenda to train professional dancers, can exert strong pressure on their female students to fit the ethereally thin mold of the prima ballerina. Second, the diversity in the types of dance for which students are being trained may determine the intensity of pressure in the body domain. In a school that trains only classical ballet dancers, the pressure will be greater than in a school that trains both for ballet and for modern dance. In modern dance settings generally there is greater diversity in female body shapes, and acceptance of athleticism and strength. This corresponds to less dichotomous gender-based roles in modern dance.

A third factor that differentiates training schools is in their overall commitment to the long-term well-being of the dancer. While some schools define their responsibility in terms of imparting dance training only, others view their role as caring for the development of the dancer in a more holistic manner. Naturally, the involvement of teachers in the prevention of eating disorders is facilitated in schools that aim to address the whole person. Often such schools enlist the support of mental health professionals who can analyze the pressures in the training setting and work with staff to address those pressures (Piran 1999). These professionals can also be used to identify trainees at risk and to provide relevant counseling. Schools that assume responsibility for the welfare of their trainees also tend to provide them with physiotherapy and body conditioning consultations and extra-curricular healthy nutrition education, body image focus groups, and relaxation training. Moreover, such schools tend to give students more room to voice their needs, and, indeed, revise school policies or training curricula in response, hence providing students with a sense of agency and power.

A fourth training site factor to consider in terms of teachers' role in prevention is the age of students. Pressures in the body domain are most damaging to prepubertal students and those in early adolescence. For example, in these young trainees appearance and weight-related pressures, and consequent weight loss, may lead to stunted growth and bone disease as well as to disruption in sexual and hormonal development. The task of learning social roles at this stage of development, an experience that commonly challenges the sense of self, may become too strenuous if students are concurrently subjected to mounting performance and appearance pressures. Girls may notice the greater sexualization and objectification of their bodies once puberty starts, and hence become more attuned to the way their bodies are treated in class. Those who experience social events that disrupt their sense of safety or positive excitement about their developing bodies at this crucial age may face later challenges in living comfortably in a woman's body. In this regard, providing respect for students' bodies and body boundaries is crucial. Considering the later onset and longer duration of puberty in boys, they may feel less physically and emotionally prepared, and therefore more taxed, by male–female pas de deux partnership training even in mid-adolescence. The process of growth during puberty involves changes in body shape and appearance, related to the timing of growth spurts. The teacher can support the acceptance of this natural process by providing a protective environment that encourages continuity of growth.

The impact of widely sanctioned prejudices on the school environment constitutes a fifth dimension to examine when one is considering the role of teachers in prevention. A school that accepts a variety of body shapes facilitates the role of its teachers in promoting a positive body image. Conversely, a teacher who himself feels criticized for putting on weight while transitioning into middle age may find it harder to support his students who are gaining weight as part of the natural process of puberty. Gender equity in terms of roles of power and influence at the school provides a good model for girls and boys as they transition into adult roles, and allows them to feel comfortable in becoming, socially and physically, young women and men. Racial attitudes in a school may be expressed through targeting body-related aspects of certain group members, leading to negative body esteem. This practice must be discouraged. The more diligently a training site addresses matters relating to weightism, sexism, racism, and other social prejudices, the more protective it will be of both teachers' and students' experiences.

To conclude, every training site has particular characteristics that either facilitate or encumber the teacher's work toward prevention of eating disorders. The teacher has to examine the context within which he or she works in order to identify the positive factors in the system and use them in the cause of prevention.

The Teacher's Own Internalized Context

Teachers carry their own professional, social, and psychological background with them into the dance studio. This background shapes the learning environment they provide for students. It is therefore of crucial importance that teachers examine what has affected their own experiences while training in dance schools, both positively and negatively, and utilize this knowledge to inform their teaching style. Toward the goal of preventing eating disorders it is of particular relevance to examine body-related experiences. Teachers who can identify elements in their training that have facilitated a positive connection with the body and a positive body image—for example, those whose own teacher was a positive role model of body acceptance and healthy eating—can then apply this knowledge to their own teaching. Teachers who identify aspects of their training that were disruptive to positive connection with the body and led to negative body esteem, such as teasing about body shape in the classroom, can learn from their experience about practices to avoid while teaching. Typically, teachers have been exposed to a large number of facilitative and disruptive experiences. The more open they are to the impact of their own training on their teaching, the greater wealth of knowledge they will have to draw on in enhancing the positive body image of their students. Sometimes teachers may develop a critical awareness of their own biases by examining their behavior in the classroom. For example, teachers may notice that they pay more attention to thin students, or that they label as "dedication" the compulsive exercise regime of a very thin student who is rapidly losing weight. These biases often reflect the impact of learned and internalized values that need to be critically examined.

The Role of Teachers in Primary Prevention

Informed by the examination of multiple contexts, the teacher needs to create an environment in his or her own classroom that will be conducive to the development of positive body and self esteem. What follows are suggestions that may help achieve this goal.

Body Functionality

Whenever she [the teacher] gave me a correction, it was about something I could change.

Research has shown that the experience of physical competence is an important aspect of body esteem, particularly among athletes (Franzoni and Shields 1984). Dance students often complain about the emphasis in their training on careful scrutiny and corrections, and the neglect of reward and praise. Consistent exposure to negative commentary erodes self and body esteem. Conversely, guiding students toward the optimal use of their bodies, accepting and working with both strengths and weaknesses, enhances their sense of competence and of a positive body connection. This rule applies especially to teachers' appearance-related corrections; comments should emphasize changes that can be achieved through proper use of the

body, rather than commentary about unchangeable body characteristics. These latter comments result in negative body esteem.

Dancing From the "Inside Out"

Sometimes she [the teacher] covered the mirrors and let us just get into the feeling.

If your focus is all the time on the outside, how can you dance? Because when you dance, you don't dance from the outside-in, you dance from the inside-out!

Both maintaining and being subjected to an ongoing critical gaze at the body and its movements take a psychological toll. As the body is objectified it ceases to be an aspect of one's subjectivity, an instrument in the personal expression of feelings, ideas, and spirit. Objectification also reduces creativity to appearance, and, sometimes, appearance to thinness. One way to maintain and nurture the importance of subjectivity in dance is to give students the opportunity to dance at least part of the time in a physical space that minimizes external gaze, like a mirror-free room. This helps connect students with their selves and with their bodies as subjective instruments of expression. Teachers may wish to engage in a dialogue with students about these subjective experiences, thus confirming the value of inner expression.

The Natural Look and Natural Transitions

I like the natural look. Everybody is different. It is an art. You can express your feelings no matter what your actual weight is. We have a right to be who we are. I don't want to change my body.

The women in that group [of dancers] looked so different from one another . . . I couldn't believe it.

I remember when I was 11 . . . I used to come home from school hungry. My mother was working, so I made myself a sandwich every day. I know that's why my body was changing. . . . My [ballet] teachers told me I was bad. I still feel guilty about it . . . I have never felt OK about my body since. (A retired dancer in her 40s)

In this modern era of high-tech communications and the ongoing manipulation of virtual images, the sense of real bodies is fading. As mentioned previously, bodies are typically considered projects to be repaired, changed, and manipulated. Natural diversity in appearance and body characteristics is rarely represented in media-generated images; rather, what is emphasized is the need to control natural developmental changes and transitions related to puberty or aging. To counteract this influence young students in dance need repeatedly to hear messages about the healthy and natural process of growth. They need the support of their teachers in order to trust, for example, that weight gain and growth spurts that occur in an uneven manner and result in sudden changes in body shape are simply the genetically determined manifestations of puberty.

Supporting Gender Equity in Dance

I applied to [a summer ballet program] . . . I didn't write the right breast size . . . my breasts are too big . . . they don't like it. . . .

He [her partner] says that I am too fat to be lifted. I feel ashamed.

Partnership [in pas de deux] is mutual. . . . Dance is like a metaphor for life.

Dance trainees often express challenges related to gender inequity. The idealized mold of female ballet dancers involves not only weight restriction, but also limitations on such matters as breast size and muscle bulk. The relative abundance of female trainees as compared with male trainees leads to a much stricter appearance code for female dancers. Male dancers, however, face other prejudices, sometimes related to allusions regarding their sexual orientation. The teacher has to be aware of these pressures, acknowledge them as problems, and deflect the tendency of dancers to feel personally ashamed or "flawed" in relation to prejudicial social expectations. While pas de deux exercises can become a deflating experience for adolescent trainees, with the female dancers typically being blamed for being "too fat" and the male dancers for being "too weak," the partnering class can be used as an occasion for challenging gender-based stereotypes and developing a pattern of mutual partnership, responsibility, and

communication. One myth, for example, to be dispelled is that a female dancer's weight, rather than her stamina, is crucial to a successful pas de deux partnership. A thin but weak female dancer is difficult to raise and maintain off the ground, as she lacks the necessary muscle strength and control to help with the lift.

A Respectful Safe Space

She [the teacher] pinched my stomach and said 'too big."

I still have blue marks on my thighs from her [the teacher] poking me because my thighs are too large.

He [the teacher] got angry because we all just didn't get it. He said, 'you are all fat."

The experience of safety and respect in the body domain is crucial to positive body and self esteem, and to a sense of personal agency, worth, and rights. Even mild violations of body boundaries are disruptive to students' body esteem. Teachers should be aware of the manner in which physical corrections are made. Clearly, harsh physical treatment of students is not acceptable. Similarly, sexualization of contact with students is highly disruptive (sexual abuse is, of course, a reportable offense). Interestingly, verbal or emotional abuse often targets the body as an easy domain for deprecation. Again, due to the sensitivity of the body domain and appearance-related pressures, verbal corrections of body movements should be made in a way that discourages their misinterpretation as affronts to body shape.

While respectful behavior by teachers is crucial for students' body and self esteem, teachers are also responsible for establishing norms of safety in their classrooms and disallowing teasing, harassment, deprecation, or any form of maltreatment by peers. Other class norms that could help increase the experience of safety in the class should be considered, such as disallowing mutual body evaluations or comparisons by peers.

The identification of teachers with favorite students may pose particular challenges in maintaining boundaries. Teachers may be so invested in some students' careers that they inadvertently attempt to dictate aspects of their lives, like eating patterns. While advice can be valuable, the respect inherent in being cognizant of boundaries and of students' right of free choice prevents long-term difficulties.

Regarding Appearance

I have to keep such a balance. To have this role, I cannot weigh more. I know that they [the dance company] would like me to lose another 10 pounds, but if I lose more weight I get really tired and I am just too weak.

Accentuated pressures for thinness currently pervade the ballet world. These pressures force a number of female ballet dancers to maintain weights that are significantly below their natural weight, and may well be associated with hormonal dysfunction and other medical complications. Teachers in "elite" training programs may feel torn between the wish to guide students toward successful ballet careers, hence transmitting and enforcing the intense standards of thinness, and supporting students in maintaining their natural body shape and guiding them to the other professional options that are available. In general, it is useful to encourage older teenagers and young adults to make an informed decision about what weight is safe and healthy for them, and to encourage them to stay at a weight that may be slightly above the "ideal."

While appearance standards are very detailed for women in ballet, students often interpret any observation regarding their body shape as a comment about their weight, perhaps because it is possible to change weight but not other body characteristics. As it is a very difficult experience for a dedicated student who is committed to the art of dance to be barred from the profession due to appearance-related considerations, it is important in these situations to be explicit about what the issues are. Otherwise, a student may tend to blame her weight for all of her difficulties.

Ideally, teachers in elite programs should work together, through ongoing activism in the ballet world, to change the current standards of thinness. A less ambitious, but equally worthwhile goal, is for teachers to work on a local basis toward "relaxing" the thinness standards of the schools in which they teach. In noncompetitive settings teachers should avoid all pressures involving body shape.

An Informed Space

If only somebody told me when I was 11 that I would stop growing if I ate too little. (An 18-year-old ex-dance student, 4 ft 11 in. [150 cm] tall)

Students rely on significant adults in their lives to either transmit relevant constructive information or guide them to reliable resources for this information. While dance teachers cannot be expected to become expert in all aspects of health and psychology, there are some areas with which teachers, especially of children and adolescents, should have some familiarity. For example, it is useful for teachers to be informed about principles of nutrition to allow for the ongoing dissemination of information in class about healthy eating, as well as to correct "nutritional myths" that students commonly hold. Similarly, a familiarity with the physiology of weight regulation and starvation, and with the risks associated with nutritional deprivation and unsupervised weight control methods, allows the teacher to share this important information as opportunities arise in discussions with students. Knowledge about the healthy process of development in puberty can help support students through this growth phase. Similarly, an understanding of the psychological and social challenges in the life of adolescents can help make teachers aware of aspects of their interactions with students or of peer interactions to which students may be particularly sensitive, like body-related teasing.

Obviously, teachers should be informed about eating disorders, and they should also know not to "describe" eating symptomatology to students, since dissemination of such information can result in iatrogenic complications. Instead, teachers should freely discuss healthy growth and development. However, should an eating disorder symptom be described *by a student* in the group context, the teacher should be prepared to explain the risks associated with this symptom, with the goal of discouraging such behavior among students. Teachers should not hesitate to state clearly their own stance against eating disorders and disordered eating patterns. Students sometimes need to hear that weight loss will not "compensate" for challenges in dance, and to witness that weight loss indeed has not changed the teacher's attitude toward a dancer.

In sum, teachers should be informed about the multiple social challenges and pressures students face in today's larger society and in the dance world. Familiarity with these pressures allows the teacher to validate them and to argue that the difficulty lies with the social and dance expectations rather than with the students themselves. This helps the students develop a critical outlook toward their social environment, rather than toward their own bodies.

The Role of Teachers in Secondary Prevention: Early Identification and Treatment

While teachers can provide a protective environment, their students may still develop strong body weight and shape dissatisfaction and resort to extreme weight control measures. It is important for teachers to recognize the multiplicity of pathways that can lead to the development of an eating disorder. These pathways can include a variety of intra-individual factors (such as temperamental tendencies), as well as a host of environmental factors (such as experiences in the family or with peers). Several strategies will aid in early identification and intervention, which are associated with a better prognosis:

Familiarity With the Early Signs of Eating Disorders

Eating disorders start with an intense preoccupation and dissatisfaction with body shape. Dysphoric mood is usually present as well. These symptoms may be followed by the onset of weight loss. Food restriction and bingeing behaviors may both be present. Purging behavior may take the form of an intense and compulsive exercise regimen; vomiting; and laxative, diuretic, or other substance use. Dance teachers should be aware of, and alert to, these manifestations of disorder.

Tendency to Observe the Well-Being of Students

In addition to providing instruction, teachers have the opportunity to observe their students' behavior closely in class. If a relationship of trust has previously developed with a weight-preoccupied student, there is some likelihood that she will approach the teacher directly, though students often attempt to keep eating disorders secret. In anorexia nervosa, secrecy helps maintain control over weight loss, while in bulimia it may be explained by symptom-related shame.

Willingness to Approach a Distressed Student

When approaching a student suspected of having developed an eating disorder it is important for the teacher to share his or her observations and invite the student to respond. The teacher should not pathologize body preoccupation and disordered eating patterns, but rather reflect an attitude that these behaviors are understandable reactions to mounting pressures. Then, the student and teacher should explore together the next steps that should be taken to connect the student with valuable resources.

Network of Mental Health Consultants

Teachers need to rely on the support of mental health professionals for consultation and treatment. It is important that they be aware of their own limits in terms of availability and training. Taking on more than one can do may prove frustrating to teacher and student.

Conclusion

Finally, as a non-dancer I would like to convey the inspiration I have received from the ballet personnel I have met over the past 15 years, who demonstrate tremendous dedication both to the training of elite dancers and to overseeing their well-being. It appears that the dance community as a whole is ready to wrestle with the challenges related not only to the prevention of eating disorders, but also to caring for its members in a holistic way. I look forward to the emergence of a new generation of empowered and healthy dancers who will make constructive changes that will benefit the community as a whole.

References

Franzoni, S.F., and S.A. Shields. 1984. The body esteem scale: Multidimensional structure and sex differences in a college population. *Journal of Personality Assessment* 48(2): 173-178.

Katzman, D. 1999. Prevention of medical complications in children and adolescents with eating disorders. In *Preventing eating disorders: A handbook of interventions and special challenges,* edited by N. Piran, M.P. Levine, and C. Steiner-Adair. Philadelphia: Brunner/Mazel (Taylor & Francis Group), 304-318.

Mrazek, P.J., and R.J. Haggerty, eds. 1994. *Reducing risks for mental disorders: Frontiers for preventive intervention research.* Washington, DC: National Academy Press.

Phelps, G.C., R. Andrea, F.G. Rizzo, L. Johnston, and C.M. Main. 1993. Prevalence of self-induced vomiting and laxative/medication abuse among female adolescents: A longitudinal study. *International Journal of Eating Disorders* 14(3): 375-378.

Pike, K.M., and R.H. Striegel-Moore. 1997. Disordered eating and eating disorders. In *Health care for women,* edited by S.J. Gallant, G.P. Keita, and R. Royak-Schaler. Washington, DC: American Psychological Association, 97-114.

Piran, N. 1999. On the move from tertiary to secondary and primary prevention: Working with an elite dance school. In *Preventing eating disorders: A handbook of interventions and special challenges,* edited by N. Piran, M.P. Levine, and C. Steiner-Adair. Philadelphia: Brunner/Mazel (Taylor & Francis Group), 256-269.

Piran, N. 2000. Eating disorders: A trial of prevention in a high risk school setting. *Journal of Primary Prevention* 20(1): 75-90.

Piran, N. 2001a. A gendered perspective on eating disorders and disordered eating. In *Encyclopedia of gender,* edited by J. Worell. San Diego: Academic Press, 369-378.

Piran, N. 2001b. Re-inhabiting the body from the inside out: Girls transform their school environment. In *From subjects to subjectivities: A handbook of interpretive and participatory methods,* edited by D.L. Tolman and M. Brydon-Miller. New York: New York University Press, 218-238.

Piran, N. 2002. Prevention of eating disorders. In *Eating disorders and obesity: A comprehensive handbook,* 2nd ed., edited by C.G. Fairburn and K.D. Brownell. New York: Guilford Press, 367-371.

Piran, N. in press. Teachers: On "being" prevention. *Eating Disorders: The Journal of Treatment and Prevention.*

Piran, N., W. Carter, S. Thompson, and P. Pajouhandeh. 2002. Powerful girls: A contradiction in terms? Young women speak about the experience of growing up in a girl's body. In *Ways of knowing in and through the body: Diverse perspectives on embodiment,* edited by S. Abbey. Welland, Ontario, Canada: Soleil, 206-210.

Pomeroy, C., and J.E. Mitchell. 2002. Medical complications of anorexia nervosa and bulimia nervosa. In *Eating disorders and obesity: A comprehensive handbook,* 2nd ed., edited by C.G. Fairburn and K.D. Brownell. New York: Guilford Press, 278-285.

Powers, P.P., and C.L. Johnson. 1999. Small victories: Prevention of eating disorders among elite athletes. In *Preventing eating disorders: A handbook of interventions and special challenge,* edited by N. Piran, M.P. Levine, and C. Steiner-Adair. Philadelphia: Brunner/Mazel (Taylor & Francis Group), 241-255.

Rodin, J., L. Silberstein, and R. Striegel-Moore. 1984. Women and weight: A normative discontent. In *Psychology and gender: Nebraska Symposium on Motivation,* edited by T. Sonderegger. Lincoln, NE: University of Nebraska Press, 267-307.

Shisslak, C.M., M. Crago, and L.S. Estes. 1995. The spectrum of eating disorders. *International Journal of Eating Disorders* 18(3): 209-219.

Smolak, L., S. Murnen, and A. Ruble. 2000. Female athletes and eating problems: A meta-analytic approach. *International Journal of Eating Disorders* 27(4): 371-380.

Stice, E. 2001. Risk factors for eating pathology: Recent advances and future directions. In *Eating disorders: Innovative directions in research and practice,* edited by R.H. Striegel-Moore and L. Smolak. Washington, DC: American Psychological Association, 51-73.

Sullivan, P.F. 2002. Course and outcome of anorexia nervosa and bulimia nervosa. In *Eating disorders and obesity: A comprehensive handbook,* 2nd ed., edited by C.G. Fairburn and K.D. Brownell. New York: Guilford Press, 226-230.

Vincent, L.M. 1979. *Competing with the sylph: Dancers and the ideal body form.* New York: Andrews & McMeel.

Recommended Readings (Editors)

Bettle, N., O. Bettle, U. Neumärker, and K.J. Neumärker. 1998. Adolescent ballet school students: Their quest for body weight change. *Psychopathology* 31(3): 153-159.

Bettle, N., O. Bettle, U. Neumärker, and K.J. Neumärker. 2001. Body image and self-esteem in adolescent ballet dancers. *Perception and Motor Skills* 93(1): 297-309.

Buckroyd, J. 2000. *The student dancer: Emotional aspects of teaching and learning dance.* London: Dance Books.

Kaufman, B.A., M.P. Warren, and L. Hamilton. 1996. Intervention in an elite ballet school: An attempt at decreasing eating disorders and injury. *Women's Studies International Forum* 19(5): 545-549.

Neumärker, K.J., N. Bettle, U. Neumärker, and O. Bettle. 2000. Age- and gender-related psychological characteristics of adolescent ballet dancers. *Psychopathology* 33(3): 137-142.

Pigeon, P., I. Oliver, J.P. Charlet, and P. Rochiccioli. 1997. Intensive dance practice: Repercussions on growth and puberty. *American Journal of Sports Medicine* 25(2): 243-247.

Robson, B.E. 2002. Disordered eating in high school dance students: Some practical considerations. *Journal of Dance Medicine & Science* 6(1): 7-13.

Robson, B.E., A. Book, and M.V. Wilmerding. 2002. Psychological stresses experienced by dance teachers: "How can I be a role model when I never had one?" *Medical Problems of Performing Artists* 17(4): 173-177.

Shapiro, S.B., ed. 1998. *Dance, power, and difference: Critical and feminist perspectives on dance education.* Champaign, IL: Human Kinetics.

Taylor, L.D. 1997. MMPI-2 and ballet majors. *Personality and Individual Differences* 22(4): 521-526.

Yannakoulia, M., M. Sitara, and A.-L. Matalas. 2002. Reported eating behavior and attitudes improvement after a nutrition intervention program in a group of young female dancers. *International Journal of Sport Nutrition and Exercise Metabolism* 12(1): 24-32.

Chapter 17

The Female Athlete Triad in Dancers

Bonnie E. Robson, MD, D.Psych, DCP, FRCP(C)

Chapter 17 discusses eating disorders as one element (with menstrual irregularities and osteoporosis) in the "female athlete triad," which the American College of Sports Medicine has been instrumental in defining and publicizing. For our purposes it has an advantage over numerous other discussions of the subject in that it takes a preventive approach.

The Position Stand on the Female Athlete Triad published by the American College of Sports Medicine (ACSM) in 1997 defines a syndrome that encompasses three serious medical conditions associated with certain athletic endeavors: disordered eating, amenorrhea, and osteoporosis (Otis et al. 1997). In defining and describing this syndrome the ACSM noted that these disorders (to which dancers have long been known to be vulnerable) cannot be viewed or treated as separate entities; recognition of any one of the components raises suspicion of the syndrome.

The ACSM Position Stand states that "pressure placed on young women to achieve or maintain unrealistically low body weight underlies the development of the Triad. . . ," especially in physically active women (Otis et al. 1997, pages i-ii). For female dancers, their body weight must in many circumstances be kept at 10% to 20% below ideal body weight (Brooks-Gunn, Warren, and Hamilton 1987). They are as vulnerable as gymnasts and figure skaters to the public demand for thinness in their sport (Ryan 1995). Teenage preprofessional ballet dancers have been found to average 87% of the expected body weight, while college-age modern dance students average 88% of expected body weight (Garner and Garfinkel 1980; Schnitt, Schnitt, and Del A'Une 1986).

This chapter is adapted from B.E. Robson, 1998, "The female athlete triad," *Journal of Dance Medicine & Science* 2(1): 42-44.

Dancers are athletes; their profession is as strenuous as ice hockey (Nicholas 1975; Shell 1986). The ACSM recognizes that all athletically active women can develop the triad, but that dance, figure skating, diving, and gymnastics (because they are subjectively scored) place their participants at higher than normal risk. The Position Stand is extremely important to dance medicine specialists, dance educators, and administrators because it recognizes that "[t]he Triad can result in declining physical performance, as well as medical and psychological morbidity [affecting a significant proportion of the dance population] and mortality [causing death]" (Otis 1997, p. i).

What's Old Is New Again

That disordered eating is associated with the dance profession is not news. L.M. Vincent discovered the first published link between dance and anorexia in a game called The Ballet Company, manufactured in 1973 by Stetson Enterprises (Vincent 1989). This is the same year that Hilda Bruch drew attention to the internal as well as the external pressures involved in the development of anorexia nervosa (Bruch 1973). Among these were traits of perfectionism and issues of control and competence (Solomon et al. 2001). Hence, it is not surprising that Garner and Garfinkel in 1980 found that 6.5% of professional ballet students had anorexia, and that the incidence of anorexia nervosa correlated with the level of competitiveness in any given dance program. Throughout the 1980s the scientific literature included studies that confirmed an unusually high incidence of eating disorders in dancers (Hamilton et al. 1987; Holderness, Brooks-Gunn, and Warren 1994; Kurtzman et al. 1990-1991), higher than in skaters or swimmers (Brooks-Gunn, Burrow, and Warren 1988), and more prevalent in those dancers who are not genetically thin (Hamilton et al. 1988).

Disordered eating not only refers to caloric restriction but also includes a wide variety of behaviors such as using diet pills, laxatives or diuretics, and purging—all associated with the psychiatric disorders of anorexia nervosa and bulimia nervosa as defined by the American Psychiatric Association *Diagnostic and Statistical Manual of Mental Disorders (DSM-IV)* (American Psychiatric Association 1994). Anorexia nervosa is seen in 0.5% to 1% and bulimia nervosa in 1%

to 4% of women aged 15 to 30. The ACSM does not make specific reference to "Eating Disorders Not Otherwise Specified" (EDNOS), which are described in the *DSM-IV*, but it might be important to take note of these disorders. Women in this category are usually of average weight and do not binge, but do purge, putting themselves at risk of electrolyte imbalance and its consequences. Some female dancers suffering from this condition might not be recognized as having one or more components of the triad, and could therefore be at risk for long-term effects. "Heavy" dancers, defined as 4% to 10% below normal weight, were found by Hamilton and colleagues to engage in more weight control behavior yet still weigh more than thinner dancers, who were 11% to 20% below normal weight (Hamilton, Brooks-Gunn, and Warren 1986).

Some dancers with EDNOS meet all the criteria for anorexia except amenorrhea. This is important as it illustrates that dancers can be extremely thin without experiencing altered menstrual function. These women may maintain their low body weight with disordered eating patterns that go unrecognized. While the ACSM does describe a full range of eating disorders, it might also be important for those assessing dancers to be cognizant of the criteria specific to EDNOS.

A Fresh Look

Some dancers may not consider their disordered eating to be aberrant. Despite the morbidity and mortality associated with anorexia, the illness is sometimes glamorously portrayed as showing the characteristics of self-denial and commitment necessary to become a "ballerina." Anna Pavlova was described as a waif or a sparrow, as ethereal as a cloud (Gordon 1983). The adulation accorded her emphasized her intense commitment to the art form; she was said to have danced many times on bleeding feet. Today it is hypothesized that this may have resulted from the dry cracked skin that is typical of anorexics.

Secondary amenorrhea, oligomenorrhea, or even primary amenorrhea may not be distressing to young dancers. These conditions may be viewed as welcome evidence of their determination, and may be underreported, especially if it is common knowledge in the school that the student with amenorrhea has been encouraged to gain weight. However, when eating disorders or amenorrhea are linked to stress fractures, dancers, their teachers, and administrators become interested in prevention. Stress fractures can be devastating and often lead to depression, as they generally require lengthy absence from dance in order to heal.

> For an extensive treatment of stress fractures in general, and the specific role of inadequate nutrition as a precipitator of this injury, see chapter 8.

As noted in the background statements of the Position Stand, exercise-associated amenorrhea (EAA) has long been recognized. In some instances it may have become an accepted part of the sport and, in fact, many coaches and advisors of athletes do not regard amenorrhea as abnormal (Otis et al. 1997). However, the ACSM statement emphasizes that amenorrhea is "neither desirable nor a 'normal' result of physical training." The ACSM draws attention to the fact that the etiology, prevalence, sequelae, and treatment of EAA are not completely known.

Menstruation has its roots in the endocrine system. A decrease of luteinizing hormone (the hormone considered responsible for ripening of the follicle and the release of the ovum during ovulation) is thought to be caused by a decrease of gonadotrophic releasing hormone (GnRH), which is secreted by the hypothalamus. The reason for the decrease in GnRH is under investigation. There are two current hypotheses: Either GnRH is decreased by exercise stress (Bullen et al. 1985; DeSouza et al. 1991; Ding et al. 1988; Loucks and Horvath 1984; Loucks et al. 1989; Rivier and Rivest 1991), or the decrease is a result of insufficient energy availability (Edwards et al. 1993; Loucks et al. 1992, 1994; Myerson et al. 1991; Williams et al. 1995; Wilmore et al. 1992). The ACSM Position Stand devotes considerable space to explaining the latter of these two issues—the imbalance in an athlete's dietary intake and energy expenditure. Simply stated, some athletes consume fewer calories than their bodies require for their level of activity. The logical result of this hypothesis is the recommendation that physically active women must practice eating patterns that match their caloric intake to their energy expenditure in order to avoid alterations in their reproductive hormones and menstrual function.

Preventing and Managing the Female Athlete Triad

Editors' note: The following passage by Professor Karen Clippinger offers some practical guidelines for prevention and management of the female athlete triad.

Dancers have a difficult challenge to achieve a very lean body while taking in enough calories to supply their increased energy needs. A dancer's diet must provide enough carbohydrates to resupply energy stores and enough protein to maintain growth of body structures and allow for recovery from training. At the same time, dancers must limit fat intake in order to maintain lean body mass (not to mention avoid the many health risks associated with high fat intake, such as increased risk of cardiovascular disease).

The U.S. Department of Agriculture's Food Guide Pyramid is a good guideline for eating a healthy diet. The pyramid emphasizes variety and encourages high intake of grains and fruits and vegetables; moderate intake of lean dairy and meat products; and low intake of foods high in calories and fat.

For a dancer to achieve a lean but healthy body, emphasis must be placed on evaluation of body composition rather than scale weight. When weight loss is indicated, techniques should be used that result in slow loss of weight and are targeted toward reducing fat intake and building lean body mass. Combining aerobic exercise and supplemental strength training with a low-fat diet provides an excellent means of achieving and maintaining desired body composition while avoiding the female athlete triad.

The importance the Position Stand gives to amenorrhea should foster early recognition of women who are at risk for developing low bone density, stress fractures, and osteoporosis. It affirms that amenorrhea is not a "natural" or "expected" accompaniment to vigorous exercise but rather a pathological condition, and thereby highlights the need for assessment and treatment of any young athlete or dancer who suffers from menstrual irregularities.

The Whole Person

In focusing on the relationship between component disorders the ACSM underlines the need for further research on osteoporosis, on dancers with eating disorders, and on EAA, and emphasizes the need for collaboration of experts from different backgrounds in conducting this research. The members of the committee responsible for drafting the Position Stand are acknowledged authorities in the field; and some, like Dr. Barbara Drinkwater, have been involved in collaborative work for many years. In 1984, she began a longitudinal study of bone mineral density in amenorrheic athletes (Drinkwater, Nilson, and Chestnut 1984). While the initial data indicated postparticipation improvement in this area, the ex-athletes never recovered full health, and it was shown that later in life their bone mineral density dropped again. Because of the risk of fractures associated with low bone mineral density this work has great relevance for dance medicine professionals (Drinkwater, Nilson, and Chestnut 1986). The Position Stand should provide impetus for similarly important longitudinal studies and further investigation of optimal training regimens.

Collaboration is necessary not only in research but also in clinical practice. Marika Molnar, a recognized dance medicine therapist, reported the case of a 17-year-old female ballet student who presented with a stress fracture. In the process she advocated for education on the risk of fractures in ballet dancers with menstrual irregularities and below average weight as a result of inadequate nutrition and the emotional and physical demands of ballet (Molnar 1997, p. 24). She noted, "Healing did not occur until both the patient and practitioner were willing to address the needs of the whole person." It is to be hoped that families, health professionals, teachers, and administrators, as well as the dancers themselves, will heed the ACSM Position Stand, which promotes exactly this type of holistic approach to healing.

Conclusion

It is unlikely that the framers of the ACSM Position Stand on the Female Athlete Triad had dancers more than peripherally in mind; nonetheless, the publication and broad distribution of that statement has potentially done the dance community a world of good by raising consciousness of a condition to which dancers are particularly susceptible. And consciousness raising is of the utmost importance, as it is the key to prevention, which is in turn by far the best and easiest way to deal with this condition. As a mental health professional this author is fully cognizant of the fact that making people conscious of their psychologically pathologic behaviors and changing those behaviors for the better are two very different things. Still, now that dancers and their teachers have before them concrete evidence of the threat confronting them there is every reason to hope that they will seek out means of combating it. The experience described by Dr. Niva Piran in the chapter preceding this one provides excellent examples of how the battle is being joined.

References

American Psychiatric Association. 1994. *Diagnostic and statistical manual of mental disorders.* 4th ed. Washington, DC: American Psychiatric Association.

Brooks-Gunn, J., C. Burrow, and M.P. Warren. 1988. Attitudes toward eating and body weight in different groups of female adolescent athletes. *International Journal of Eating Disorders* 7(6): 749-757.

Brooks-Gunn, J., M.P. Warren, and L. Hamilton. 1987. The relation of eating problems and amenorrhea in ballet dancers. *Medicine and Science in Sports and Exercise* 19(1): 41-44.

Bruch, H. 1973. *Eating disorders: Obesity, anorexia nervosa, and the person within.* New York: Basic Books.

Bullen, B., G.S. Skrinar, I.A. Beitinn, G. von Mering, B.A. Turnbull, and J.W. McArthur. 1985. Induction of menstrual disorders by strenuous exercise in untrained women. *New England Journal of Medicine* 312(21): 1349-1355.

DeSouza, M.J., M.S. Maguire, C.M. Maresh, W.J. Kraemer, K.R. Rubin, and A.B. Loucks. 1991. Adrenal activation and the prolactin response to exercise in eumenorrheic and amenorrheic runners. *Journal of Applied Physiology* 70(6): 2378-2387.

Ding, J-H., C.B. Sheckter, B.L. Drinkwater, M.R. Soules, and W.J. Brenner. 1988. High serum cortisol levels in exercise-associated amenorrhea. *Annals of Internal Medicine* 108(4): 530-534.

Drinkwater, B.L., K. Nilson, and C.H. Chestnut III. 1984. Bone mineral content of amenorrheic and eumenorrheic athletes. *New England Journal of Medicine* 311(5): 277-281.

Drinkwater, B.L., K. Nilson, S. Ott, and C.H. Chestnut III. 1986. Bone mineral density after resumption of menses in amenorrheic athletes. *Journal of the American Medical Association* 256(3): 380-382.

Edwards, J.E., A.K. Lindeman, A.E. Mikesky, and J.M. Stager. 1993. Energy balance in highly trained female endurance runners. *Medicine and Science in Sports and Exercise* 25(12): 1398-1404.

Garner, D.M., and P.E. Garfinkel. 1980. Socio-cultural factors in the development of anorexia nervosa. *Psychological Medicine* 10(4): 647-656.

Gordon, S. 1983. *Off balance: The real world of ballet.* New York: Pantheon Books.

Hamilton, L., J. Brooks-Gunn, and M.P. Warren. 1986. Nutritional intake of female dancers: A reflection of eating problems. *International Journal of Eating Disorders* 5(5): 925-934.

Hamilton, L., J. Brooks-Gunn, M.P. Warren, and W.G. Hamilton. 1987. The impact of thinness and dieting on the professional ballet dancer. *Medical Problems of Performing Artists* 2(4): 117-122.

Hamilton, L., J. Brooks-Gunn, M.P. Warren, and W.G. Hamilton. 1988. The role of selectivity in the pathogenesis of eating problems in ballet dancers. *Medicine and Science in Sports and Exercise* 20(6): 560-565.

Holderness, C.C., J. Brooks-Gunn, and M.P. Warren. 1994. Eating disorders and substance use: A dancing vs a nondancing population. *Medicine and Science in Sports and Exercise* 26(3): 297-302.

Kurtzman, F.D., J. Yager, J. Landsverk, E. Wiesmeier, and D.C. Bodurka. 1990-1991. Eating disorders and associated symptoms among dancers and other student populations at UCLA. *Kinesiology and Medicine for Dance* 13(1): 16-32.

Loucks, A.B., E.M. Heath, K. King, D. Morrall, M. Verdum, and J.R. Watts. 1994. Low energy availability alters luteinizing hormone pulsatility in regularly menstruating, young exercising women. Endocrine Society Meeting, Abstract 822.

Loucks, A.B., and S.M. Horvath. 1984. Exercise-induced stress responses in amenorrheic and eumenorrheic runners. *Journal of Clinical Endocrinology and Metabolism* 59(6): 1109-1120.

Loucks, A.B., G.A. Laughlin, J.F. Mortola, L. Girton, J.C. Nelson, and S.S. Yen. 1992. Hypothalamic-pituitary-

thyroidal function in eumenorrheic and amenorrheic athletes. *Journal of Clinical Endocrinology and Metabolism* 75(2): 514-518.

Loucks, A.B., J.F. Mortola, L. Girton, and S.S. Yen. 1989. Alterations in the hypothalamic-pituitary-ovarian and the hypothalamic-pituitary-adrenal axes in athletic women. *Journal of Clinical Endocrinology and Metabolism* 68(2): 402-411.

Molnar, M. 1997. Stress fracture of the second metatarsal: A case report. *Journal of Dance Medicine & Science* 1(1): 22-26.

Myerson, M.B., B. Gutin, M.P. Warren, M.T. May, I. Contento, M. Lee, F.X. Pi-Sunyer, R.N. Pierson Jr., and J. Brooks-Gunn. 1991. Resting metabolic rate and energy balance in amenorrheic and eumenorrheic runners. *Medicine and Science in Sports and Exercise* 23(1): 15-22.

Nicholas, J.A. 1975. Risk factors, sports medicine and the orthopedic system: An overview. *Sports Medicine* 3(5): 243-258.

Otis, C.L., B. Drinkwater, B.M. Johnson, A. Loucks, and J. Wilmore. 1997. American College of Sports Medicine Position Stand: The Female Athlete Triad. *Medicine and Science in Sports and Exercise* 29(5): i-ix.

Rivier, C., and S. Rivest. 1991. Effect of stress on the activity of the hypothalamic-pituitary-gonadal axes: Peripheral and central mechanisms. *Biology of Reproduction* 45(4): 523-532.

Ryan, J. 1995. *Little girls in pretty boxes.* New York: Doubleday.

Schnitt, J.M., D. Schnitt, and W. Del A'Une. 1986. Anorexia nervosa or thinness in modern dance students: Comparison with ballerinas. *Annals of Sports Medicine* 3(1): 9-13.

Shell, C.G., ed. 1986. *The dancer as athlete: The 1984 Olympic Scientific Congress Proceedings.* Champaign, IL: Human Kinetics.

Solomon, R., J. Solomon, L.J. Micheli, J.J. Saunders, and D. Zurakowski. 2001. Personality profile of professional and conservatory student dancers. *Medical Problems of Performing Artists* 16(3): 85-93.

Vincent, L.M. 1989. *Competing with the sylph: Dancers and the pursuit of the ideal body form.* Kansas City, MO: Andrews & McMeel. (1979. 2nd edition. Princeton, NJ: Princeton Book Company.)

Williams, N.I., J.C. Young, J.W. McArthur, B. Bullen, G.S. Skrinar, and B. Turnbull. 1995. Strenuous exercise with caloric restriction: Effect on luteinizing hormone secretion. *Medicine and Science in Sports and Exercise* 27(10): 1390-1398.

Wilmore, J.H., K.C. Wambsoans, M. Brenner, C.E. Broeder, I. Paijmans, J.A. Volpe, and K.M. Wilmore. 1992. Is there energy conservation in amenorrheic compared to eumenorrheic distance runners? *Journal of Applied Physiology* 72(1): 15-22.

Recommended Readings (Editors)

Bass, M., L. Turner, and S. Hunt. 2001. Counseling female athletes: Application of the stages of change model to avoid disordered eating, amenorrhea, and osteoporosis. *Psychological Reports* 88(3) Part 2: 1154-1160.

Beals, K.A., R.A. Brey, and J.B. Gonyou. 1999. Understanding the female athlete triad: Eating disorders, amenorrhea, and osteoporosis. *Journal of School Health* 69(8): 337-340.

Garner, D.M., L.W. Rosen, and D. Barry. 1998. Eating disorders among athletes: Research and recommendations. *Child and Adolescent Psychiatric Clinics of North America* 7(4): 839-857.

Joy, E., N. Clark, M.L. Ireland, J. Martire, A. Nattiv, and S. Varechok. 1997. Team management of the female athlete triad Part I: What to look for, what to ask. *Physician and Sportsmedicine* 25(3): 95-110.

Joy, E., N. Clark, M.L. Ireland, J. Martire, A. Nattiv, and S. Varechok. 1997. Team management of the female athlete triad Part 2: Optima; treatment and prevention tactics. *Physician and Sportsmedicine* 25(4): 55-69.

Lebrun, C.M. 2001. Female athlete triad. In *Sports medicine for specific ages and abilities,* edited by N. Maffulli, K.M. Chan, R. MacDonald, R.M. Malina, and A.W. Parker. Edinburgh: Churchill Livingstone, 177-185.

Myszkewycz, L., and Y. Koutedakis. 1998. Injuries, amenorrhea and osteoporosis in active females: An overview. *Journal of Dance Medicine & Science* 2(3): 88-94.

Nattiv, A., K.Yeager, B. Drinkwater, and R. Agostini. 1994. The female athlete triad. In *Medical and orthopedic issues of active and athletic women,* edited by R. Agostini. Philadelphia: Hanley & Belfus, 169-174.

Putukian, M. 1998. The female athlete triad. *Clinics in Sports Medicine* 17(4): 675-696.

Sabatini, S. 2001. The female athlete triad. *American Journal of the Medical Sciences* 322(4): 193-195.

Sanborn, C.F., M. Horea, B.J. Siemers, and K.I. Dieringer. 2000. Disordered eating and the female athlete triad. *Clinics in Sports Medicine* 19(2): 199-213.

Dance Glossary

Alexander Technique—A body therapy system designed to make the participant aware of use and misuse of the body, particularly with reference to posture, mechanical efficiency, and emotion.

arabesque—A movement in which the body weight is supported by one leg. The supporting leg may be straight or half bent, while the gesturing leg is straight and extended to the rear. The arms are normally placed to provide the longest possible line from fingertips to toes. There are a number of arabesque positions.

assemblé—A ballet step in which one foot slides along the floor and into the air. The supporting foot then pushes off from the floor, joins the other in the air, and the two feet land together in fifth position.

attitude—A position in which the body weight is supported on one leg. The supporting leg may be straight or bent, with the arm on the same side opened front, side, or back. The other leg is extended to the back and bent 90° at the knee, while the corresponding arm is raised above the head.

barre—Generally a cylindrical piece of wood that is fastened horizontally to the walls of the dance studio at a height of approximately 3 ft 6 in. (107 cm) from the floor. Warm-up exercises are done at the barre at the beginning of every ballet class.

contraction—A concave curving of the lumbar and thoracic spine through use of the psoas and abdominal muscles. Throughout this action the knees bend and the shoulders remain over the hips, with the body as elongated as possible.

demi-plié—A bending or flexing of the knees only to the point where the heels are still on the floor. Demi-plié can be performed in all five ballet positions, and in parallel.

demi-pointe—Position in which the weight of the body is supported on the balls of the feet and plantar aspect of the toes; also known as half pointe.

développé—The unfolding movement described for développé à la seconde can be performed in other directions—to the front, the back, and in parallel position—without turning out at the hip.

développé à la seconde—A movement in which the gesturing leg is raised until the thigh is at a right angle to the body, with the toe at the knee of the supporting leg. From this point the gesturing leg gradually extends (straightens) to the side of the body.

en avant—Any movement to the front of the body.

en ayer—Any movement to the rear of the body.

en dedans—An inward movement in which the gesturing leg or the body turns toward the supporting leg.

en dehors—An outward movement in which the gesturing leg or the body turns away from the supporting leg.

entrechat—A springing movement into the air, beginning and ending in fifth position, in which the legs are straight and criss-cross while in the air. The feet are pointed downward. The legs criss-cross a varying number of times, depending on the type of entrechat being performed. In an entrechat quatre, for example, the legs and feet go through four positions: the beginning and finish in fifth and one criss-cross in the air.

extension—A movement in which the gesturing leg is extended out from the body. This term has also come to mean the height to which a dancer can raise the leg above waist level.

floor work—Movement performed while sitting or lying on the floor (especially prevalent in modern dance technique).

fouetté—A variety of ballet steps characterized by a whipping action of the foot or leg out to an open position and quickly back in again. This whipping action can also propel the dancer into a series of turns known as fouetté rond de jambe en tournant.

grand battement—A movement in which the gesturing leg is raised from the hip into the air and brought down again. Grand battement is performed with both knees straight. It can be done front, side, or to the back, and usually starts and finishes in fifth position.

grand plié—A bending at the knees in which the dancer begins in an erect position and slowly flexes the knees until the heels come away from the floor. The back remains straight, with the shoulders over the hips. The grand plié passes through demi-plié and can be performed in all five ballet positions and parallel. In grand plié in second position the heels remain on the floor, although the movement is larger than demi-plié à la seconde.

jeté—A jump from one leg to the other. The change of weight is preceded by a brushing or throwing action of the gesturing leg.

parallel position—In modern and jazz dance, a position in which the feet are placed side by side, in line with the hip sockets, with the toes of both feet pointing straight ahead.

passé—A transitional movement in which the foot of the gesturing leg passes the knee of the supporting leg as it goes from one position to another.

Pilates exercises—A series of exercises developed by Joseph Pilates, designed to strengthen specific muscle groups. Many of these exercises are performed on specially designed apparatus that utilizes springs to provide resistance.

pirouette—A ballet turn in which the body is whirled or spun around on one foot, either on pointe or demi-pointe. Pirouettes can be performed en dedans or en dehors. Momentum for the turn comes from a plié and arm movement. The head is whipped around so that it is last to turn and first to arrive at front facing. There are many types of pirouettes.

plié—Bending movement of the knee or knees; perhaps the most basic ballet movement (see demi-plié and grand plié).

pointe—Position in which the dancer moves or balances on the tips of the toes, with the aid of the toe (pointe) shoe.

port de bras—A movement or series of movements made by passing the arm or arms through various positions. This term also refers to a group of exercises designed to develop grace and harmony of arm movement.

relevé—The action of raising the body onto pointe or demi-pointe. Relevé can be performed smoothly and continuously or with a springing movement.

rond de jambe—A circular action of the gesturing leg. It moves from first position through fourth front, second, and fourth back, and then passes through first position again. It can be performed with the toe of the gesturing leg on the floor (rond de jambe à terre) or in the air (rond de jambe en l'air). This exercise can be done en dedans or en dehors.

saut de basque—A jumping and traveling step in ballet, in which the dancer turns in the air with one foot drawn up to the knee of the other leg.

tendu—An action in which the foot and leg are stretched away from the body. In battement tendu the gesturing leg is opened to the front, side, or back, while the toe rests lightly on the floor. Then it is returned to a closed position.

tour jeté—The technical name for this ballet step is grand jeté dessus en tournant. In this step the dancer is propelled into the air as in a leap, but in midair the body is turned quickly to face the direction from which the step originated. While the dancer is airborne, both legs pass closely together (i.e., exchange positions) with the knees straight. Then the step is landed in demi-plié in arabesque position.

turnout—The ability of the dancer to stand and move with the legs externally rotated at the hip so that the toes are directed diagonally away from the midline of the body.

Medical Glossary

abductors—Muscles that draw a body part away from the median line.

acetabulum—A cup-shaped socket on the external surface of the pelvis, in which the ball-shaped head of the femur sits and articulates.

Achilles tendon—Heel tendon; the tendon of insertion of the triceps surae (gastrocnemius and soleus) into the tuberosity of the calcaneus.

acromioclavicular—Denoting the articulation between the clavicle and the scapula and its ligaments.

adductors—Muscles that draw a body part toward the midline of the body; in dance, often synonymous with "groin muscles."

afferent neuron—A structure that passes messages or impulses from one part of the body to another by way of an electrochemical process. In particular, afferents carry nerve impulses from the peripheral sensory receptors toward the central nervous system, into the spinal cord, or into the brain.

allograph—A graft of tissue between two genetically dissimilar individuals of the same species, such as a tissue transplant between two humans.

alpha motor neuron—The final common pathway for transmission of motor impulses from the central nervous system to the skeletal muscles. These motor neurons innervate extrafusal muscle fibers.

amenorrhea—Absence or abnormal cessation of the menses.

annulus—A ring-shaped structure, such as the outer edge of an intervertebral disc.

anorexia nervosa—A personality disorder characterized by prolonged refusal to eat, resulting in life-threatening weight loss, amenorrhea, and emotional disturbance concerning body image.

anterior cruciate ligament—Internal ligament of the knee, which originates on the lateral femoral condyle and inserts on the anterior aspect of the tibia; a primary control of back-to-front motion and rotation of the knee.

anterior tibialis—Muscle that originates on the lateral condyle, surface of the tibia, and interosseous membrane, and inserts at the bases of the second to fourth metatarsal bones and tarsal bones except for the talus. It dorsiflexes and inverts the foot.

anteversion (femoral)—Position of the femoral neck relative to the femoral shaft in the horizontal plane; a forward turning; in dance, refers primarily to inward rotation of the femur in the hip socket.

arthrography—A method of radiographically visualizing the inside of a joint, using contrast solution ("dye") to define soft tissue.

arthroscopic surgery—A technique for diagnosis or surgical treatment within a joint, performed by passing surgical instruments through a rigid metal tube containing a light and fiber optics (an endoscope).

arthrosis—Disease of a joint.

autogenic reflex—The simplest functioning unit of the nervous system; a reflex that operates automatically. This particular reflex serves the role of triggering muscular relaxation to protect a muscle from excessive tension.

avulsion—The separation, by tearing, of any body part from the whole.

basal ganglia—A group of nuclei or cluster of cell bodies within the brain that are located in the inner layers of the cerebrum surrounding the lateral portions of the thalamus. These structures project a rich supply of nerve fibers to the spinal cord, and also up to the motor cortex. Collectively, the basal ganglia are part of the system that organizes motor activity.

biceps brachii—A muscle of the arm; arising in two heads from the scapula, inserts on the tuberosity of the radius and flexes and supinates the forearm.

biceps femoris—One of the hamstring muscles, with two heads at its origin. It flexes the leg and extends the thigh, rotating it laterally.

bulimia—A disorder characterized by an insatiable craving for food, often resulting in episodes of continuous eating followed by purging, depression, and self-deprivation.

bursa—A fibrous sac between tendons and the bones beneath them. Lined with a synovial membrane that secretes synovial fluid, the bursa acts as a small cushion that allows the tendon to move over the bone as it contracts and releases.

calcaneus—The heel bone; the largest of the tarsal bones. It articulates proximally with the talus and distally with the cuboid.

capsule—A membranous structure that envelops an organ, a joint, or any other body part.

cavus (foot)—A highly arched foot.

cerebellum—A structure lying behind and below the cerebrum that has two hemispheres and a very convoluted appearance. Knowledge about the precise functioning of various parts of the cerebellum is incomplete; generally, it seems to be important in the coordination and monitoring of complex patterns of skilled motor activity.

cerebral cortex—The outermost layer of the cerebrum, or large umbrella-like dome of the brain. The cerebrum is divided into two hemispheres by the longitudinal fissure or groove. The cortex is about 1/4 in. (0.6 cm) thick and composed mostly of tightly packed neuron cell bodies. The cerebral cortex receives and interprets sensory information, organizes complex motor behaviors, and stores and utilizes learned experiences.

chondral—Pertaining to cartilage.

chondromalacia—Degeneration or softening of cartilage, most commonly on the undersurface of the patella.

circumduction—One of four basic movements allowed by various joints of the skeleton. It is a combination of abduction, adduction, extension, and flexion. The circular movement of a limb.

coccyx—The small bone at the end of the vertebral column, formed by the union of four (sometimes five or three) rudimentary vertebrae; articulates with the sacrum.

collagen—The main protein of connective tissue, cartilage, and bone.

computed tomography (CT)—A radiographic technique that produces a film representing a detailed cross section of tissue structure. It is 100 times more sensitive than conventional radiography.

concentric contraction—A form of muscle contraction in which the muscle fibers shorten as tension develops.

condyle—A rounded articular surface at the extremity of a bone that anchors muscle ligaments and articulates with adjacent bones.

coracoacromial—Pertaining to the coracoid process and the acromium of the scapula. The coracoid process is the thick curved extension of the superior border of the scapula to which the pectoralis major is attached.

corticospinal tracts—Neurons having axons and nerve fibers that originate in the cerebral cortex and descend to the spinal cord, making up a motor transmission network. The axons of this system are some of the longest in the body. This structure is also known as the "pyramidal system."

cuboid, cuboidal—Pyramidal bone on the lateral side of the foot, in front of the calcaneus; articulates with the calcaneus, lateral cuneiform, fourth and fifth metatarsal bones, and occasionally the navicular.

cuneiform—Three bones of the foot—intermediate, lateral, and medial—on the distal row of the tarsus.

differential diagnosis—The determination of which of two or more diseases or injuries with similar symptoms is the one from which the patient is suffering.

disc—A structure between the bodies of adjacent vertebrae, composed of an outer fibrous part that surrounds a central gelatinous mass.

dorsiflexion—Turning of the foot or toes upward.

dysphoria—A disorder or affect characterized by depression or anguish.

dysphoric mood—A mood characterized by feelings of unpleasantness or discomfort.

eccentric contraction—A type of muscle contraction that involves lengthening of the muscle fibers against resistance.

efferent neuron—A neural structure that transmits impulses from the central nervous system out to effector organs, such as muscles or glands.

effusion—The escape of fluid from the blood vessels or lymphatics into the tissues or a cavity.

elastin—A yellow elastic fibrous mucoprotein; a major connective tissue protein of elastic structures.

endomysium—The sheath of delicate reticular fibrils that surrounds each muscle fiber.

enzyme—A protein secreted by cells that acts as a catalyst to induce chemical changes in other substances.

epidemiology—The study of the determinants of disease or injury in a population.

eversion—A turning outward, such as a turning of the foot outward at the ankle.

excursion—Any movement from one point to another with a return to the original position.

extensor digitorum longus—A muscle that originates on the lateral condyle of the tibia and anterior margin of the fibula; inserts by tendons to the dorsal surfaces of the bases of the second to fifth toes; serves to extend the four lateral toes.

extensor hallucis longus—Long extensor muscle of the great toe; originates on the lateral surface of the tibia and interosseous membrane; inserts at the base of the distal phalanx of the great toe.

external rotators—Muscles by which a part can be turned externally; of special concern to dancers are the hip rotators (see chapter 11).

extrafusal—Muscle fibers that make up the main skeletal muscles (in comparison to intrafusal fibers, which are located in muscle spindles).

extra-pyramidal—Referring to the part of the motor system that constitutes a second motor pathway, including all of the motor axons not found in the pyramidal tract. It is believed that the extra-pyramidal neurons modify some of the operations of the pyramidal system by refining and smoothing out movements, and carrying a large part of the impulses for postural adjustment and reflex movements.

facet—A small, smooth-surfaced spinous process for articulation.

fascia—A sheath of fibrous tissue that encloses muscles and muscle groups and separates their several layers.

female athlete triad—A syndrome that encompasses disordered eating, amenorrhea, and osteoporosis (see chapter 17).

femoral anteversion—See anteversion.

femoral condyle(s)—A rounded projection at the distal end of the femur; articulates with the tibia; affords attachment to the cruciate ligaments.

femur—The thigh bone; the longest and largest bone in the body. The head of the femur fits into the acetabulum of the pelvis.

fibroblast—A stellate or spindle-shaped cell. It is present in connective tissue and is capable of forming collagen fibers, fibrous tissues in the body, tendons, aponeuroses, and supporting and bending tissues of all sorts. Such cells also proliferate at the site of chronic inflammation.

fibrocartilage—A variety of cartilage that contains visible collagenic fibers.

fibula—The lateral and smaller of the two bones of the lower leg, lateral to and smaller in diameter than the tibia.

flexor digitorum longus—A muscle that originates on the posterior surface of the tibia and inserts by tendons into the bases of the four lateral toes; flexes the second to fifth toes.

flexor hallucis brevis—A muscle that originates on the medial surface of the cuboid and middle and lateral cuneiform bones, and inserts by two tendons. The medial tendon inserts on the medial side of the base of the proximal phalanx of the big toe. The lateral tendon inserts on the lateral side of the same, both via sesamoids. It flexes the metatarsophalangeal joint of the big toe and supports the medial longitudinal arch.

flexor hallucis longus—A muscle that originates on the posterior surface of the fibula; inserts at the base of the great toe; flexes the great toe (see chapter 4).

fluoroscopy—Examination of the tissues and deep structures of the body by X ray, using a fluoroscope. The technique offers immediate serial images that are invaluable in many clinical procedures.

fusiform muscle—A spindle-shaped muscle; one that has a fleshy belly, tapering at either extremity.

gamma efferent pathway—Motoneurons that begin in the gray matter of the spinal cord and that have axons passing through spinal nerves to the specialized fibers of the muscle spindles.

gamma (stretch) reflex—The reflex that results when the extrafusal fibers are suddenly stretched. The muscle spindle will be stretched and spindle afferents will be activated, which will then reflexively produce extrafusal contraction to reduce the stretch.

gastrocnemius—A two-headed muscle that originates from the popliteal surface of the femur, upper part of the medial condyle, and capsule of the knee; combines with the soleus to form the tendocalcaneus (Achilles tendon), which inserts into the lower half of the posterior surface of the calcaneus; plantarflexes the foot and flexes the knee joint.

gemellus inferior—A muscle that originates on the tuberosity of the ischium; blends with the tendon of the obturator internus and inserts into the inner surface of the greater trochanter; rotates the thigh laterally.

genu recurvatum—A condition of hyperextension of the knee.

genu valgum—A deformity characterized by the legs curving inward so that the knees are close together with the ankles widely separated; "knock-knees."

genu varum—A deformity characterized by one or both legs being bent outward at the knee; "bowlegs."

glucose—Dextrose, or starch sugar; it is the product of complete hydrolysis of cellulose, starch, and glycogen.

gluteals—The muscle group that includes the gluteus maximus, medius, and minimus.

gluteus maximus—A muscle that originates on the dorsal aspect of the ilium, the posterior surface of the sacrum and coccyx, and the sacrotuberous ligament; inserts on the iliotibial band of the fascia lata and the gluteal ridge of the femur; extends, abducts, and rotates the thigh laterally.

gluteus medius—A muscle that originates on the lateral surface of the ilium; inserts at the greater trochanter of the femur; abducts and rotates the thigh.

glycogen—Animal or liver starch; found in most tissues of the body, especially those of the liver and muscles; the principal carbohydrate reserve, it is readily converted into glucose.

Golgi tendon organ—A muscle receptor that detects and signals tension on a tendon. It is usually found at the origin or insertion of a muscle, rather than in the tendon itself.

gonadotrophic releasing hormone (GnRH)—A hormone secreted by the hypothalamus. It stimulates release of gonadotropin hormone by the anterior pituitary gland.

gracilis—The most superficial of the five medial femoral muscles. It originates near the pubis symphysis and inserts on the shaft of the tibia, below the medial tuberosity. It functions to adduct the thigh and flex the leg and to assist in the medial rotation of the leg after it is flexed.

greater trochanter—A broad, flat process on the femur, at the upper end of its lateral surface, to which the following muscles are attached: gluteus medius and minimus, piriformis, obturator internus and externus, and gemelli.

groin muscles—The muscles attached at the junctional region between the abdomen and the thigh.

hamstrings—Inner hamstring comprises the tendons of the gracilis, sartorius, semimembranosus, and semitendinosus muscles; outer hamstring is the tendon of the biceps femoris muscle.

hip flexors—Generally considered to include the psoas, rectus femoris, sartorius, and iliacus muscles.

humerus—The bone of the arm, articulating with the scapula above and the radius and ulna below.

hyperextension—Extension of a limb or body part beyond the normal limit.

hypertonia—The condition of having an abnormally high degree of muscular tension.

hypothalamus—A portion of the brain, forming the floor and lateral wall of the third ventricle. It activates, controls, and integrates the peripheral autonomic nervous system, endocrine processes, and many somatic functions, such as body temperature, sleep, and appetite.

hypotonia—The condition of having an abnormally low degree of muscular tension.

iatrogenic—Caused by treatment or diagnostic procedures. Denoting an unfavorable response to therapy, induced by the therapeutic effort itself.

idiopathic—Denoting a disease of unknown cause.

iliac crest—The lateral, flaring portion of the pelvis.

iliacus—A muscle that originates on the iliac fossa; inserts into the psoas tendon on the lesser trochanter of the femur and capsule of the hip joint; flexes the thigh and trunk.

iliocostalis—The lateral division of the erector muscle of the spine, having three subdivisions: lumborum, which extends, abducts, and rotates lumbar vertebrae; thoracis, which does the same for the thoracic vertebrae; and the cervicis, which similarly services the cervical vertebrae.

iliofemoral ligament—A Y-shaped ligament that covers the anterior and superior portions of the hip joint. It is attached above to the lower part of the anterior–inferior spine of the ilium and diverges to form two bands; inserts on the intertrochanteric line.

iliopectineal—Relating to the ilium and the pubis.

iliopsoas—A compound muscle consisting of the iliacus and the psoas major.

iliotibial band—A band of connective tissue that extends from the iliac crest to the knee and links the gluteus maximus to the tibia.

ilium—The broad flaring portion of the pelvis; joins the pubis and ischium to form the acetabulum.

induction—The appearance of an electrical impulse as a result of the presence of another electric current or field nearby.

internal rotators—Muscles by which a body part can be turned internally—for example, semitendinosus and popliteus at the leg, and pectineus at the thigh.

interneuron—A neural structure that originates and ends totally within the central nervous system; interneurons make up 95% of all neurons in the nervous system.

intrafusal—Denoting muscle fibers that are not part of the main skeletal muscle, but are located in muscle spindles and have specialized sensory and motor functions.

intrinsic muscles of the foot—First plantar layer: flexor digitorum brevis, abductor digiti minimi, abductor hallucis; second plantar layer: quadratus plantae, lumbricales; third plantar layer: flexor hallucis brevis, adductor hallucis, flexor digiti minimi brevis; first dorsal layer: extensor digitorum brevis, extensor hallucis brevis.

inversion—A turning inward.

irradiation—The dispersion of a nervous impulse beyond the normal path of conduction.

ischial apophysitis—Inflammation of the bony outgrowth (process, or tuberosity) on the lower posterior portion of the hip bone.

ischial tuberosity—Bony projection at the junction of the lower end of the body of the ischium and its ramus.

isometric—Denoting a form of muscular contraction in which the muscle is engaged in a static contraction against resistance. This condition can be contrasted to isotonic muscular contraction, in which movement occurs through range of motion against resistance.

kyphosis—Posterior convexity in the curvature of the thoracic spine.

labrum (acetabular)—A fibrocartilaginous rim of tissue surrounding the acetabulum.

lamina(e) (vertebral)—The flattened posterior portion of the vertebral arch from which the spinous process extends.

lateral collateral ligament—The cordlike band of fibrous tissue that passes from the lateral epicondyle of the femur to the head of the fibula; serves to stabilize the knee laterally.

lateral meniscus—A crescent-shaped fibrocartilage in the knee joint attached to the lateral border of the upper articular surface of the tibia. In combination with the medial meniscus it helps to absorb shock.

lesser trochanter—A short conical process on the posteromedial part of the femur, below its neck. It receives the insertion of the psoas major and iliacus (iliopsoas) muscles.

ligament—A band or sheet of fibrous tissue binding joints together and connecting two or more bones, cartilages, or other structures.

limbic system—A network of subcortical structures located in the forebrain that are connected to other structures in the brain and are also interconnected. Recent studies indicate that parts of the limbic system are involved in arousal.

Lisfranc joint—A junction between the medial cuneiform bone and the proximal head of the second metatarsal in the foot.

longissimus (thoracis)—A muscle that originates from the transverse and articular processes of the lower thoracic vertebrae; inserts by lateral slips between transverse processes of all thoracic vertebrae and 9 or 10 lower ribs; extends thoracic vertebrae.

lordosis—A concave posterior curvature of the lumbar spine ("hollow back," "swayback").

lumbar—The part of the back between the thorax and the pelvis.

lumbar pedicle—Arch of a vertebrae.

lumbodorsal fascia—The extensive subdivision of the vertebral fascia that sheaths the sacrospinalis muscle.

luteinizing hormone—The hormone considered responsible for ripening of the follicle and the release of the ovum during ovulation.

macrotrauma—The prefix "macro-" denotes large. In this usage it means a single large impact to a site, causing injury.

malleolus—A rounded process on either side of the ankle joint.

medial collateral ligament—The broad fibrous band that passes from the medial epicondyle of the femur to the medial margin and medial surface of the tibia; serves with the lateral collateral ligament to stabilize the knee for side-to-side motion.

medial meniscus—A crescent-shaped fibrocartilage in the knee joint attached to the medial upper articular surface of the tibia.

medulla—One part of the brainstem. It is the superior extension of the spinal cord and contains sensory nerve tracts ascending to the brain, descending motor tracts that extend toward muscles and glands, and another collection of neurons and nerve tracts that regulate vital processes like respiration and blood pressure.

menarche—Beginning of the menstrual function.

meniscus—Crescent-shaped fibrocartilage found in certain joints, such as the knee.

metatarsal—Distal portion of the foot, between the instep and the toes; consists of the five long bones articulating proximally with the cuboid and cuneiform bones and distally with the phalanges.

microtrauma—The prefix "micro-" indicates a unit of smallness. In this usage it means small repetitive traumas to a specific site.

multifidus—Referring to the state of being cleft into many parts.

myotatic reflex—The automatic response of muscular contraction when a muscle is stretched. A common example of this type of reflex is the knee jerk that occurs when the patellar tendon is hit, causing the quadriceps muscle to be stretched and thus to contract in response.

navicular—A bone at the medial side of the foot; articulates with the head of the talus, the cuneiform bone, and occasionally the cuboid.

neuroanatomy—The anatomy of the nervous system.

neuromuscular spindle—A structure located in skeletal muscles that contains both sensory receptors and muscle fibers. It consists of a fluid-filled capsule tapering at both ends.

neurophysiology—The physiology of the nervous system.

obturator externus and obturator internus—Two of the muscles that insert on the greater trochanter, near the upper extremity of the femur, and serve to rotate the thigh laterally.

oligomenorrhea—Abnormally light menstruation.

orthotic—An external appliance designed to promote a specific motion or to correct musculoskeletal deformities.

osseous—Bony.

osteochondritis—A disease of the epiphyses, or bone-forming centers of the skeleton, beginning with necrosis and fragmentation of the tissue followed by repair and regeneration. Inflammation of a bone with its cartilage.

osteoid osteoma—A small, benign, but painful tumor of bone occurring especially in the bones of the extremities and vertebrae, most often in young persons.

osteopenia—Decreased calcification or density of bone.

osteophyte formation—A bony outgrowth secondary to degenerative processes; "bone spur."

osteoporosis—A disorder characterized by abnormal loss of bone density.

os trigonum—An anomalous bone growth found just posterior to the talus.

paraspinal muscles (erector spinae)—A name applied to the fibers of the more superficial of the muscles of the back, originating from the sacrum, spines of the lumbar and the 11th and 12th thoracic vertebrae, and the iliac crest, which split and insert as the iliocostal, longissimus, and spinalis muscles; extend the vertebral column.

paratenon—The material, fatty or synovial, between a tendon and its sheath.

paresthesia—The state of having an abnormal sensation.

pars interarticularis—A supporting bar of bone between the superior and inferior facet on each side of the vertebral arch (see chapter 7).

patella—The kneecap.

patella alta—A kneecap that rides unusually high.

patellofemoral—Pertaining to the kneecap and the femur.

pathologize—To denote a state of disease or abnormality.

pectoralis major—A muscle that originates at the clavicle, sternum, the six upper ribs, and the aponeuroses of the external oblique and rectus abdominis; inserts at the head of the humerus; adducts, flexes, and medially rotates the arm.

pedicle(s)—One of the paired parts of the vertebral arch that connect a lamina to the vertebral body (see chapter 7).

pennate muscle—A feather-shaped muscle (see chapter 5).

peroneus brevis—The shorter of the peroneal muscles. It originates on the lateral surface of the fibula and inserts at the base of the fifth metatarsal. With the peroneus longus it helps to evert, abduct, and plantarflex the foot.

peroneus longus—The longest peroneal muscle; originates at the lateral condyle of the tibia and the lateral surface of the fibula; it inserts by a tendon passing behind the lateral malleolus and across the sole of the foot to the medial cuneiform and base of the first metatarsal; plantarflexes, everts, and abducts the foot.

peroneus tertius—Originates at the anterior surface of the fibula and the interosseous membrane; inserts at the base of the fifth metatarsal; assists in dorsiflexion of the foot.

pes planus—A condition characterized by the flattening out of the arch of the foot.

phalanges—The long bones between joints of the fingers or toes.

piriformis—A muscle of the hip; originates at the greater sciatic notch of the ilium and second to fourth lumbar vertebrae; inserts on the upper border of the great trochanter; rotates the thigh laterally.

plantar fasciitis—A painful condition of the foot, secondary to tightness or inflammation of the plantar fascia, the thick central portion of the fascia investing the plantar muscles.

plantarflexion—A toe-down motion of the foot at the ankle; "pointing" the foot.

plantaris (the aponeurosis plantaris)—Radiates toward the toes from the medial process of the calcaneal tuberosity and gives attachment to the short flexor muscle of the toes.

plica—A general term for a ridge or fold, commonly found on the inside of the knee joint capsule.

plyometrics—Bounding or high-velocity exercise that entails eccentric and rapid concentric contractions, such as jumping or throwing and catching a weighted ball.

popliteus—A muscle that originates at the lateral condyle of the femur and inserts on the posterior surface of the tibia; flexes the knee and rotates the leg medially.

posterior cruciate ligament—Is stronger but shorter and less oblique than the anterior. It attaches behind the spine of the tibia, to the popliteal notch, and inserts into the inner condyle of the femur, stabilizing the knee.

pronation—Eversion and abduction of the foot, causing a lowering of the medial edge; "rolling in" (see chapter 14).

proprioception—The collection of sensations coming from the body, including those from the skin, joints, muscles, and vestibular apparatus.

prostaglandins—Physiologically active substances present in many tissues that stimulate contractility of smooth muscle; lower blood pressure; and regulate acid secretions, body temperature, and platelet aggregation. They also control inflammation.

proteoglycan—A group of glycoproteins found primarily in connective tissue.

psoas (major)—A muscle that originates at the bodies of the vertebrae and intervertebral discs from the 12th thoracic to the 5th lumbar; inserts on the lesser trochanter of the femur; flexes the thigh. Psoas minor originates at the bodies of the 12th thoracic and 1st lumbar vertebrae and discs; assists with flexion of the spine (see chapter 9).

pyramidal—The motor transmission network made up of neurons beginning in the cerebral cortex with axons descending to the spinal cord. The name comes from the wedge-shaped bulges the fibers of this system form on the surface of the medulla. This system is also known as the corticospinal tract.

quadratus femoris—A muscle of the thigh that originates at the tuberosity of the ischium; inserts on the intertrochanteric crest and quadrate tubercle of the femur; adducts and rotates the thigh laterally.

quadratus lumborum—Quadrate muscle of the loins; originates at the iliac crest, iliolumbar ligament, and transverse process of the lower lumbar vertebrae; inserts at the 12th rib and transverse process of the upper lumbar vertebrae; flexes the lumbar vertebrae laterally.

quadriceps femoris—Quadriceps muscle of the thigh; originates by four heads: rectus femoris, vastus lateralis, vastus intermedius, vastus medialis; inserts by a common tendon that surrounds the patella and ends on the tuberosity of the tibia; extends the leg and flexes the thigh by the action of the rectus femoris.

reciprocal reflex—An automatic response that acts as a protective reflex to prevent muscle injury. When a given muscle contracts maximally the antagonist muscle or muscles are reciprocally inhibited from contracting. Also known as reciprocal inhibition.

rectus abdominis—Straight muscle of the abdomen; originates on the crest and symphysis of the pubis; inserts on the xiphoid process and fifth to seventh costal cartilages; flexes the vertebral column and draws the thorax downward.

rectus femoris—A muscle of the thigh; originates on the ilium and upper margin of the acetabulum; inserts to a common tendon of the quadriceps femoris at the base of the patella, on the tuberosity of the tibia; extends the leg and flexes the thigh.

reticular formation—A formation consisting of a netlike mass of interwoven neurons extending from the brainstem up to the thalamus. This formation has both ascending and descending axons, with neurons extending throughout the central nervous system. Evidence has shown that the reticular formation is important in arousal or attention, sensory integration, and motor aspects of neural function.

reticulospinal tracts—The nerve fibers of the reticular formation, extending between that formation and the spinal cord.

retinaculum—A strong fibrous band. The patella has both a lateral and a medial retinaculum, which attach to the tibia.

retrocalcaneal bursa—A fibrous sac lined with a synovial membrane that secretes synovial fluid and acts as a small cushion allowing the tendon to move over the bone. It lies between the Achilles tendon and calcaneus.

retroversion—Position of the femoral head relative to the femoral shaft in the horizontal plane; a backward turning; in dance, refers primarily to outward rotation of the femur in the hip socket.

rhomboid—The greater rhomboid muscle originates from the spinous processes and supraspinalis ligaments of the second, third, fourth, and fifth thoracic vertebrae; inserts on the medial border of the scapula; draws the scapula toward the vertebral column.

rotator cuff—A muscle group of the shoulder consisting of the subscapularis, supraspinatus, infraspinatus, and teres minor; holds the ball of the shoulder joint against the socket.

rubrospinal tract—The nerve tract extending from the red nucleus to the spinal cord.

sacrum—The wedge-shaped segment of the vertebral column forming part of the pelvis; formed by the fusion of five originally separate sacral vertebrae; articulates with the last lumbar vertebra, the coccyx, and the hip bone on either side.

sartorius—A muscle that originates on the anterior superior spine of the ilium; inserts at the medial surface of the tibial tuberosity; flexes the thigh and leg.

scapular humeral joint—The joint at which the shoulder blade articulates laterally with the bone of the upper arm (humerus).

sciatica—Pain in the lower back and hip radiating down the back of the thigh into the leg (see chapter 7).

scoliosis—A lateral deviation (curvature) in the vertical line of the spine. It includes rotation (see chapter 7).

semispinalis—The superficial part of the transversospinalis muscles; composed of the capitis, cervicis, and thoracis; serves to extend and rotate the head and vertebral column.

sequelae—A morbid condition following as a consequence of a disease.

serratus anterior—A muscle that originates on the first eight or nine ribs; inserts at the medial border of the scapula; draws the scapula forward and rotates it to raise the shoulder in abduction of the arm.

soleus—The deeper of the two major muscles of the leg (with the gastrocnemius). It originates from the shaft of the fibula and middle third of the tibia and is joined by the Achilles tendon to the calcaneus; plantarflexes the foot.

spinal fusion—A surgical procedure involving fixation of an unstable segment of the spine, usually done with a bone graft, a synthetic device, or both.

spinalis muscles—Spinal muscles of the head, neck, and thorax, originating on the spinous process of the respective vertebrae; serve to extend the vertebral column.

spinous process—A prominence or projection of bone; part of the vertebrae projecting backward from the arch, giving attachment to muscles of the back.

spondylolisthesis—A forward displacement of a vertebra over a lower segment, usually due to a defect in the pars interarticularis (see chapter 7).

spondylolysis—A degenerative lesion or stress fracture of the pars interarticularis.

static stretches—A form of stretching achieved by holding the body in a position that elongates the target muscle or muscles, usually for a period of 30 to 60 seconds.

stenosis—A constriction or narrowing of an opening, passageway, or body structure.

sternoclavicular joint—One of the joints at which the medial aspect of the clavicle articulates with the sternum.

sternum—The breastbone, forming the middle of the anterior wall of the thorax and articulating with the clavicles and cartilages of the first seven ribs.

stress fracture—A fatigue fracture, caused by repeated, prolonged, or abnormal stress.

subluxation—Incomplete or partial dislocation.

subtalar—Below the talus (ankle bone); second largest of the tarsal bones; as in subtalar joint (see chapter 13).

supination—Inversion and abduction of the foot, causing elevation of the medial edge.

supraspinatus—A muscle that originates on the supraspinous fossa of the scapula and inserts at the greater tuberosity of the humerus. It abducts the arm.

synapse—A submicroscopic gap between the end of one nerve cell and the cell membrane of another; the point at which one neuron affects the firing rate of another cell by the release of a transmitter substance.

synovial fluid—A transparent alkaline viscid fluid (joint "oil"), secreted by the synovial membrane; contained in joint cavities, bursae, and tendon sheaths.

synovial joints—A specialized form of articulation permitting more or less free movement; bony elements covered by articular cartilage, and surrounded by a capsule lined with synovial membranes and containing synovial fluid.

talus—The "ankle bone"; second largest of the tarsal bones; articulates with the tibia and fibula to form the ankle joint.

tarsus—The "instep"; the seven bones of the foot: talus, calcaneus, navicular bone, three cuneiform bones, and the cuboid.

tectum—The structure that makes up the roof of the midbrain. It is composed of the superior and inferior colliculi, or rounded elevations on either side of the midbrain.

tendinopathy—A tendon abnormality resulting from an ischemic (lacking in blood supply) or degenerative process rather than inflammation.

tenosynovitis—Inflammation of a tendon and its enveloping sheath.

tensor fascia lata—A muscle that originates on the iliac crest and inserts at the iliotibial band of the fascia lata; serves to flex, abduct, and rotate the thigh medially.

tibia—The inner and larger bone of the leg below the knee. It articulates with the femur and head of the fibula and with the talus below.

tibialis posterior—A muscle that originates on the tibia, fibula, and interosseous membrane; inserts at the bases of the second to fourth metatarsal bones and tarsal bones, except the talus; plantarflexes and inverts the foot.

tibial torsion—Twisting of the larger bone of the lower leg.

tibia vara—See genu varum.

transcutaneous electrical muscle stimulation—A therapeutic procedure in which mild electrical stimulation is applied by electrodes in contact with the skin over a painful or weak area.

transverse process—A prominence on either side of the vertebrae projecting laterally from the junction between the lamina and the pedicle.

transversus abdominis—A muscle of the abdomen that originates at the cartilages of the six lower ribs, the thoracolumbar fascia, and the iliac crest; forms the conjoint tendon that inserts with the rectus sheath into the pubic crest; compresses abdominal viscera.

trapezius—The "cowl muscle"; originates on the occipital bone, the nuchal ligament, and the spinous processes of the seventh cervical and all thoracic vertebrae. It inserts at the clavicle, acromion, and spine of the scapula; draws the head to one side or backward and rotates the scapula.

triceps surae—Muscles of the calf; gastrocnemius and soleus considered as one muscle.

trochanter—One of the two bony prominences on the proximal end of the femur that serve as the point of attachment of various muscles.

trochlear groove—A smooth articular surface of bone upon which the patella glides.

vascular—Relating to or containing blood vessels, or indicative of a copious blood supply.

vastus medialis—A thigh muscle that originates on the medial aspect of the femur; inserts at the tibial tuberosity by a common tendon of the quadriceps femoris and patella ligament; extends the leg.

vestibular apparatus—A structure that contributes to the collection of proprioceptive sensations. It is located adjacent to the inner ear and is sensitive to positions of the head in space and to sudden changes in direction of body movement.

Index ∿

Note: The italicized *f* and *t* following page numbers refer to figures and tables, respectively.

A

abdominal muscles 31, 66, 82*f*, 84*f*, 86*t*, 87, 94, 139, 140
  external oblique 82
  internal oblique 82
  isometric contraction 86
  pyramidalis 31
  rectus abdominis 31, 82
  strengthening 66
  transversus abdominis 31, 82
  weak 87
abdominal strengthening exercises 88
abductors
  of hip 30*t*
  overused 31
  rotation of proximal joints 30*t*
  shoulder joints 30*t*
Ace bandage 66
acetabulum 113, 136, 149
Achilles tendon 112, 112*f*
  description 47, 47*f*, 48
  evaluation of 24
  flexibility 42
  rupture 48
  stretching 42
  tendinitis 39, 48-49
    diagnosis 48
    etiology 48
    rehabilitation 49
    treatment 48, 48*f*, 49
  tendinopathy 13*t*
  triceps surae 47*f*, 147
ACSM Position Stand 213, 214
adolescence 204, 207
  growth-dependent risk factors 87
  growth spurt 85, 87
  idiopathic type of scoliosis 90
  malalignment 62
  puberty 203, 204, 206, 207
adductors
  of hip 30*t*
  overactive 32
  rotation of proximal joints 30*t*
  shoulder joints 30*t*
  tension 31
  tightness 34
aerobic dance 79
  biomechanics, lower extremity analysis 129, 130-131
  foot realignment 130
  injury rates 130
  plantar fasciitis: case study 131-134
  risk factors 130
  shoes 130, 133
age
  risk of injury 15
  senior dancers 15
air-cast walking brace 41, 42, 43, 48, 48*f*, 49, 100, 102
Alexander Technique 29, 94
alignment 94. *See also* malalignment; posture
  anatomic 19
  basic 24, 25*f*
  corrected 21, 22*f*
  distortion in 32
  foot 131
  improving 26
  knee 32
  lateral distortion 32
  of lower extremities 60
  problems 24, 25*f*, 77
allograft 69
amenorrhea 87*t*, 90, 99, 211, 212-213, 214
  exercise-associated amenorrhea (EAA) 213

analgesics 92
anatomical measurements 15
ankle. *See also* subtalar joint; talus
  bones of 40, 40*f*
  combined actions with tarsus 169, 170, 170*f*
  dorsiflexion 10*t*, 132, 133*f*, 169
  equinus deformity 133, 133*f*
  evaluation of 23, 24
  exercises 43
  joints 40, 41, 131, 168-170, 170*f*, 186, 186*f*
  ligaments 12, 40
  mortise 40
  plantarflexion 10*f*, 63, 169
  pronation (roll in) 24, 24*f*, 25*f*
  range of motion 15, 42, 43, 49, 50
  sprains 11, 13*t*, 23, 23*f*, 39, 40, 40*f*
  stabilization 41, 42
  supination (roll out) 23, 24, 24*f*, 25*f*
  weights 143
ankle injuries 15, 39, 50
  Achilles tendinopathy/strain 13*t*
  anterior tibialis tendinopathy 13*t*
  etiology 40, 41
  flexor hallucis longus tendinopathy/strain 13*t*
  os trigonum/post-op 13*t*
  os trigonum removal 13*t*
  peroneal strain 13*t*
  plantar fasciitis 13*t*
  posterior tibialis tendinopathy 13*t*
  sprain 11, 13*t*, 23, 23*f*, 39, 40, 40*f*
ankle sprains
  air-cast 41
  balance board 43
  barre work 43
  bleeding 41
  contrast baths 43
  dance surfaces 41
  gel-cast ankle brace 41-42
  grades of injury 41
  massage 43
  open *versus* closed management 43
  prevalence of 40
  previous ankle sprains 41
  rehabilitation 41, 42-43
  resistance exercises 43
  swelling 41
  swimming pool exercises 43
  treatment 41-42
  warm up 43
annulus fibrosus 82, 82*f*
anorexia nervosa 100, 208, 212
anterior cruciate ligament 12, 65, 69. *See also* ligament, anterior cruciate
  reconstruction 69
anterior labral tears 75
anterior superior iliac crest. *See* iliac crest, anterior superior iliac crest
anterior talofibular ligament (ATF) 40, 41
anterior tibialis 13*t*
anti-inflammatory medications 44, 48, 87, 91, 92, 93, 131. *See also* nonsteroidal anti-inflammatory drugs
anxiety 195, 197-198
arabesque 86, 86*t*, 87*t*, 88, 91, 105
arousal
  component of stress 194
  reduction 196
  stress management 194
arthritis. *See also* osteoarthritis
  degenerative 69
  facet 79
  great toe joint 41
  hip 75
arthroscopy 62, 66
asthma 12, 15

ATF ligament. *See* anterior talofibular ligament
attitude 86*t*, 88, 91, 142
autogenic inhibition 152, 153*f*, 155, 157, 157*f*
autogenic training 196

B

back. *See also* spine
   deep back muscles 82
   discogenic back pain 92
   dorsal back pain 93
   flexibility exercises 94
   injury rate 4, 79
   low back 79, 88, 91, 92, 93
   low back pain, mechanical 13*t*, 93
   lower back problems 31, 33
   muscles 87
   pain 88, 89, 90, 91, 93, 105, 114
   problems 12, 15
   rehabilitation 94
   strain 89
   upper back injuries 79, 93
   upper back muscles 94
Baitch, Stephen P. 129
balance board 43. *See also* BAPS
ballet barre 42, 43, 94, 102, 146
   exercises 59, 66, 94, 137
BAPS (biomechanical ankle platform system) 42
Bartenieff Fundamentals 29
   arm circle exercise 30*t*, 32, 33*f*
   body half exercise 30*t*, 34, 35, 35*f*
   description of 30, 30*t*
   forward pelvic shift exercise 30*t*
   heel rock exercise 30*t*
   injury potential, assessing 34
   knee reach exercise 30*t*
   Laban Movement Analysis System 30, 32
   lateral pelvic shift exercise 30*t*
   lower limbs 32
   "thigh lift" exercise 30, 30*t*, 31*f*
   training in 36
   upper body analysis 32-34
   "X" rolls exercise 30*t*
basal ganglia 154, 154*t*
Baum, Jessica 3
biceps brachii 152
biceps femoris 58
bingeing 208
biomechanics 109
   aerobic dance 129
   aerobic dancer's lower extremities 130-131
   ankle joint 186, 186*f*
   biomechanical cause of injury 15
   body mechanics 94
   knee 54-58, 54*f*-57*f*
   meniscus 58
   patellofemoral joint 60
   principles 111
   pronation 186, 187*f*
   spine 79, 80-85
   turnout 135, 142-148
bladder 21
body dissatisfaction 201, 202
body esteem 202, 205, 206
body image 204, 205
   shape 205, 206, 207
Body-Mind Centering 29
body type analysis 21-25, 22*f*-26*f*
bone
   calcaneus 40*f*, 47, 47*f*, 48
   coccyx 31
   cuboid 40*f*
   cuneiform 40*f*, 101, 101*f*
   fibula 40, 40*f*
   foot 165, 166*f*
   fragments 104
   greater trochanter 30
   health 15
   humerus 32, 34
   iliac cres 22
   ilium 11*t*
   impingements 34
   malleoli 40, 40*f*

   metatarsals 40, 40*f*
   navicular 40*f*, 166*f*, 168
   patella 24
   phalanges 40*f*
   sacrum 30, 31
   scan 104
   scapula 21, 23*f*, 30, 32-34
   sesamoid 100, 101*f*
   spurs 50
   talus 40, 40*f*, 41
   tarsal 24, 40*f*
   tibia 40, 40*f*, 47
bone mineral density 214
bone scan 45, 88, 91, 91*f*, 93, 98, 101, 101*f*, 102, 102*f*, 103*f*
   stress fractures 45
bone spurs 50, 91, 91*f*. *See also* osteophyte formation
brace 87, 92, 93, 94, 100, 105
   anti-lordotic brace 91, 91*f*, 93
   Boston brace 88, 89*f*
   jumper's knee 65
   knee 61, 69
   scoliosis 90
bracing. *See* brace
breathing 94, 118, 120, 121, 154, 158, 159, 196
   breath support 30*t*, 34
   sounds 115
bulimia nervosa 208, 212
bunions 188
bursa 34, 47, 75
   femoral head 76
   iliopectineal 75
   retrocalcaneal 48. *See also* bursitis
bursitis 9, 76, 98

C

calcaneofibular ligaments 41, 44*f*
calcaneus 40*f*, 41, 47*f*, 48, 132, 132*f*, 166*f*, 168, 186, 186*f*, 187, 187*f*, 188. *See also* heel
calcium 14, 15
cartilage
   articular 58, 66, 81
   growth 87, 90
   hyaline 186
   meniscal problems 53, 53. *See also* meniscus
cerebral cortex 154, 154*t*
   limbic system 152, 153*f*, 154
cervical spine 80, 80*f*, 82*f*
   cervical spondylolysis 94
   flexibility 86
   injuries 79, 94
   strength 86
chondromalacia 45, 187
Clippinger, Karen S. 135
coccyx 31, 80
cognitive, restructuring 196-197
collagen 65
   ligament failure 55
   ligaments 69
   meniscus 58
   tendon 57
compression 41, 42, 63. *See also* RICE
computed tomography (CT) 91, 91*f*, 93
concentric muscle contraction 57
conditioning 197
   body 204
   elasticity 171
   insufficient 172
   muscular endurance 171
   principles 171-172
contrast baths 48
coracoacromial arch 34
cortisone
   corticosteroid injections 44, 48, 49, 65, 76, 131
cruciate ligament. *See* ligament
cycling 100

D

dairy intake 13-14
dance class
   conditioning 171
dance surface 41, 87, 99. *See also* floor

dance teacher
    approach to training 202
    eating disorders prevention 201-209
    positive role model 204-205
Dancing on My Grave (Kirkland) 193
degenerative arthritis. *See* arthritis, degenerative
deltoid ligaments 40, 44*f*
demi-plié. *See* plié
demi-pointe 40, 41, 42, 47, 49, 49*f*, 62, 69, 157
depression 195, 202
développé 57, 66, 75, 114, 138, 146
développé à la seconde 145*f*
d'Hemecourt, Pierre A. 3
diabetes 21
diet 197
    dietary intake 213
    dieting 100
    pills 212
disc 87, 93
    discectomy 93
    discogenic back pain 91
    herniation 79, 85, 85*f*, 87, 88, 89*f*, 91, 92, 93
        computed tomography (CT) 92*f*
        description of 91, 92
        prevalence of 91
        treatment 9 2-93
    inflammation 91
    intervertebral 80, 81, 81*f*, 82, 82*f*
    pain 13*t*, 92
    pressure 92
    protrusion 91
    rupture 91
discectomy 93
disordered eating. *See* eating disorder
diuretics 208, 212
dorsal spine. *See also* thoracic spine
    back pain 93
    kyphosis 93
dorsiflexion 42
    ankle 132, 133*f*, 169, 170*f*
    great toe 43
    toes 49
drawer sign 41. *See also* Lachman's Test

E

eating disorders
    anorexia nervosa 100, 208, 212
    bulimia 100, 208, 212
    disordered eating patterns 202, 207
    history form 21
    risk factor for injury 15
    role of dance teachers 201-209
    social withdrawal 202
"Eating Disorders Not Otherwise Specified" (EDNOS) 212
eccentric muscle contraction 86
    spine 85
    tendinitis 57
electrical muscle stimulation 44, 46, 48, 49, 62, 63, 65, 87, 90, 93
electrolyte imbalance 212
electromyography 84, 85
elevation 41, 42, 63. *See also* RICE
energy expenditure 213
entrechat six 41
epidemiological studies 3, 15
epilepsy 21
equinus deformity 133, 133*f*
erector spinae 31, 83
estrogen 100
eversion 42
    heel 132
    range of motion 131, 132
exercise-associated amenorrhea (EAA) 213
extension 142
    and flexion of hip 31
    and flexion of knee 57-58
    and flexion of spine 30*t*
    contracted quadriceps muscles 14, 113, 113*f*, 114*f*
    glenoid-humeral joint 30*t*
    hip 30*t*, 137
    incorrect extension in second position 114, 114*f*
    shoulder joints 30*t*
extensor digitorum longus 170*f*, 171*f*

extensor hallucis longus 170*f*
external oblique muscles 82, 84*f*
external rotation. *See also* turnout
    full 140
    hip 60, 62, 63, 66, 77, 84, 135, 136, 140-141, 141*f*, 142
    knee 55
    lower extremities 58, 59, 60
    strengthening 140, 140*f*
    test for 10*t*
    tibia 61
external tibial torsion 61
extrafusal muscle fibers 158*f*
extrapyramidal system 153*f*
extrinsic risk factors. *See* risk factors for dance injuries

F

facet
    arthritis 79, 82
    arthrosis 88, 89*f*, 91, 91*f*
    inferior L4 facet 91, 91*f*
    joint 81, 82, 86, 87, 91, 93
    joint capsule 82
    joint stress 93
    lumbar facet joint 82
    subtalar joint 186
fascia 48
    lumbar 85, 86*t*, 88
    lumbodorsal 87, 88, 93
    plantar fascia (PF) 49, 49*f*, 50
    tensor fascia lata 114, 128
fatigue 29, 41, 106, 197
Feldenkrais Method 29, 94
Female Athlete Triad 100, 211
    Amenorrhea 211
    eating disorders 211-214
    osteoporosis 211
    preventing and managing 213
femur 84
    bursa at femoral head 76
    femoral anteversion 22, 23, 61, 62, 86*t*, 87, 87*t*, 99*t*, 136, 137*t*
    femoral condyles 47, 61
    femoral insertion in acetabulum 113
    femoral neck 61
    femoral neck retroversion 136, 137, 137*f*
    internal rotation 136, 137*f*
    knee joint 54
    menisci function 58
    patellofemoral compression force 56, 57, 57*f*
    stress fractures 104, 105
    stretching frog position 137
    trochanter 84*f*
fibro-osseous tunnel 43, 44, 44*f*. *See also* flexor hallucis longus (FHL)
fibrous annulus 92
fibula 40, 40*f*, 47, 186*f*, 187*f*
    distal 102
    head 47*f*
    pain 102
Fitt, Sally Sevey 165
flexibility 197
    Achilles tendon 42
    adolescent growth spurt 87
    anti-lordosis strengthening and flexibility program 85, 85*f*, 93
    biomechanical factors 159-160
    cerebral cortex 152, 154
    cervical region 86
    conditioning 167-168
    description of 151
    factors 153*f*
    gains 137
    growth spurt 86*t*, 93
    hamstring 34, 94, 138
    iliopsoas 88
    increasing 26
    inflexibility 35
    ligamentous 10*t*
    limbic system 152, 154
    lumbar region 86, 94
    motor activity and 152-160, 153*f*-159*f*
    overall, maintaining 42
    quadriceps 62
    range of motion 151
    stretching techniques 151
    thoracic region 86

flexibility, selected exercises
    adductors 160, 161, 161f
    calf stretch 162, 162f
    hamstring stretches 161, 161f, 162
    purpose of 151-152
    standing deep calf stretch 162, 163, 163f
flexion
    and extension of hip 31
    and extension of knee 57-58
    and extension of spine 30t
    glenoid-humeral joint 30t
    hip 30t, 31
    lateral 83
    lumbar spine 83
    shoulder joints 30t
flexor digitorum longus 43, 44f, 170f, 171f
flexor hallucis brevis 44, 45, 45f, 46f, 47
flexor hallucis longus (FHL) 170f, 171f
    anatomy of 43, 44, 44f
    tendinopathy 13t
flexor hallucis longus (FHL) tendinitis
    ankle and foot injuries 39, 43, 44, 44f
    etiology of 43, 44
    pronation 43
    treatment 44
floor 130
    wood 131
    work 77, 88, 100, 115
fluoroscopy 76
foot
    abnormal foot mechanics 131
    alignment 131
    arch, test for 10t
    bones 40, 40f, 165, 166f
    cavus 10t
    hypermobility 132
    injuries 39, 50
    joints 131
    malalignment 131
    Morton's foot 10t, 43
    pain 101, 102
    podiascope 25
    pronation 24, 48, 49, 59, 61, 131
    range of motion 50
    realignment 130
    sickling 41
    strapping and padding 188
    supination 24, 40, 41, 48
    type 10t
    wear 130
forefoot 24, 25f, 132
fouettés 43
fracture 63, 67. See also stress fracture
    ankle and tarsus 174
    avulsion 12
    compression 82
    fifth metatarsal 45
    frank 47
    inferior L4 facet 91, 91f
    insufficiency 100
    navicular 102
    non-union 101
    sesamoids 45, 47
    spiral 104
    stress 47, 82, 87, 89, 188
fusiform muscle 57

G

Gallwey, Timothy 195
gamma efferent pathway 153f, 155, 155f, 158, 159, 159f
gamma motor neurons 152
gamma reflex pathways 152
    conditioned 115
    loss 92-93
    quadriceps inhibition 61, 66
ganglion cysts 45
Garrick, James 9
gastrocnemius. See gastroc-soleus muscle
gastroc-soleus muscle 47, 47f, 133, 151, 157, 170f
gel-cast ankle brace 41-42
gender. See also male dancer
    equity 204, 206
    inequity 206

    risk of injury 15
    sexism 204
    sexual orientation 204
    stress fractures 99
genu recurvatum 22, 86t
genu valgum (knock-knees)
    evaluation for 22, 23, 99t
genu varum (bowlegs)
    evaluation for 22, 23f
glenoid-humeral joint 30t. See also shoulder
gluteal muscles 30, 31
    gluteus maximus 86, 143
    hypercontracted 31
    overuse 35
    spasm 34
Golgi tendon organs (GTOs) 153f, 157
gonadotrophic releasing hormone (GnRH) 213
gracilis 31
Graham contraction 86
grand battements 138, 146
grand plié. See plié
greater trochanter 30, 73, 140
great toe 40. See also hallux
    distal phalanx 47
    dorsiflexion 43
    triggering and snapping 44
growth 204
    cartilage 87, 87t, 90
    phase 207
    spurt 86t, 87t, 93, 204, 206
gymnastics 14

H

hallux 40, 41, 43
hamstrings 93
    balanced usage 31
    flexibility 34, 138
    flexibility exercises 94
    knee 57-58
    muscles 67, 86
    overuse 35
    pain 34
    strengthening 62, 63, 69
    stretching 88, 93, 138, 138f
    tendinitis 64
    tendons 58
    tightening 85, 87, 88, 93
    weakness 69
heart disease 21
heat 87, 93, 94.
heel
    cord stretching 49
    eversion 132
    fat pad 49
    lift 48
    pain 131, 132, 133, 187
    spur syndrome 188
height 10t
herniation. See disc herniation
hip 30t, 31
    abductors 30t, 146
    adductors of 30t
    arthritis 75
    clicking and popping 73, 114
    extension 30t, 31, 137
    extensors 86
    external rotation 10t, 23, 24f, 60, 84, 135, 136, 140-142
    external rotators 62, 63, 66, 77, 151
    flexion 30t, 31, 84, 86t
    flexor flexibility 138, 139, 139f
    flexor flexibility (Thomas test) 11t
    flexors 146, 147f
    flexors, stretching 140
    flexor strength 143
    hyperextension 137
    internal rotation 10t, 35, 61, 84, 138
    internal rotators, stretching 139, 140
    internal snapping 73, 74, 76
    joint 64, 137
        injuries 31
        pain 31
        patterning 34
        rotation of 30t

hip *(continued)*
    ligaments 137
    medial snapping hip 76
    muscle imbalances 76
    pain 75
    popping sounds 114
    range of motion 15, 136
    snapping 73, 74, 76, 77
    socket 113, 114*f*
    stretching 66
    tendon 113
    tight hip flexors 86*t*
hip flexor. *See* iliopsoas
history form 20-21. *See also* screening
hormones
    disorders 12, 15
    gonadotrophic releasing hormone (GnRH) 213
    hormonal changes 203
    hormonal development 204
    hormonal dysfunction 207
    imbalance 12, 100
    luteinizing 213
humerus
    graduated rotation 34
    head of 32
    range of motion 32
hyaline cartilage 44, 186
hyperestrogenism 90
hyperextension. *See* knee, hyperextension; spine, hyperextension
hyperlordosis 77, 79. *See also* lumbar spine hyperlordosis
hypermobility, foot 132
hypertonia 152, 158
hypertrophy
    contralateral pedicle 89
    lamina 89
hypoestrogenism 87*t*, 99, 100

I

ice 41, 42, 43, 44, 49, 63, 66, 69, 87, 94. *See also* RICE
Ideokinesis 29
iliac crest 83, 84
    anterior superior iliac crest 22
    anterior superior iliac spine (ASIS) 11*t*
iliacus 74*f*, 84, 128
iliocostalis 82, 82*f*
iliofemoral ligament 60, 62, 137, 138, 139*f*
iliopsoas. *See also* psoas
    contraction 84
    description of 84
    flexibility 84, 88
    flexion of leg 31
    function 30
    hip flexor 139
    muscle 64
    muscle-tendon 74
    provocative hyperflexion test 75, 76*f*
    rehabilitation 77
    strength 84, 88, 146, 147, 147*f*
    tendinitis 73-77, 74, 75, 76. *See also* snapping hip
    tendons 74, 76, 84, 84*f*, 114. *See also* hip, flexor
iliopsoas tendinitis. *See also* tendinitis
    diagnosis 75, 75*f*
    history and etiology 73, 74, 74*f*, 75
    terms, anatomical location 74
    treatment 76
iliotibial band 61, 62, 73
    Ober's test 11*t*
    patella 62
    stretching 63
    tightness 11*t*
ilium 11*t*
incontinence 92
infection 93
inflexibility 35. *See also* flexibility
injuries
    aerobic dance 130
    ankle 15, 50
    ankle and tarsus 173-174
    back 79
    back injury rate 79
    brachial plexus 94
    brachial plexus 94

chondral 63
collateral ligament 68
coping 197-198
cruciate ligament 69
duration of 9, 11
foot 50
hip 73
history 15
knee 31-32
knee ligament 67
lower extremities 134
neck 79, 94
neurological 94
overuse 9, 11*t*, 12, 34, 39, 64, 99, 99*t*
-prone locations 31
rib cage 13*t*
sesamoid 39
severity of 11, 13, 14
types 11*t*
upper back 93
injury rates 3-4, 12, 13, 14, 15
injury survey 3-16
internal oblique muscles 82, 84*f*
internal rotation. *See* hip internal rotation
International Association for Dance Medicine & Science 109
interneuron. *See* neuron
intrinsic risk factors. *See* risk factors for dance injuries
isokinetic
    exercises 69
    strength testing 14
isometric contraction 62, 63, 66, 158
    abdominal muscles 86
    spine 85
    strength 167
isometric exercise 62, 94
isotonic exercises 62, 63, 65, 69

J

joint
    abduction 30*t*
    acromioclavicular 30*t*
    adduction 30*t*
    ankle 40, 41
    glenoid-humeral 30*t*
    hip 30*t*, 31
        injury-prone location 31
        pain 31
        patterning 34
        rotation of 30*t*
    interphalangeal 45*f*
    knee 31-32
    metatarsophalangeal (MTP) 45*f*, 46, 47
    mortise 41
    rib-sternum 34
    rotation of 30*t*
    scapulohumeral 32
    scapulo-thoracic 30*t*
    shoulder 30*t*, 32, 33
    subtalar 40*f*
    talocrural 40*f*
joint fluid 81
jumper's knee 64
    brace 65
jumps 3, 48, 62, 65, 66, 104
    assemblés 47
    jetés 47
    landing from 57, 59, 65-66, 67, 112, 166
    patellar tendinitis 64
    performing 186
    poor technique 41
    repetitive stresses 3
    saut de basque 67
    stress fractures 99
    in swimming pool 49
    tour jeté 67

K

kinetic chain short arc exercises 62, 63
Kinney, Susan A. 3
Kirkland, Gelsey 193

knee
    alignment 32
    biomechanics 54-58, 54f-57f
    biomechanics of 54-58, 54f-57f
    brace 69
    evaluation of 22, 23
    extension 57-58
    external rotation 55
    femoral anteversion (lack of external rotation) 22, 23
    flexion 56, 57-58, 61
    flexion and extension 53, 66
    genu recurvatum 22
    genu valgus (knock-knees) 22, 23
    genu varum (bowlegs) 22, 23, 23f
    hyperextension 21, 22, 24, 62, 63, 67
    immobilizer 63
    internal rotation 55
    joint 31, 32, 53, 54, 55
    lateral release 13
    ligaments 54, 55, 55f, 67
    muscles 57-58
    pain 61, 66, 67, 130-131
    patellofemoral joint 53
    Q-angle, test for 11t
    quadriceps stabilization of knee 31
    range of motion 66
    rate of injury 53, 54t
    rehabilitation 42
    screwing the knee 66
    sleeve 62
    strengthening 66
    synovial tissue 54
    tendons 57-58
knee, strain
    correct technical training 60, 60f, 61f
    definition of 58
    etiology of 58, 59, 59f
    external rotation of hip 60
    microscopic tear 58
    pain 60
    symptoms 60
    treatment 60, 60f
    turnout 59, 59f, 60f
knee injuries 4, 31-32, 53, 67
    biomechanics of 54-58
    medical problems 58-69
    rate of 53
    terms for anatomical location 55
knee joint
    anterior cruciate ligament 54, 54f, 59f
    biceps femoris 54, 54f
    coronary ligament 59f
    fibular collateral ligament 54, 54f
    iliotibial band 59f
    lateral meniscus 59f
    medial meniscus 59f
    patellar ligament 54, 54f, 59f
    popliteus tendon 59f
    posterior cruciate ligament 54, 54f, 59f
    quadriceps femoris tendon 54, 54f
    tibia 54
    tibial collateral ligament 54, 54f
    transverse ligament 54, 54f, 59f
Kravitz, Steven R. 185
kyphosis 80, 80f
    dorsal 93
    thoracic 80, 93

L

Laban Movement Analysis 29, 32, 36. *See also* Bartenieff Fundamentals
labrum, tears 73
Lachman's test 68, 68f
lateral femoral condyle 54f, 55, 55f, 58
Lauffenburger, Sandra Kay 29
laxatives 208, 212. *See also* eating disorders
leg. *See* lower extremities
lifting 93, 94
    disc herniation 91, 92
    posture 85, 85f, 86t
    technique 92
ligamentous laxity 60

ligaments 67
    ankle 12, 40
    ankle and tarsus 168
    ankle ligament reconstruction 12
    ankle sprains 41
    anterior cruciate (ACL) 12, 54, 54f, 55, 55f, 58, 59, 65, 67
        reconstruction 69
        rupture 68
    anterior ligament, head of fibula 54, 54f
    anterior talofibular (ATF) 41
    biceps femoris 54, 54f, 55f
    calcaneofibular 41
    collagen 69
    collateral 58, 67, 67f
    collateral ligament injuries 68
    coronary 59f
    deltoid 40
    fibula 54f, 55f
    fibular collateral 54, 54f, 55f
    flexibility, test for 10t
    hip 137
    iliofemoral 60, 62, 137
    injuries 41, 67-69
    knee 54, 55, 55f, 67
    Lachman's test 68, 68f
    lateral capsular 65
    lateral collateral (LCL) 55, 67
    ligamental laxity 62, 137
    ligament tear 68
    medial collateral (MCL) 32, 55, 58, 67
    medial patellofemoral ligament 63
    patellar ligament 54, 54f, 55f, 59f
    patellofemoral ligament tears 63
    posterior cruciate (PCL) 54, 54f, 55f, 58, 59f, 68
    posterior inferior tibio-fibular 44f
    posterior talo-fibular 44f
    sprain 12, 87, 93
    strength 55
    support of spine 82-85
    talo-fibular 44f
    tear 67
    tenderness 68
    tibial collateral 54, 54f, 55f
    tibio-fibular 44f
    transverse 54, 54f, 55f, 59f
Likert scale, severity of injuries 9, 11, 13, 14-15
limbic system, cerebral cortex 152, 153f, 154
limb length discrepancy. *See* lower extremities
Lisfranc fractures 101f
longissimus 82, 82f
longitudinal studies, screening exams 15
lordosis 80, 92, 93. *See also* lumbar spine
    anti-lordosis strengthening and flexibility program 85, 85f, 92, 93
    anti-lordotic bracing 88, 89f, 91, 93
    anti-lordotic exercises 76, 77, 91
    anti-lordotic rehabilitation 89, 93
    cervical 86
    correcting 24
    hyperlordosis 84, 85, 86t, 87, 87t, 88, 92, 93, 94
    lordotic posture 93
    lordotic spine 114-115
    lumbar 60, 74, 80, 82, 83, 84, 85, 85f, 86, 87, 87t
    lumbar anti-lordotic strengthening 93
    rehabilitation 85
    stabilization 86
low back. *See* lumbar spine
lower extremities 98
    alignment 60
    biomechanics of 129, 130-131
    extensors 152
    external rotation 58, 59, 60
    injuries 83, 134
    injury rate of 53, 54t
    leg length 11t, 87t
    limb length discrepancy 87t
    malalignment 60-61, 79
    stress 87
Luke, Anthony C. 3
lumbar hyperlordosis. *See* lordosis
lumbar spine 74, 80f, 83, 84, 87, 91, 105. *See also* lordosis
    anatomy 81f
    articulation 115, 116

asymmetry 90
fascia 85, 88
flexibility 86
flexion 115
hyperextension 31, 82, 88, 91
hyperlordorsis 79
hypertension 87t
injuries 31, 79
lumbar erector spinae 31
lumbar extensor muscles 30
pedicles 105, 106f
strain 13t
strength 86
vertebrae 80, 81f

M

macrotrauma injury 104
magnetic resonance imaging (MRI) 63, 66
malalignment 94. *See also* alignment
    adolescent dancer 62
    anterior knee pain 61
    pronation 43
    foot 131
    lower extremities 60-61, 79, 131
    patella 130-131
    pelvis 79
    postural 94
    rib cage 115
    spinal 31
male dancers 6, 13, 14, 53, 101, 102, 104, 206. *See also* gender
    disc herniation 91, 92
    eating disorders 203
    injury rates 15
    torn menisci 53
malleolus
    lateral 10t, 47f, 186f, 187f
    medial 11t, 40, 40f, 43, 44f, 47f, 186f
march fractures 98, 188
Marshall test 10t
massage 43, 93, 94, 196
    deep friction 46, 49
    ice 46, 48, 65, 93, 133
medial knee strain 58, 59, 59f
medial plica. *See* plica
medial tibial stress syndrome (MTSS) 173
meditation 196
menarche 87t, 99
    delayed 87
    scoliosis 90
meniscus
    articular cartilage 58
    biomechanical behavior 58
    collagen 58
    description of 58
    knee joint 58, 59f
    knee lubrication 58
    lateral 58, 59f, 65
    medial 55, 55f, 58, 59, 65
    meniscal problems 53
        etiology 65-66
    meniscal tears 53, 58, 65, 66, 69
    menisci function 58
    symptoms of injury 66
    treatment 66
menstruation 15, 21, 99, 100, 213, 214. *See also* amenorrhea; menarche;
        oligomenorrhea
metatarsals 166f
    cortical thickening 101
    fifth 10t, 40, 45
    first 25, 45f, 101
    metatarsalgia (pain in ball of foot) 131
    metatarsophalangeal (MTP) joint 45f, 46, 47, 59, 59f
        first MTP angle 10t
        great toe 43
        pseudo hallux rigidus 43
    second 101
    stress fractures 188
    third 101
Micheli, Lyle J. 3, 73, 79, 97
microfracture 98. *See also* stress fracture
microtrauma. *See* overuse injury
mid-tarsal joint. *See* tarsal joint, mid-tarsal

Morton's foot 10t, 43
motor cortex 154, 154t
motor system
    basal ganglia 154, 154t
    cerebellum 154, 154t
    cerebral cortex 154, 154t
    components 154, 155, 155f
    descending motor tracts 154, 154t, 155, 155f
    motor cortex 154, 154t
    motor movement patterns 154, 154t
muscle
    abdominal 31, 66, 82, 82f, 83, 84f, 86, 86t, 87, 94, 139, 140
    abductor 31, 32
    activation, turnout 146, 147
    adductor 34
    ankle joint 40
    back 87
    biceps femoris 58
    collagen 57
    concentric muscle contraction 85
    eccentric muscle contraction 85
    erector spinae 31
    flexibility 152, 153f, 154
    flexor digitorum longus 43, 44f
    flexor hallucis brevis 44, 45f, 46f, 47
    flexor hallucis longus (FHL) 43, 44, 44f
    fusiform 57
    gastrocnemius 47, 47f, 48
    gastroc-soleus 133, 133f
    gemellus inferior 142f
    gemellus superior 142f
    gluteal 30, 31, 86
    gracilis 31
    groups, combining 175
    hamstrings 57-58, 67, 86
    iliopsoas 64, 84-85
    imbalance 29, 31, 32, 76, 80, 87, 175
        tone 29
    impingements 34
    internal oblique 82, 84f
    intrinsic 170f
    lumbar extensor 30
    multifidus 82
    obturator externus 142f
    obturator internus 142f
    paraspinal 82
    paraspinous muscle spasm 88
    pectoralis major 34
    pennate 57
    peroneal 40, 41, 42
        peroneus brevis 40
        peroneus longus 40
    piriformis 142f
    plantaris 47f
    popliteus 47f
    psoas 74f, 84, 84f, 94, 112, 113, 115, 116, 125, 152
    pyramidalis 31
    quadratus femoris 142f
    quadratus lumborum 31
    quadriceps 57
    rectus abdominis 31
    rectus femoris 31, 35, 64
    relaxants 92
    rhomboids 34
    rotator cuff 32, 34
    semimembranosus 58
    semispinalis 83
    semitendinosus 58
    serratus anterior 33
    shoulder joint 32, 33
    soleus 47
    spasms 31, 114, 165
    strain 93
    strengthening, after tendinitis 65
    support of spine 82-85
    supraspinatus 34
    tendon imbalance 99
    tibialis posterior 40, 41, 42
    tone 29, 158
    transversus abdominis 31
    trapezius 33, 34
    triceps surae 47, 47f, 151

upper back 94
vastus medialis 62
muscle tone 158
musculoskeletal
problems 59, 61
system, tissues 64
musculotendinous structures 137
musculotendinous unit 57
myotatic reflex 153f, 155, 156, 156f, 157

N

navicular 166f, 168
neck 81
injuries 4, 79, 94
injury rate 4
problems 33
-shoulder tension 33
nerve
endings 42
roots 81, 82f, 91, 92
sciatic nerve pain 34
neural foramen 82f
neural sac 92
neurological injury 11t, 90, 94
neuromuscular
action 35
connectivity 34
patterns 35
spindles (NMS) 153f, 155, 156 158f
neurons
alpha motor efferent 156, 156f, 157
efferent 156f
interneuron 155-156
motor 158f
sensory 158f
sensory afferent 156, 156f
nonsteroidal anti-inflammatory drugs (NSAIDs) 65
Norris, Richard N. 39
Novaco, Raymond W. 193
nucleus pulposus 82
numbness 92
nutrition 4, 99, 106, 204, 207, 214. See also diet

O

oligomenorrhea 212
oral anti-inflammatories 49-50
oral contraceptives 12, 100
orthopedic exam 22
orthotics 44, 88, 89f, 131, 134
for balance 22
character or jazz shoes 22
overuse injuries 188
pointe 22
pronation 49
rigid shoe insert 101
semirigid orthotic devices 131, 133
soft ballet shoes 22
Springlite carbon fiber footplate 49, 49f
street shoes 22
osteoarthritis 45, 91
osteochondritis 45
osteoid osteoma 89
osteopenia 12, 202
osteophyte
excision 91
formation 91, 91f. See also bone spurs
osteoporosis 211, 214
os trigonum 9, 12, 13, 13t
overuse injuries 9, 11t, 12, 39, 99, 99t. See also microtrauma
causes of 64
definition of 64
improper turnout 135
inefficient patterns 29
patellofemoral pain 60
poor training 64
pronation 185-188, 188
spinal 86-88
symptoms 64
technique 64
training 29, 64
treatment 87-88
variety 95
Owen, Michael 3

P

pain 62
ankle sprains 41
back 89, 90, 105
chronic 45
discogenic back 13t, 91, 92
dorsal back 93
dorsum 101, 102
evaluation of 172-174
fibula 102
first metatarsal 45
foot 101, 102
forefoot 101
functional analysis 173
heel 131, 132, 133, 187
hip joint 31
knee 31, 61, 66, 67, 130-131
localization 173
lower back 91, 92, 105, 114
malalignment 62
management 195-196
mechanical low back 13t, 79, 93
medial knee strain 60
nature of 173
patellofemoral joint 9, 53, 60, 69
pelvis 87
sacral area 31
scale 14
sciatica 34, 91
shin 131
spondylolysis 89
synovial band 54
tendon 65
thoracic spine 13t, 114
paratenon 48, 58
paresthesia 92
par interarticularis 81, 82, 87, 88, 88f, 105, 105f. See also spondylolysis
patella 24, 55, 55, 56f, 63
dislocation 62, 63, 67
patellofemoral compression forces 61, 62
patellofemoral ligament tears 63
patellofemoral pain 61, 62, 69
Q-angle, test for 11t
restraining braces 63
subluxation 53, 61, 62, 63
tendinitis 53, 64-65, 65
tendon 11t, 56, 56f, 58, 64
patellae, subluxating and dislocating
etiology 62-63
femoral anteversion 62
symptoms 63
treatment 63
patellofemoral joint 61, 62
description of 55, 56, 56f
femur 55, 56, 57f
iliotibial band 56f
iliotibial expansion 56, 56f
lateral collateral ligament 56, 56f
patellar retinacular attachments 56, 56f
patellofemoral ligament 56, 56f, 63
quadriceps 55, 56, 56f
rectus femoris tendon 56, 56f
trochlear groove 55, 56
vastus lateralis tendon 56, 56f
patellofemoral joint pain 9
bracing 61
etiology of 60-61, 61f
knee problems 60
symptoms 61
treatment 61-62
pectoralis major 34
pedicle 81, 81f, 89
pelvis 112, 136, 139
malalignment 79
pain 87
pelvic rocks 118
pelvic tilt 31, 77, 80, 94, 139
pelvis lift 147
stabilization 31
strengthening exercises 88, 105
performance anxiety 193, 195. See also stage fright
peripheral nervous systems 151

periscapular injuries 93
peroneus
    brevis 40, 44f, 170f, 171f
    longus 23, 23f, 40, 44f, 170f, 171f
    peroneal muscles 40, 42
    peroneal tendons 43
    strain 13t
    tertius 170f, 171f
phalanges 166f. *See also* toe
    first toe bone 49
    proximal 49, 49f
    proximal and distal 168
physical screening. *See* screening
physiotherapy 204
Pilates 49, 62, 64, 104
Piran, Niva 201
piriformis syndrome 91
pirouettes 43, 62, 67, 155
plantar fascia (PF)
    avulsions 49
    fasciitis 13t, 49, 49f, 50, 131-134
    ruptures 49
    stretching 134
plantarflexion 42, 48
    ankle 63, 169, 170f
    heel pain 187
    talus 187
plantaris 47f, 170f
Plastino, Janie Gudde 19
Plica 54, 61
plié 60, 61, 62, 66, 102, 143, 147
    demi-plié 59, 112f, 142
    grand plié 43, 143-144, 147
    lateral meniscus 65-66
    medial knee strain 58, 59, 59f
    quadriceps muscle 64
    tibialis anterior 112
plumb line 21. *See also* posture
plyometrics 65
podiascope
    evaluation of turnout 25, 26f
    negative aspect of 5
pointe work 3, 6, 48, 49, 62, 69, 101, 184
    ballet 53
    demi-plié 59, 112f
    demi-pointe 40, 41, 42, 47, 49, 49f, 62, 69, 157
    orthotics 22
    pointe 48, 49, 62, 69, 101, 186
popliteal angle 10t, 13, 15
popliteus 47f
popping sounds 113, 114
posterior cruciate ligament (PCL) 54, 54f, 55f, 58, 59f, 68. *See also* ligaments
posterior spinous process 82
posterior tibial
    nerve 44f
    vessels 44f
posterior tibialis 42, 43. *See also* tibialis posterior
    muscle 40, 44f
    tendinopathy 13t
posture 84. *See also* alignment
    awareness 85f
    corrected 21, 22f
    errors 80
    evaluation 20, 21
    grid 21
    lifting 85, 85f, 86t
    lordotic 93
    malalignment 94
    plumb line 21
    postural mechanics 94
    sleeping 94
    spinal problems 79
posture exam. *See* screening
pronation 24, 25f, 42, 48, 129, 132, 132f, 133
    aerobic dancers 131
    angle 134
    ankles 24, 24f, 25f
    biomechanics 186, 187, 187f
    excessive 187, 187f
    flexor hallucis longus (FHL) tendinitis 43
    foot 24, 48, 49, 59, 61, 131

injurious effects 187-188
    overuse injuries 185-188
    pain 42
    peroneus longus 171f
    preventing 188
    subtalar joint 186, 187, 187f
    tarsus 169, 170f
proprioception 50, 153f, 155
exercises 69
    fibers 69
    flexibility exercises 152
    input 57, 69
    proprioceptive endings 42
    proprioceptive information 58
    proprioceptive neuromuscular facilitation (PNF) 62, 137, 138, 138f, 140, 151, 158, 159
    proprioceptive rehabilitation 42
    training 69
prostaglandins 65
psoas 84, 84f, 112, 113, 115, 116, 152. *See also* iliopsoas
    major 74f
    minor 74f
    strengthening 94, 125
    weak 86t
psychology
    history form 21
    psychological resources 193
    sport 193, 195
puberty 204, 206, 207
    eating disorders 203
    prepubertal students 204
pulmonary function 90
purging. *See* bulimia nervosa 212
pyramidal system 153f

Q

Q (quadriceps) angle 61, 62
    knee stabilization 31
    strains 61
    test for 11t
quadratus lumborum 31, 82f, 83
quadratus plantae 44f
quadriceps 56, 57, 63, 64, 65, 67, 128
    contraction 62
    eccentric, work 65
    exercises 69
    flexibility 62
    muscle during plié 64
    muscles 56, 57, 63, 65
    muscles in extension 113, 113f, 114, 114f
    rehabilitation program 63
    strength 57, 66
    tendon 55
quadriceps femoris 152

R

racism 204
radiograph 88, 88f, 91, 93, 101f, 102, 102f, 103f, 104f, 105f
reciprocal inhibition 152, 153f, 155, 157, 158f
rectus abdominis 31, 82
rectus femoris 62, 64, 128, 139
    flexion of leg 31
    stabilization 35
reflex. *See* gamma reflex pathways
rehabilitation 39, 65, 69, 93, 198
    Achilles tendinitis 49
    ankle sprain 42-43
    barre work 43
    iliopsoas tendinitis 77
    injured back 94
    knee 42, 63
    lumbar hyperlordosis 85, 93
    program 77, 92
"Rehabilitation of the Injured Ankle" (Molnar) 42
relative rest 76, 100
relaxation 158, 159, 196
    techniques 94, 152, 154
    training 204
relevé 46f, 47, 48
    ankle sprains 41
    sesamoid problems 45

rest 1, 63, 65, 66, 91, 92. *See also* RICE
reticular formation 156
reticulospinal tracts 155
retinaculum
   lateral 62, 63
   structures 63
   tears 63
rhomboids 34
rib cage
   injury 13*t*
   lifted 114-115
   malalignment 115
   placement 114
   rib-sternum joints 34
RICE (rest, ice, compression, and elevation) 41, 42, 43, 49
risk factors for dance injury 10*t*-11*t*, 13-14
   aerobic dance injuries 130
   age 15
   amenorrhea 87*t*
   bone health 15
   calcium intake 15
   disordered eating 15, 202
   duration of training 15, 87*t*
   extrinsic 4, 9, 12, 13-14, 15, 130
   femoral anteversion 87*t*
   flexibility 87*t*
   floor 130
   growth cartilage 87*t*
   growth spurt 87, 87*t*
   intensity of training 87*t*
   intrinsic 4, 12, 15
   lifting 87*t*
   limb length discrepancy 87*t*
   lumbar hyperlordosis 87*t*
   male dancers 15
   menarche 87*t*
   menstrual irregularities 15
   poor impact absorption 87*t*
   range of motion 15
   sex 15
   shoewear 130
   spike heels 87*t*
   training techniques 87*t*, 130
Rist, Rachel 19
Robson, Bonnie E. 211
rolfing 29
rond de jambe 114, 142, 152
rond de jambe en l'air 75
rotator cuff. *See* shoulder, rotator cuff

S

sacrum 30, 31, 82
sartorius 139
scapula
   arm movement 32
   mobility 32, 33
   overstabilization 32
   rotation of 30*t*, 34
   scapulae discrepancy 21, 23*f*
   scapular prominence 90
   scapulohumeral joints 32
   scapulohumeral rhythm 32, 33
   scapulo-thoracic joints 30*t*
Scheurmann's disease 93
sciatica 81
   description of 86*t*, 88, 91
   pain 91
   sciatic nerve 34, 91
   treatment 91
scoliosis 79, 84, 87, 95. *See also* lumbar spine, thoracic spine
   adolescent idiopathic type 90
   brace 90
   dance career 90, 90*f*
   description of 89, 90*f*
   determining magnitude of 90
   indications of 21, 22, 23*f*
   lumbar asymmetry 90
   menarche 90
   prevalence 90
   screening 90
   test for 10*t*
   thoracic rib hump 89

screening 3, 6, 8, 19, 20
   body type analysis 20
   description of 20
   findings, access to 20
   history form 5*f*-6*f*, 20-21
   injury history 20
   for injury potential 36
   kinesiologist, consultation with 20
   model program 19
   observations following 26
   physical exam, description of 19-20
   posture exam 20, 21-25, 22*f*- 26*f*
   preparticipation dance history 15
   program (UC Irvine) 20
   psychological issues 21
   results 20
screwing the knee 61, 62, 65, 147
second position grand plié 143-144
self-esteem 90
semimembranosus 58
semispinalis muscles 82
semitendinosus 58, 69
senior dancers. *See also* age
   risk of injury 15
sensory pathways 155
sensory receptors 153*f*
sesamoids 166*f*
   anatomy, etiology, and diagnosis 44, 45, 45*f*
   bipartite 45, 46*f*
   bones 100, 101*f*
   description of 44, 45, 45*f*
   ethnic dances 45
   fracture 47
   injuries 39, 44-47
   lateral 45*f*, 46*f*
   medial 44, 45, 46*f*
   "pad" 46, 46*f*
   sesamoidectomy 47
   sesamoiditis 46, 46*f*, 47
   stress fractures 47
   treatment and rehabilitation 45-46, 46*f*, 47
sex. *See* gender
sexism 204
sexual abuse 206
sexual orientation 206
shin, pain 131
shinsplints 98, 112, 165, 173
   posterior 188
   tibialis posterior muscle 187-188
shoes 64
   aerobic dance 130, 131, 133
   ballet 22
   character or jazz 22, 48
   cushioning 131
   heel lift 48
   high-heeled 87, 87*f*, 133, 133*f*
   modified 45*f*
   orthotics 22, 44, 49, 49*f*, 88, 89*f*, 131, 134
   pointe 43, 48
   "rocker" sole 49
   running 49
   shock absorbent 64
   Springlite carbon fiber footplate 49, 49*f*
   street 22
   wear 130
   wooden-soled, rocker-bottom 46*f*
shoulder
   dislocations 32
   glenoid-humeral joint 30*t*
   joint 30*t*, 32, 33
   mobility 32
   -neck tension 33
   rotation/circumduction 30*t*
   rotator cuff 32, 34
   serratus anterio r 33
shoulder, rotator cuff
   muscles 32
   tear 34
sickled foot 41
slipped disc. *See* disc
snapping hip 73, 76, 77. *See also* iliopsoas tendinitis
   internal 74
   medial 73, 74, 76
   tendon 74

soleus 47f
spine 84. See also cervical spine; dorsal spine; lumbar spine; thoracic spine
    basic reflex pathway 155, 156f
    biomechanics 79, 80-85
    concentric muscle contraction 85
    curvature of (scoliosis) 21, 22, 23f
    eccentric muscle contraction 85
    electromyographic studies 85
    erector spinae 31, 82, 82f
    facet arthrosis 91, 91f
    flexion/extension of 30t, 31, 74, 82, 91
    injury-prone location 31
    injury rate 79
    lordotic 114-115
    lumbar 74, 91
    lumbar hyperlordosis 79
    malalignment 31
    and muscular control 85, 86
    overuse injuries 86, 87, 87t, 88
    pain 13t
    paraspinal muscles 82
    paraspinous muscle spasm 88
    poor posture 79
    posterior spinous processes 82
    rotation of 30t, 82
    specific problems 88-94
    spinal column 80, 80f
    spinal cord 81, 154, 155-159, 156f-159f
    spinal cord reflex pathways 152, 153f
    spinal curves 80
    spinal fusion 89, 90, 91, 94
    spinalis 83, 83f
    spinous process 81, 86
    spondylolysis 88, 88f, 89, 89f
    stability 85
    stabilization 82
    stress fracture 105-106
    thoracic 80f
spondylolysis 13t, 79, 87, 93, 105, 105f
    description of 88, 88f
    older dancers 89
    pain 89
    prevalence of 88
    spondylolisthesis 91
    symptoms 88
    treatment 88, 89, 89f
sprains 11, 11t, 98
    ankle 13t, 23, 23f
    ankle, bleeding 41
    ankle and tarsus 174
    ligament 12, 87
    ligament sprain secondary to lordotic posture 93
    lower leg 165
stabilization
    ankle 41, 42
    lordosis 86
    spine 82, 85
stage fright. See also performance anxiety 193
stenosing tenosynovitis 74
sternum
    rib-sternum joints 34
    sternoclavicular joints 30t, 32, 34
    sternoclavicular mobility 33, 34
steroid injection 44, 48
strain 11t, 13t, 98
    acute 12
    ankle and tarsus 174
    back 89
    low back 91
    lower leg 165
    lumbar 13t
    muscle 93
    periscapular 93
strength 174-176, 197
    abdominal muscles 66
    Achilles tendinitis, rehabilitation 49
    ankle and tarsus 165-183
    anti- lordotic strengthening and flexibility program 85, 85f, 88, 92, 93
    bones of foot 165, 166t
    cervical spine 86
    common conditioning practices 167-168, 171-172
    elasticity 179-180
    exercises 76, 100, 101, 174-179, 176f-178f, 180-182, 180f-183f
    FHL tendinitis, rehabilitation 44
    flexibility exercise program 88, 93
    hamstring 62, 63, 69
    hip flexor 143
    iliopsoas 88, 94, 125, 146, 147f
    increasing 26, 174-176
    injuries 166-167
    isometric contractions 167
    lower leg and foot 171
    lumbar spine 86
    muscle, after tendinitis 65
    muscle groups 170, 170f, 171, 171f
    pain 172-174, 175f
    pelvis 105
    peroneal muscles 42
    range of motion 174, 175f
    restoration of 50
    strength, how much is enough? 179
    stretching after 175-176
    testing, isokinetic 14
strength exercises, ankle and tarsus
    all combined actions 176, 176f
    ankle/tarsus series 176
    dorsiflexors of ankle 176, 177, 177f
    intrinsic muscles of foot 177, 177f
    plantarflexors of ankle 178, 178f, 179
stress fracture 37, 45, 47, 82, 87, 89, 98, 112, 173, 188, 213, 214
    bilateral 101, 103
    case studies 100-105
    cause 97-98
    description of 97
    diagnosis 97-98
    femur 104
    fibular 101, 102
    frank fracture 97, 98
    history 98
    lower extremities 99
    march fractures 98
    pars interarticularis 89
    pedicle 89
    pronation 188
    risk factors 99-100
    spinal stress fractures 105-106
    tibia 103, 104
    treatment 100
stress, psychological 13
    coping skills 193
    management 194-195
    -mitigating factors 198
    preventive strategies 196
    regulatory techniques 196
    reduction 193, 197
    remediation procedures 196
stretching. See also flexibility; range of motion
    Achilles tendinitis, rehabilitation 49
    after strengthening 175-176
    ballistic 138
    exercises 100, 101, 154, 176
    FHL tendinitis, rehabilitation 44
    guidelines 179-180
    hamstring 88, 93, 138, 138f, 139f
    heel cord 49
    hip adductors 138, 139f, 140
    hip extensors 140
    hip flexors 66, 138, 139, 139f, 140
    hip internal rotators 138, 139f, 139, 140
    iliofemoral ligaments 62
    lumbodorsal fascia 88
    methods of 137-140, 138f-140f
    muscle 158
    peri-pelvis 76
    plantar fascial tissue 134
    plastic stretch 153f
    proprioceptive neuromuscular facilitation (PNF) 137, 138f
    standing or supine passé stretch 140
    static 137
    straddle stretch 138
    techniques 151

stretching, ankle and tarsus 165-183
subluxation, patella 62, 63
subtalar joint 40t, 61, 132, 132f, 133, 134, 186, 186f
    inversion, range of motion 131, 132
    pronation 188
supination (roll out) 23, 24, 24f, 25f, 40, 41, 42, 48, 169, 170f
    pain 42
supine barre 63
supraspinatus 34
surgical tubing 143, 146
swimming 42, 92, 94, 100, 102, 104
synovial band
    fluid 58, 69
    joints 32, 81
    pain 54
    plicae 54
    sheaths 58
    thickening 54
    tissue 54

T

Tai Chi 196
talocrural joint 40f
talus 166f, 168, 186f, 187, 187f
    ankle sprains 40, 40f
    tilt sign 41
tarsal joint, mid-tarsal 132, 133
tarsus
    combined actions with ankle 169, 170, 170f
    joints 165, 166f, 168-170, 170f
    neutral position of 169
    pronation 169
    supination 169
    turnout, evaluation of 24, 25f
teacher. *See* dance teacher
technique 111, 130
    aerobic 79
    altering 14, 76
    assessing 62
    ballet 6, 58
    Bartenieff Fundamentals 29-36
    Changes 106
    class 115
    classical ballet 6
    correct 76
    East Indian 45
    errors 80
    faulty 60, 61, 62, 70, 80, 88
    faulty and FHL tendinitis 43
    flamenco 45
    floor 64
    folk dance 53, 66
    inefficient patterns 29
    jazz 87, 100, 138, 149
    jumps, landing from 41
    lumbar hyperextension 91
    modern dance 6, 77, 79, 99, 149, 203, 211
    modifying 14-15
    overuse injury 64
    poor 61, 70, 88
    relaxation 94
    spinal problems 79
    torn menisci 53
    training 99
Teitz, Carol 53
tendinitis 76, 98, 114, 165, 173
    Achilles 39
    Adductor 75
    Chronic 48
    concentric muscle contraction 57
    decription of 64-65
    eccentric muscle contraction 57
    etiology 64
    flexor hallucis brevis 45
    flexor hallucis longus (FHL) 39, 43
    foot 166
    hamstring 64
    iliopsoas 73, 74, 75, 76
    muscle strengthening 65
    patella 64, 65
    peroneus brevis 23, 23f

symptoms 64-65
    treatment 65
tendinitis. *See* iliopsoas tendinitis
tendo calcaneus 44f
tendon. *See* tendinitis
    abductor hallucis 44, 44f, 45f
    Achilles 112, 112f
    adductor hallucis 44
    collagen 57
    flexor hallucis brevis 45f
    flexor hallucis longus 44, 44f
    gastrocnemius 47f
    hamstring 58
    hip socket 113
    iliopsoas 74, 76, 84, 84f, 114
    pain 65
    paratenon 58
    patellar 58
    plantaris 47f
    popliteus 58, 59f
    quadriceps 113
    quadriceps femoris tendon 54, 54f
    range of motion 57
    snapping 73, 74, 76, 77
    supraspinatus 34
    synovial sheaths 58
    tendinopathy 13t
    tendo calcaneus 44f
tensor fascia lata 31, 73
Theraband 42, 175
thigh
    abduction 31
    adductors 62, 63
    angle 11t
    muscle imbalance 31
Thomas test 11t
thoracic outlet syndrome 94
thoracic spine 80, 82, 93. *See also* dorsal spine
    flexibility 86
    hyperkyphosis 86t
    pain 13t
    scoliosis 79
    vertebrae 93
tibia 40, 40f, 47, 61, 186f
    external rotation 61
    knee joint 54
    menisci function 58
    posterior tibialis 170f
    stress fracture 103
    stress fractures 97
    tibialis anterior 112, 112f, 170f, 171f
    tibialis posterior 42, 43, 170f, 171f
    tibial malleolus 187f
    tibial torsion 61
    tibial varum (bowing) 131, 132
    turnout, evaluation of 24
    vara 99t
tibialis anterior 112, 112f, 170f
tibial torsion 61
toe. *See also* phalanges
    description of 168
    dorsiflexion 10t, 49, 49f
    first 10t, 49, 49f
    great toe 40, 41, 43, 44, 47
    second 10t
tomogram 105, 106f
tomography 98
training 106, 109
    considerations 64
    injures 29
    duration of 15, 64
    eating disorders 202
    overuse injuries 29
    participation 64
    poor 64
    proprioception 69
    risk factors 87t
    schedules 61
    techniques 130
Transcendental Meditation (TM) 196
transcutaneous electrical muscle stimulation. *See* electrical muscle
    stimulation

transverse processes 81, 82, 82*f*, 83
transverse tibio-fibular ligaments 44*f*
transversus abdominis muscles 31, 82, 84*f*
trapezius
   lower 33
   middle 34
   overuse of upper 33
Trepman, Elly 79
triceps surae 47, 47*f*, 152
trochanter
   of femur 84*f*
   greater 114
   lesser 113
trochlear grooves 62, 63
tubercle 166*f*
tumors 93, 98
turnout 3, 58, 59, 60, 65, 66, 135-149
   anatomical constraints 136, 137, 137*f*
   biomechanics of 135, 144*f*, 147, 148
   biomechanical constraints 142-143, 149
   bony, musculotendinous, and ligamentous constraints 136, 137, 137*f*
   correct 58,60, 60*f*,135, 136, 136*f*, 143, 145*f*, 148, 148*f*, 149
   degree of external rotation 149
   description of 136, 136*f*
   excessive rotation 147, 148
   evaluation of 23, 24
   forced 49, 87*t*, 135, 147, 148, 148*f*
   improper 43, 59, 61, 115, 135, 147-149
   improving 62, 66, 135, 137, 138, 139, 142, 143, 144, 146, 149
   lack of 23, 43, 61, 86*t*, 144, 140
   measuring 24, 140-142, 149
   and medial knee strain 59, 59*f*, 60, 60*f*
   optimal 136
   strengthening rotators 142, 143, 147
   stretching methods 137-140, 143
   extreme torsional stress 147
   skill development 147, 148
turns 62. *See also* pirouette

U

ultrasound 44, 46, 48, 49, 76, 87, 93, 94
upper back. *See* back; dorsal spine; thoracic spine

V

vastus medialis (VMO) 62
   contraction 62
vertebra. *See also* spine
bodies 82
   compression 31
   description of 80-81
   fifth lumbar (L5) 84
   lower thoracic 82
   lumbar 80, 82, 82*f*, 83
   12th thoracic 84
   vertebral arch 81
vestibular system 153*f*, 155*f*
visualization 152, 154, 158, 197, 198
vocalization 94, 115
vomiting. *See* eating disorders; purging

W

Walaszek, Arleen 79
warm up 94, 111, 117, 160
   dance classes 171
   exercises 115-128, 116*f*-127*f*
   principles 115
   technique class 115
warm-up exercises 1, 115-127
Warren, Michelle 99
Washington, Ernest 1
weight 207, 211
   body 201, 202
   control methods 207, 208
   distribution 59. *See also* medial knee strain
   measurement 10*t*
   and shape dissatisfaction 208
weightism 204
weight training 94
wobble-type board 42. *See also* BAPS (Biomechanical Ankle Platform System)
wooden-soled, rocker-bottom shoes 46, 46*f*

Y

yoga 196

Z

Zen in the Art of Archery (Herrigel) 111

About the Editors

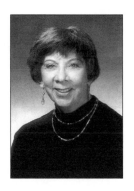

Ruth Solomon, Professor Emerita, has been a distinguished performer and choreographer in the modern dance idiom for many years. Also a dance educator of note, she cofounded the dance department at New York University Tisch School of the Arts and directed the dance program at the University of California at Santa Cruz from 1970 until her retirement in 2000. Her articles on dance have appeared in all major periodicals in the field, and her research in dance medicine has resulted in articles in medical journals and chapters in medical texts. She was the National Dance Association's Scholar of the Year in 1992, Dance Professional of the Year in 1998, and Heritage Honoree in 2003. She serves on the board of directors of the International Association of Dance Medicine & Science and on the editorial board of the *Journal of Dance Medicine & Science.*

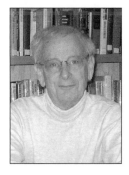

John Solomon, PhD, is a freelance editor who has coauthored or edited numerous texts in the field of dance medicine and science. He is cocompiler of the *Dance Medicine & Science Bibliography* (1996, 2001, 2004) and "Abstracts from the Current Literature," a regular feature of the *Journal of Dance Medicine & Science.* He is also coeditor of the groundbreaking book *East Meets West in Dance: Voices in the Cross-Cultural Dialogue* (1995).

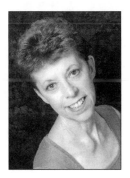

Sandra Cerny Minton, PhD, was professor and dance director at the University of Northern Colorado from 1972 to 1998. She has also been a dance specialist in the Arts Infusion Program in Denver Public Schools. She frequently presents workshops for teachers, conducts research, and writes. Her books include *Body & Self* (1989), *Modern Dance: Body & Mind* (1991), *Dance Mind & Body* (2003), and *Choreography, Second Edition: A Basic Approach Using Improvisation* (1997). Dr. Minton's research has focused on the behavior of dance teachers, the role of imagery in dance teaching, and the effects of dance on self-esteem and creative thinking. Dr. Minton's work has been published in many dance journals. In 1999 Dr. Minton was selected as the National Dance Association Artist/Scholar, and in 2001 she taught in Finland as a Fulbright Scholar.

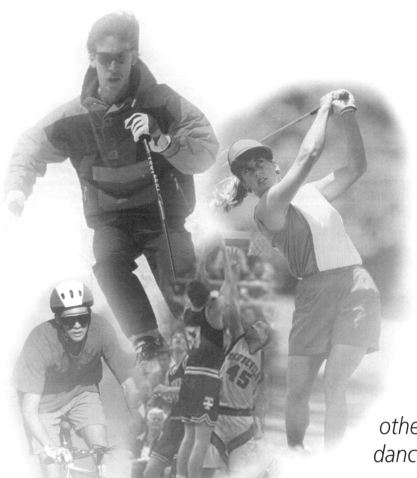